Telemedicine and Technological Advances in Dermatology

Keyvan Nouri
Editor

Telemedicine and Technological Advances in Dermatology

Springer

Editor
Keyvan Nouri
Leonard M. Miller School of Medicine
University of Miami
Miami, FL, USA

ISBN 978-3-031-69090-7 ISBN 978-3-031-69091-4 (eBook)
https://doi.org/10.1007/978-3-031-69091-4

This Springer imprint is published by the registered company Springer Nature Switzerland AG
The registered company address is: Gewerbestrasse 11, 6330 Cham, Switzerland

Dedication and Acknowledgements

I would like to dedicate this book to all my patients, your trust and presence in my care have been a profound privilege, shaping both my life and mission. My heartfelt gratitude extends to my loving family and friends for their unwavering support. Also, a special dedication to my professors, mentors, colleagues, students, residents, and fellows, as learning from each of you has been an absolute honor. My appreciation also goes to the dedicated medical, nursing, and administrative staff who've worked closely with me throughout the years.

A sincere thank you to my fellows, Daphne G. Eckembrecher, Francelia J. Eckembrecher, Fabio Frech, Loren Elizabeth de la Caridad Hernandez, and Isabella Dreyfuss for their time and dedication. Lastly, thank you to the publishers at Springer Nature, Grant Weston, Ram Prasad Chandrasekar, and all the diligent authors who contributed to crafting this excellent book.

Keyvan Nouri, MD, MBA

Foreword

While the role of technology in dermatology has often been a controversial subject in our field, the rapid advancement of technology in our world is finally taking hold throughout the dermatology landscape. Whereas teledermatology was not long ago relegated to rather underutilized areas of our country and specialty, a global pandemic brought the need for technological innovation to the forefront. Overnight, practices were transformed from bustling locales seeing high volumes of patients to empty offices. Those first steps into teledermatology were challenging for many, but as we are apt to do, dermatologists adapted quickly and designed workflows and systems to efficiently see patients in the safety of their own homes. People became very interested in the subject and I have had the honor of lecturing around the world on applications of technology in teledermatology, helping dermatologists along the way adapt to a new practice modality.

However, this rapid adoption of a new technology also revealed that many aspects of telemedicine as a whole were ill-suited to dermatology, likely because our adoption of telehealth had been quite slow prior to the pandemic. Many telemedicine platforms buckled under the strain of a plethora of new users. Blurry, grainy videos with poor lighting were the norm. Nearly every dermatologist has a story of trying to conduct a video visit with a patient who was actively driving. All the technology that seemed to be applicable in other arenas of life—such as being able to watch a crystal-clear HD video of someone making their dog do tricks halfway across the globe in real time—seemed to have passed us up in medicine. Even worse, dermatology seemed to be one of the few specialties that actually cared about video or image quality and technology didn't catch up quickly. So then, the hard work of designing technology for a new use case really began.

We now stand on the precipice of a revolution in dermatology, where novel therapeutics are meeting new technological innovations, coming together to enhance—rather than detract from—patient care. For all the complaints and struggles with electronic medical records and other technology-based hassles, we can now deliver high-quality care asynchronously and treat patients with psoriasis while achieving the same objective improvements as in-person care. The rapid adoption of AI in other facets of life is now facing dermatology, both in ways both helpful and expected (ChatGPT helping to create handouts and answering patient queries) and potentially more insidious (publications claiming that an AI system can diagnose skin conditions as well as a dermatologist). What is particularly important, though, is that dermatologists remain at the forefront of discussing these issues and deciding how to implement technological advancements. This is why this book is so relevant to our field now and serves as a gateway between what has been developed and where we are headed.

In this book, you will learn about the remarkable advancements in teledermatology and technology that pioneers in our field have been championing. Important issues in teledermatology, such as its use in skin of color and its role in expanding access to care, will be discussed, along with specific use cases for every possible application of this technology, spanning areas such as teledermatopathology, telecosmetics, teledermatological surgery, and teledermatology for hair disorders, from leaders in these respective fields.

Of course, a discussion of technology in dermatology would not be complete without addressing some of the novel imaging technologies that have become available. If we think back to the world of dermatology prior to dermoscopy, it seems hard to imagine any trainee graduating these days without having been trained in using such a device. However, it bears remembering that this technology is not an old one, with the initial manuscript introducing dermoscopy published in 1989 and the first non-contact polarized handheld dermatoscope being introduced after 2000. It may not be long before optical coherence tomography, reflectance confocal microscopy, and ultrahigh-resolution ultrasonography become part of the mainstream, especially with smaller device sizes and easier-to-use interfaces being developed.

Lastly, you will be able to evaluate the development of many novel technologies in dermatology such as AI, nanotechnology, and stem cell therapy, among others. Whether or not we believe our expertise is unique and irreplaceable, the age of artificial intelligence is upon us and a timely discussion about the limitations and ethical considerations of the use of AI in dermatology seems particularly important.

This book serves as an anchor for our specialty—a tribute to all that has been explored in telemedicine and technology within dermatology, but always with an eye forward to what is coming next. Such a comprehensive and thoughtful, intentional project has never been undertaken in our specialty, and I am deeply grateful to Dr. Nouri for taking the time and energy to put this publication forward. No stone is left unturned in delving into the latest and most interesting developments in dermatology, and you will almost certainly finish this book having learned much about the uses and potential of technology in dermatology and excited about the future of our specialty!

New York, USA George Han, MD, Ph.D.

Preface

In the rapidly evolving landscape of healthcare, telemedicine stands out as a transformative force, revolutionizing the way dermatological care is delivered and received. As we delve into the pages of "Telemedicine and Technological Advances," the reader is invited on a comprehensive journey through the intricate intersection of dermatology and cutting-edge technologies.

The world of teledermatology unfolds in the opening chapters, guiding readers through the basics with "An Introduction to Teledermatology" and then immersing them into the specialized realms of inflammatory skin conditions, hair disorders, skin cancer, wound care, surgical procedures, and pathology—all accessible through the lens of telemedicine.

Beyond the clinical scope, this book explores the expanding horizons of telemedicine, extending its reach into education, research, and global healthcare. "Tele-education in Dermatology" and "Conducting Clinical Research Remotely Through Technology" shine a light on the educational and investigative aspects, while "Geriatric Teledermatology" addresses the unique needs of elderly populations.

Photography, dermoscopy, optical coherence tomography, reflectance confocal microscopy, and high-resolution ultrasonography form a comprehensive arsenal of imaging technologies discussed in detail, providing a holistic view of the tools that empower dermatologists. Furthermore, artificial intelligence takes center stage, exploring its applications in dermatology and pondering the ethical considerations and limitations associated with this powerful technology.

As technology continues to advance, so does the array of treatment options available to dermatologists. Chapters on lasers, aesthetic dermatology, three-dimensional printing, nanotechnology, and stem cell therapy illustrate the continuous integration of innovation into the field, offering novel approaches to enhance patient care.

This book is not just a compilation of technological advancements; it is a collaborative effort of experts, researchers, and practitioners who strive to optimize dermatologic care. The goal is not merely to explore these advancements but to pave the way for their ethical implementation, ensuring that patients receive the highest quality of care in an ever-evolving healthcare landscape.

As we embark on this enlightening journey through the realms of telemedicine and technological advances in dermatology, we invite readers to engage with the content and envision a future where the fusion of medicine and technology transcends boundaries, making quality dermatologic care accessible to all.

Miami, USA Keyvan Nouri, MD, MBA

Contents

Teledermatology

An Introduction to Teledermatology 3
Nicole Levin and Keyvan Nouri

Telemedicine for Inflammatory Skin Conditions 15
Fabio Stefano Frech, Yasmine Nousari, Ali Rajabi-Estarabadi, and Carlos Nousari

Telecosmetics and Lasers 27
Loren Elizabeth de la Caridad Hernandez, Noreen Mohsin, Daphne G. Eckembrecher, Francelia J. Eckembrecher, and Keyvan Nouri

Teletrichology for Hair Disorder Consultations 49
Adaeze Nwosu, Mariya Miteva, and Antonella Tosti

Skin Cancer Telemedicine 59
Kayla D. Mashoudy, Sofia M. Perez, and Keyvan Nouri

Telewound Care 79
Divya Chopra, Neil Seth, Noreen Mohsin, and Hadar Lev-Tov

Teledermatological Surgery 95
Soraya Azzawi and Keyvan Nouri

Teledermatopathology 115
Samantha Ouellette, Phillippe Hans Jean-Pierre, Shelley Uppal, and Babar K. Rao

Optimizing Care with Teledermatology 127
Daphne G. Eckembrecher, Francelia J. Eckembrecher, Sofia M. Perez, Shrey Patel, Zoe Tsoukas, and Keyvan Nouri

Tele-Education in Dermatology 137
Soraya Azzawi and Keyvan Nouri

Teledermatology in Skin of Color 149
Jacob Beer, Francelia J. Eckembrecher, Daphne G. Eckembrecher, Hemali Shah, and Heather Woolery-Lloyd

The Effect of Teledermatology on Access to Care 155
Edward Hadeler and Keyvan Nouri

Global Dermatology and Telehealth 161
Bianca Sanabria and Carrie Kovarik

Conducting Clinical Research Remotely Through Technology 179
Edward Hadeler and Keyvan Nouri

Geriatric Teledermatology 185
Jaya Manjunath and Carrie Kovarik

Imaging Technology

Digital Photography 205
Loren Elizabeth de la Caridad Hernandez, Kayla Mashoudy, Daphne G. Eckembrecher, Francelia J. Eckembrecher, Noreen Mohsin, and Keyvan Nouri

Teledermoscopy 219
Shelley Uppal, Akhil Gupta, and Giovanni Pellacani

Optical Coherence Tomography in Dermatology 235
Charlotte Gust, Cristel Ruini, Fabia Daxenberger, Sandra Schuh, Elke Sattler, and Julia Welzel

Reflectance Confocal Microscopy 253
Isabella Dreyfuss, Francelia J. Eckembrecher, Daphne G. Eckembrecher, and Keyvan Nouri

The Application of High-Resolution Ultrasound in Dermatology 259
Jalal Maghfour, Betty Nguyen, and Iltefat H. Hamzavi

AI and Tech Advances

Artificial Intelligence: Applications in Dermatology 275
Dennis H. Murphree, Yong-hun Kim, Michael Z. Zhang, Anirudh Choudhary, Puneet K. Bhullar, and Nneka I. Comfere

Ethical, Legal, and Social Issues in Digital Dermatology 287
Carlo Botrugno, Bonnie Kaplan, and Gabrielle DiBartolomeo

Technological Advancements in Lasers 317
Betty Nguyen, Fabio S. Frech, and Michael Abrouk

Advances in Aesthetic Dermatology ... 329
Loren Elizabeth de la Caridad Hernandez, Francelia J. Eckembrecher, Daphne G. Eckembrecher, Noreen Mohsin, Shelley Uppal, Marwa Hakimi, Ashley Vander Does, and Keyvan Nouri

Three-Dimensional Printing in Dermatology ... 367
Isabella Dreyfuss, Daphne G. Eckembrecher, Francelia J. Eckembrecher, Amanda Ramnot, and Keyvan Nouri

The Applications of Nanotechnology in Dermatology ... 375
Noreen Mohsin, Loren Elizabeth de la Caridad Hernandez, Francelia J. Eckembrecher, Daphne G. Eckembrecher, and Keyvan Nouri

Stem Cell Therapy in Telemedicine and Technological Advances in Dermatology ... 387
Michael Kaiser and Evangelos V. Badiavas

Index ... 399

Teledermatology

An Introduction to Teledermatology

Nicole Levin and Keyvan Nouri

Abstract Teledermatology (TD) encompasses the interpretation of a patient's clinical history in conjunction with electronically transmitted images, in order to make a diagnosis and provide appropriate treatment recommendations. Three main platforms are currently being utilized: *synchronous* (real-time video consultation), *asynchronous* (store-and-forward [SAF]), and *hybrid*. The main advantage provided by the use of telemedicine in dermatology is easier access to specialized medical care, especially for underserved patients and those limited by geographical barriers. TD can also be a useful tool for triaging patients, as well as a valuable asset in training residents and physicians. Furthermore, teledermatology consultations can be used in both the outpatient and inpatient setting, with many studies supporting its reliability and accuracy when compared to in-person consultations. Some barriers for its use to consider include the dependence on image/video quality, limited interaction between patients and physicians, medicolegal implications, and ethical concerns surrounding the shift of a patient-centered approach to a technology-centered one.

Keywords Teledermatology · Dermatology · Telemedicine

Learning Objectives

- Understand the history of telemedicine and the origins of teledermatology.
- Recognize the platforms and practice models being utilized in teledermatology.
- Examine the application of teledermatology in various dermatological conditions and its advantages and limitations.

N. Levin (✉)
FAU Charles E. Schmidt College of Medicine, Boca Raton, FL, USA
e-mail: nicolelevinmd@gmail.com

K. Nouri
Dr. Phillip Frost Department of Dermatology and Cutaneous Surgery, University of Miami Miller School of Medicine, Miami, FL, USA

K. Nouri (ed.), *Telemedicine and Technological Advances in Dermatology*,
https://doi.org/10.1007/978-3-031-69091-4_1

1 Introduction

Living in an ever-changing world, we find ourselves constantly evolving and adapting to different circumstances and situations. During these unprecedented times, new innovations in telemedicine have made technology and medicine more integrated than ever before. A quick search for "teledermatology" (TD) on Pubmed will reveal that more articles were published in 2020 regarding this topic than any other year on record. Although the COVID-19 pandemic may have spiked newfound interest in this subject matter, teledermatology will continue to expand and improve for many years to come.

We hope this book provides helpful insight into the utilization of teledermatology for a wide variety of dermatological conditions, with the goal of providing the best patient care possible. Teledermatology has the potential to not only improve the quality of patient care, but also to improve access to specialized physicians despite geographical barriers, and reduce healthcare costs for patients [1].

2 Delivery Methods

Teledermatology involves the interpretation of a patient's clinical history in conjunction with electronically transmitted images, in order to obtain a diagnosis and provide treatment recommendations.

There are currently three main platforms being utilized in teledermatology [1, 2].

- *Synchronous* (real-time video consultation): Employs live videoconferencing between the patient and dermatologist. The advantages of this method include the ability to establish a relationship between the patient and physician, directly provide patient education, clarify any clinical history, and explain treatment options. The main disadvantage is the reliance on the quality of internet connectivity. The image quality of live video is inferior to the quality of captured images. Another drawback to consider is the need to account for potentially different time zones between the patient and physician.
- *Asynchronous* (store-and-forward [SAF]): Clinical and dermoscopic images are obtained from the patient and digitally stored. These specialized images are then forwarded for consultation to the responding dermatologist, who can analyze and review these images along with the accompanying patient history. The main advantage of this method in comparison to the synchronous modality is the superior image quality, which is of particular importance in a specialty heavily reliant on accurate visual recognition. There is also no constraint among different time zones. This data can be conveniently shared on computers, tablets, smartphones, online portals, and/or apps. Although this modality is the most popular among the three, its main downside is that supplemental information cannot be immediately obtained. Additional coordination with either the consulting physician or patient would be required, which may delay the clinical process.

- *Hybrid*: A combination of the synchronous and asynchronous platforms. Although this platform overcomes certain restrictions of the aforementioned modalities, it isn't as frequently utilized. It requires a large amount of bandwidth and storage space.

3 Consultation and Triage

There are currently 4 recognized practice models for teledermatology, including: consultative, triage, direct care, and follow-up [3].

The consultative model depends on the collaboration between the referring doctor and dermatologist. The consulting dermatologist can give advice and make recommendations. However, the patient remains under care of the referring physician and the referring physician must assume all responsibility for any recommendations that are implemented. The consultative model can be utilized using live videoconferencing or the store-and-forward method. This is currently the most commonly used teledermatology model in the United States [3].

The triage model is very useful for prioritizing patients based on the severity of their condition and can determine whether or not an in-person evaluation is required. This method ensures that patients are seen in a timely manner due to the decrease in both unneeded referrals and number of patients on waiting lists. Triage can be particularly helpful in underserved areas and places with limited resources.

The direct care model establishes a convenient connection between patients and dermatologists. Patients can photograph their skin condition and send these images directly to their physician. This method is considered to be the most flexible, however, it may be more difficult for providers to accurately diagnose a patient's skin condition without a previously established therapeutic relationship. Another disadvantage is the potential reluctance of providers to prescribe certain medications without an in-person consultation. SAF still remains the preferred modality for direct patient care [4].

The follow-up model is a subset of the direct care model. It allows for virtual long-term monitoring of chronic skin conditions, such as psoriasis or stasis ulcers. This method is normally utilized when there has been previously established in-person care. Chronic conditions often require frequent visits to the clinic, and remote follow-up care can save patients both time and money [3].

4 History

One of the first uses of telemedicine was in the early 1900s to help ship captains obtain medical advice through ship to shore radio [5]. The basis of many currently utilized telemedicine platforms originates from the telemetry research conducted by the National Aeronautics and Space Administration (NASA). Their research demonstrated that astronauts' vital signs and physiological functions could be monitored by physicians on earth through advanced telecommunication systems [6].

Another major contribution towards the advancement of telemedicine was the development of the television [3]. It was the first device that allowed for accurate visual transmission of data. However, the quality of images shared over video teleconferencing is inferior to captured images. Therefore, it wasn't until the creation and ubiquitous use of the internet, that the store-and-forward application of teledermatology was made possible. Moreover, technological advancements such as the advent of smartphones and mobile apps have been integral in linking diverse patient populations with specific providers, further increasing the means of connectivity between patients and physicians. As of 2013, there were 229 dermatology-related apps, approximately 50% of which were targeted towards patient use [7].

The United States Department of Defense (DoD) has also paved the way for the improvement and further development of TD. Up to 75% of outpatient visits in combat zones are the result of dermatological conditions and 40% of military telemedicine consultations are skin-related [8].

In 1992, the military employed telemedicine for the first time in order to assist a major humanitarian relief mission in Somalia. In 1996, the first military teledermatology service was created through the combined efforts of the National Naval Medical Center and dermatologists from the Uniformed Services University. Their online server was based on a SAF platform, and it allowed dermatologists to answer consults from field units, aircraft carriers, ships, and even a submarine. Since these physicians could access patient information at any moment and reply from any location, their response time was relatively quick, usually within 12 h. Over the course of 2 years, this system successfully delivered 89 teledermalogical consultations [8].

Consequently, in 2004, TD consults were approved by the DoD through a system that could be accessed by all active duty, reserve, and National Guard soldiers. This service continues to be used today along with other telemedicine services that have been added over the years [8].

Today, the rapid development of TD may be partially explained by recent healthcare precautions imposed by the COVID-19 pandemic, an unequal geographical distribution of dermatologists, and technological advances [9].

5 Conditions Examined

5.1 Acne

Acne is a chronic inflammatory skin condition involving the pilosebaceous unit. Its pathophysiology includes hyperseborrhea, altered follicular keratinization, and the proliferation of Propionibacterium acnes bacteria [10]. It is estimated that acne affects around 9.4% of the global population, which makes it the eighth most common disease worldwide [11].

Ruggiero et al. were the first to analyze the grade of satisfaction among patients using telemedicine during COVID-19 for acne consultations [12]. 52 patients (24 male, 28 female) between the ages of 18 and 27 years old were surveyed regarding their teledermatology experience. 92.3% of patients rated the dermatologist's attention to their condition as favorable, 71% were satisfied with the treatment they received, and 80.7% reported high well-being after treatment [12].

Another analysis regarding the use of teledermatology among patients with mild to moderate acne also demonstrated positive outcomes [13]. 72 patients (26 male, 46 female) with a median age of 22.3, all reported to be satisfied with TD. During video consultations, physicians were able to comfortably evaluate the clinical severity of the patient's skin disease, as well as provide education and additional information on treatment continuation. Patients were also able to upload high-resolution images of their acne, making it easier for dermatologists to better evaluate the severity of their condition and prior treatment efficacy. Furthermore, out of the 72 patients in this study, less than 10 required additional in-person office visits. Limitations of TD noted were the inability to conduct procedures such as chemical peels and microneedling [13].

Khosravi et al. compared the follow-up rates for acne patients between TD and outpatient dermatology visits [14]. The median time to follow-up was 45.5 days in the TD group and 64 days for the in-person group ($p < 0.001$). This significant difference in timing suggests that TD may provide easier access to care and shorter waiting times. 30.8% of TD follow-ups were virtual and 69.2% were face-to-face. Whereas, 100% of face-to-face follow-ups chose an in-person follow-up. The overall rate of follow-up was lower in the TD group than the in-person group, 13% versus 31% ($p < 0.0001$), respectively [14].

The discrepancy in the rate of follow-ups between the two groups may be partially explained by the increased use of stronger oral medications in the TD group than in-person group. 43% of TD patients versus 28.5% of in-person patients were treated with oral antibiotics with or without topical therapy or OCPs. 18.5% of TD patients versus 12.5% of in-person patients were treated with oral spironolactone with or without topical agents or OCPs. If greater acne control was obtained in the TD group, then these patients may be less inclined to consider a follow-up appointment. There was no significant difference in insurance status between patients, therefore this factor unlikely influences the follow-up rates between TD and in-person patients [14].

A randomized controlled trial conducted by Fruhauf et al. compared the treatment efficacy, safety, and patient satisfaction for the treatment of facial acne between TD and outpatient dermatology visits [15]. Both groups had excellent and almost identical therapeutic outcomes, with fewer adverse reactions in the TD group. Moreover, all of the patients seen by virtual consultation were pleased with mobile services alone and did not request additional in-person consultations [15].

It appears that TD is particularly useful for the treatment of skin diseases like acne, given the visual nature of this condition and relative ease of diagnosis. Most importantly, patient satisfaction is high with the utilization of teledermatology for acne consultations. Even if TD isn't solely used for the consultation and treatment of patients, it can at least be a very beneficial adjunct to outpatient care.

5.2 *Wounds*

Teledermatology has been utilized for a wide range of skin conditions, including wound care. A large-scale systematic review focusing on telemedicine in dermatology discussed 11 studies specifically focused on wound care [9]. The wounds evaluated included pressure ulcers, diabetic foot ulcers, diabetic foot infections, leg ulcers, nonhealing surgical wounds, and other chronic wounds [16–26]. All studies demonstrated similar outcomes between TD and in-person wound care consultations, and the authors of the review suggested that TD may become a critical tool for nursing homes and home care [9].

Pressure ulcers result from constant pressure on skin over a bony prominence, causing tissue breakdown and necrosis [27]. They are relatively common, affecting around 3 million adults yearly in the United States [27]. Pressure ulcers are a preventable condition and dermatologists play an integral role in the early recognition and treatment of these wounds. Hill et al. evaluated the use of telemedicine for pressure ulcers, and compared to in-person consults, 97% of video consults were able to detect the presence of a pressure ulcer [18]. The diagnosis of ulcer staging over video was almost identical to that of an in-person visit [18]. A study by Phillips et al. evaluating the diagnosis of pressure ulcers in newly injured spinal cord patients post-discharge demonstrated that the group utilizing telemedicine had the greatest number of reported and identified pressure ulcers when compared to telephone and in-person consultations [16].

Diabetic-related foot complications, such as ulcers, are considered the most common cause of morbidity among patients with diabetes [28]. Frequent screening is necessary among diabetic patients because the majority of diabetic foot ulcers are asymptomatic until non-healing ulcers appear. Proper preventative care can reduce unwanted and often debilitating complications [28]. The application of teledermatology for the management of diabetes-related foot ulceration was evaluated in a study by Wilbright et al. [17]. The time to healing of forefoot ulcers between patients treated in-person at a diabetes foot program and those treated through telemedicine was compared. No significant difference in healing times was noted between the two groups [17].

Foot infections are a related and relatively common complication among diabetic patients. The utilization of teledermatology for the diagnosis of foot infections was assessed by Hazenberg et al. Their study demonstrated that the diagnosis of foot infections remotely through photographs was highly specific (> 85%) but not sensitive. The use of infrared thermography to detect hotspots was very sensitive (> 90%) but not specific (< 25%). However, diagnosis using both pictures and thermography was sensitive (> 60%) and specific (> 79%). These results support the use of telemedicine for convenient at home monitoring of diabetic foot infections. TD can serve an important role in the early detection of both diabetic foot ulcers and infections.

Furthermore, Braun et al. verified that telemedical wound care consultation of leg ulcers had high concordance between virtual consultation (images sent through email) and face-to-face evaluations [22]. The use of TD for wound care in nursing homes has also been studied [20]. Utilizing telemedicine in this setting improves cost-efficiency through better selection of wound dressings, decreases unnecessary patient referrals, and even reduces the time to wound healing among nursing home patients [20].

Another prospective study demonstrated the efficacy of TD for the management of chronic wounds [25]. Wound healing was compared after one year between patients receiving care through telemedicine and those receiving in-person conventional care. The one-year follow-up demonstrated that complete wound healing was seen in 70% of patients in the telemedicine group compared to 45% in the conventional group [25]. The main difference in wound healing results from patient education on proper wound care provided by experts during teleconsultations [25].

5.3 Cancer

Skin cancer is the most common type of cancer [29]. Skin cancer can be categorized into melanoma and nonmelanoma. The most common types of nonmelanoma cancer include squamous cell (SCC) and basal cell carcinoma (BCC). BCC originates from the basal layer of the epidermis and is the most common type. It is normally slow-growing and rarely metastasizes. SCC originates from the uncontrolled proliferation of epidermal keratinocytes and is the second most common type of skin cancer, accounting for about 20% of nonmelanoma skin cancers [29]. Melanoma is considered the most aggressive type of skin cancer and is characterized as a malignant neoplasm derived from melanocytes, which are found in the basal layer of the epidermis. The 4 major subtypes of invasive melanoma include: superficial, nodular, lentigo maligna, and acral lentiginous. Although melanoma only accounts for about 2% of all skin cancer, it causes the most skin cancer deaths [29].

Early recognition of melanoma is critical as it may significantly improve the patient's prognosis. The greater the depth of invasion of the cancer, the worse the prognosis. A Breslow thickness < 1 mm, non-ulcerated melanoma has a 5-year survival rate of approximately 95%, compared to a > 4 mm ulcerated melanoma with lymph node metastasis that has a 5-year survival rate of 24% [30].

A comprehensive study analyzing 143 US dermatology practices covering 4.7 million patients across 13 states, estimated that due to reduced access to care as a result of the COVID-19 pandemic, there was an average diagnostic delay of 2.1 months for cutaneous SCCs, 1.9 months for BCCs, and 1.8 months for cutaneous melanomas [31].

A systematic review conducted by Eissing et al. reviewed the use of teledermatology for skin cancer [9]. Of the 204 publications that met their inclusion criteria, 52 specifically focused on the use of TD for the diagnosis of skin cancer, atypical nevi, and neoplasms. Of the 52 articles analyzed, 36 articles determined TD to be a reliable/effective modality. In comparison to in-person dermatology consults, 3 studies demonstrated TD to be equivalent, 8 studies determined TD to be superior, and 5 showed TD to be inferior. Another comparative study by Arzberger et al. regarding the evaluation of high-risk melanoma patients, determined that the identification of melanomas was equivalent between face-to-face and teledermatology consults [30].

Inadequate in-person access to dermatologists due to geographical barriers, restrictions from the COVID-19 pandemic [31], or any other reason can delay timely skin cancer diagnosis and potentially increase associated morbidity and mortality, as a result. However, teledermatology for the diagnosis of skin cancer seems to offer a reliable, accurate, and cost-effective alternative.

5.4 Hair

The use of telemedicine for the diagnosis of hair disorders is known as teletrichology [32]. Patients are instructed to part their hair in the middle and take pictures of their frontal and temporal hairline. If a patient is concerned with patchy alopecia, then it is suggested that they take images at the center and periphery of the patchy area [32]. The main drawback with this modality is the dependence on image quality as well as the patient's adherence to instructions.

6 Benefits and Risks

1. Accuracy and Advantages

The adoption of any new healthcare delivery method requires its careful examination in order to ensure that high standards of care are upheld. First among these standards is the accuracy of TD. Systematic review has found primary diagnostic accuracy rates to be 11% greater in-person when compared to TD [33]. This comparison of diagnostic concordance between the two modalities is deemed acceptable. Furthermore, the comparison of clinical management concordance ranges from moderate to very good [33]. The differentiation between diagnostic accuracy and clinical management is relevant because often times, subsequent management may have a greater effect on clinical outcomes than the accuracy of the original diagnosis. For example, the decision to biopsy a lesion thought to be malignant may reveal that it is actually benign. On the other hand, the decision to forego biopsy on a lesion considered to be benign, that is actually malignant, would result in a worse outcome for the patient.

When comparing the likelihood of an in-clinic dermatologist agreeing with the diagnosis and follow-up of a TD session, one must also compare the rates of agreement in context of the likelihood for two different dermatologists coming to the same conclusion in-person. A comprehensive analysis on the accuracy of TD concluded that teledermatologists and clinical dermatologists completely agreed with each other in 41–94% of cases and had partial agreement in 50–100% of cases [34]. A study evaluating the diagnostic accuracy of the histopathology analyzed from pigmented lesions revealed an accuracy rate of 92% and 86% among clinical dermatologists and teledermatologists, respectively. However, the clinical dermatologists missed two cases of melanoma, whereas the teledermatologists did not miss any [34]. In addition, research shows that the reliability of TD increases with the inclusion of extra information. When dermoscopy was included along with standard images, accuracy increased [35]. Additionally, patient satisfaction with TD remains high and comparable to in-patient visits according to a systematic review of 23 studies conducted in 2021 [36].

Widespread access to electronic devices has also allowed TD to be used as a valuable training tool among residents and physicians. This modality provides increased exposure to a variety of dermatological conditions, on a multitude of skin tones and types [3]. TD can also provide additive value as a source of second opinions for patients who seek consultation from physicians with a higher familiarity of their skin type, especially those without geographic access to inpatient dermatologists [37].

2. Cost Effectiveness

Given the widespread use and availability of the TD model, its cost effectiveness must be considered for both providers and patients. Zakaria et al. found a statistically significant mean cost savings of $140.12 per patient referred to TD services at the Zuckerberg San Francisco General Hospital and Trauma Center compared to a conventional inpatient model [38]. The cost effectiveness of TD further increases when considering additional externalities imposed on patient access to in-person providers. Some examples in favor of TD include: inadequate access to transportation required to reach an in-person setting, inability to schedule accommodations to account for travel time, faster time to biopsy or excision, reduction of in-person referrals, and reduced overhead fees for providers [14]. However, certain studies regarding cost-effectiveness had more mixed results, stating that the cost effectiveness was minimized when TD was used for services which would then require a follow up appointment in-person for procedures such as biopsy screens [39].

3. Barriers

As teledermatology continues to evolve, new barriers arise along with its development. Some challenges include the inability to perform procedures or conduct additional testing, decreased patient–physician interaction, lower reimbursements for physicians, and lack of familiarity with technical aspects [40]. There are also ethical concerns that telemedicine will shift the focus of medicine by changing a patient-centered approach to a more technologically-centered one [35]. Moreover, legal implications of TD are also a consideration. The safety and security of electronically transmitted patient data is a real concern, and the American Academy of Dermatology Association emphasizes that providers must secure health information through the use of encryption. Additionally, firewall-protected servers should be used to store confidential medical information. Patients should also be well-informed regarding how their information will be stored and who will be able to access it [36]. In addition, the confidence of a physician to make a diagnosis remotely instead of during in-person inspection introduces an element of subjectivity that can vary from physician to physician. Concerns over limitations of camera quality and holistic assessment must also be considered [41].

7 User Attitudes

A recent survey conducted among 184 practicing dermatologists shed light on the prevalence of teledermatology as well as physician's opinions on particular aspects [40]. 88.5% reported utilizing teledermatology. The majority (51.5%) were practicing in metropolitan or Tier 1 cities. The virtual platform most commonly used was WhatsApp, followed by audio calls, and different video calling softwares. When asked to compare the difficulty of TD to traditional consults for making a diagnosis, 71.1% of physicians reported TD to be slightly difficult, 9.2% felt there was no significant difference and 3.6% considered TD to be easier [40].

The ease of diagnosis with teledermatology also varied depending on skin condition. Acne was considered the easiest to diagnose, followed by tinea, alopecia, bacterial infections, eczema, viral infections, and pigmentary disorders. Inflammatory dermatitis was most difficult to diagnose. When asked about the use of teledermatology after COVID-19, over 70% of dermatologists stated that they plan to use TD in combination with physical consultations moving forward [40].

8 Conclusion

The prevalence of skin diseases in the United States collectively exceeds that of obesity, hypertension, and cancer [42]. Meanwhile, the average waiting time for an appointment with a dermatologist in 2009 was around 34 days but varied from 20 to 73 days, depending on location [35]. Due to the COVID-19 pandemic, it was not possible for many individuals to receive specialized medical care. As a result, telemedicine is currently being utilized more than ever before. The rapid development of technology combined with the expertise of medical professionals is paving the way for easier accessibility to high-quality care. Teledermatology is a valuable and cost-effective option for all patients, especially those who are underserved and have little or no access to specialty care.

References

1. Lee JJ, English JC 3rd. Teledermatology: a review and update. Am J Clin Dermatol. 2018;19(2):253–60.
2. Pasquali P, Sonthalia S, Moreno-Ramirez D, et al. Teledermatology and its current perspective. Indian Dermatol Online J. 2020;11(1):12–20.
3. Coates SJ, Kvedar J, Granstein RD. Teledermatology: from historical perspective to emerging techniques of the modern era: part I: history, rationale, and current practice. J Am Acad Dermatol. 2015;72(4):563–74; quiz 575–66.
4. Pathipati AS, Lee L, Armstrong AW. Health-care delivery methods in teledermatology: consultative, triage and direct-care models. J Telemed Telecare. 2011;17(4):214–6.
5. Wootton R. Recent advances: telemedicine. BMJ. 2001;323(7312):557–60.
6. Zundel KM. Telemedicine: history, applications, and impact on librarianship. Bull Med Libr Assoc. 1996;84(1):71–9.
7. Brewer AC, Endly DC, Henley J, et al. Mobile applications in dermatology. JAMA Dermatol. 2013;149(11):1300–4.
8. Rosenbaum BE, Campion CH, Cohen JM, Latkowski JA. The Department of Defense: pioneers of early teledermatology. Dermatol Online J. 2017;23(2).
9. Trettel A, Eissing L, Augustin M. Telemedicine in dermatology: findings and experiences worldwide—a systematic literature review. J Eur Acad Dermatol Venereol. 2018;32(2):215–24.
10. Dreno B. What is new in the pathophysiology of acne, an overview. J Eur Acad Dermatol Venereol. 2017;31(Suppl 5):8–12.
11. Tan JK, Bhate K. A global perspective on the epidemiology of acne. Br J Dermatol. 2015;172(Suppl 1):3–12.
12. Ruggiero A, Megna M, Annunziata MC, et al. Teledermatology for acne during COVID-19: high patients' satisfaction in spite of the emergency. J Eur Acad Dermatol Venereol. 2020;34(11):e662–3.
13. Villani A, Annunziata MC, Abategiovanni L, Fabbrocini G. Teledermatology for acne patients: how to reduce face-to-face visits during COVID-19 pandemic. J Cosmet Dermatol. 2020;19(8):1828.
14. Khosravi H, Zhang S, Siripong N, Moorhead A, English III JC. Comparing acne follow-up: teledermatology versus outpatient dermatology visits. Dermatol Online J. 2020;26(4).
15. Frühauf J, Krock S, Quehenberger F, et al. Mobile teledermatology helping patients control high-need acne: a randomized controlled trial. J Eur Acad Dermatol Venereol. 2015;29(5):919–24.
16. Phillips VL, Temkin A, Vesmarovich S, Burns R, Idleman L. Using telehealth interventions to prevent pressure ulcers in newly injured spinal cord injury patients post-discharge. Results from a pilot study. Int J Technol Assess Health Care. 1999;15(4):749–55.
17. Wilbright WA, Birke JA, Patout CA, Varnado M, Horswell R. The use of telemedicine in the management of diabetes-related foot ulceration: a pilot study. Adv Skin Wound Care. 2004;17(5 Pt 1):232–8.
18. Hill ML, Cronkite RC, Ota DT, Yao EC, Kiratli BJ. Validation of home telehealth for pressure ulcer assessment: a study in patients with spinal cord injury. J Telemed Telecare. 2009;15(4):196–202.
19. Terry M, Halstead LS, O'Hare P, et al. Feasibility study of home care wound management using telemedicine. Adv Skin Wound Care. 2009;22(8):358–64.
20. Vowden K, Vowden P. A pilot study on the potential of remote support to enhance wound care for nursing-home patients. J Wound Care. 2013;22(9):481–8.
21. Hazenberg CE, van Netten JJ, van Baal SG, Bus SA. Assessment of signs of foot infection in diabetes patients using photographic foot imaging and infrared thermography. Diabetes Technol Ther. 2014;16(6):370–7.
22. Braun RP, Vecchietti JL, Thomas L, et al. Telemedical wound care using a new generation of mobile telephones: a feasibility study. Arch Dermatol. 2005;141(2):254–8.

23. Houghton PE, Kincaid CB, Campbell KE, Woodbury MG, Keast DH. Photographic assessment of the appearance of chronic pressure and leg ulcers. Ostomy Wound Manage. 2000;46(4):20–6, 28–30.
24. Stern A, Mitsakakis N, Paulden M, et al. Pressure ulcer multidisciplinary teams via telemedicine: a pragmatic cluster randomized stepped wedge trial in long term care. BMC Health Serv Res. 2014;14:83.
25. Zarchi K, Haugaard VB, Dufour DN, Jemec GBE. Expert advice provided through telemedicine improves healing of chronic wounds: prospective cluster controlled study. J Invest Dermatol. 2015;135(3):895–900.
26. Bowling FL, King L, Paterson JA, et al. Remote assessment of diabetic foot ulcers using a novel wound imaging system. Wound Repair Regen. 2011;19(1):25–30.
27. Mervis JS, Phillips TJ. Pressure ulcers: pathophysiology, epidemiology, risk factors, and presentation. J Am Acad Dermatol. 2019;81(4):881–90.
28. Lim JZ, Ng NS, Thomas C. Prevention and treatment of diabetic foot ulcers. J R Soc Med. 2017;110(3):104–9.
29. Linares MA, Zakaria A, Nizran P. Skin cancer. Prim Care. 2015;42(4):645–59.
30. Arzberger E, Curiel-Lewandrowski C, Blum A, et al. Teledermoscopy in high-risk melanoma patients: a comparative study of face-to-face and teledermatology visits. Acta Derm Venereol. 2016;96(6):779–83.
31. Marson JW, Maner BS, Harding TP, et al. The magnitude of COVID-19's effect on the timely management of melanoma and nonmelanoma skin cancers. J Am Acad Dermatol. 2021;84(4):1100–3.
32. Randolph M, Al-Alola A, Tosti A. Diagnosis of hair disorders during the COVID-19 pandemic: an introduction to teletrichoscopy. J Eur Acad Dermatol Venereol. 2021;35(3):e167–8.
33. Warshaw EM, Hillman YJ, Greer NL, et al. Teledermatology for diagnosis and management of skin conditions: a systematic review. J Am Acad Dermatol. 2011;64(4):759–72.
34. Levin YS, Warshaw EM. Teledermatology: a review of reliability and accuracy of diagnosis and management. Dermatol Clin. 2009;27(2):163–76, vii.
35. Pala P, Bergler-Czop BS, Gwizdz JM. Teledermatology: idea, benefits and risks of modern age—a systematic review based on melanoma. Postepy Dermatol Alergol. 2020;37(2):159–67.
36. Hadeler E, Gitlow H, Nouri K. Definitions, survey methods, and findings of patient satisfaction studies in teledermatology: a systematic review. Arch Dermatol Res. 2021;313(4):205–15.
37. Lozzi GP, Soyer HP, Massone C, et al. The additive value of second opinion teleconsulting in the management of patients with challenging inflammatory, neoplastic skin diseases: a best practice model in dermatology? J Eur Acad Dermatol Venereol. 2007;21(1):30–4.
38. Zakaria A, Miclau TA, Maurer T, Leslie KS, Amerson E. Cost minimization analysis of a teledermatology triage system in a managed care setting. JAMA Dermatol. 2021;157(1):52–8.
39. Barbieri JS, Yang X, Kovarik CL. Evaluating the cost-effectiveness of teledermatology. J Am Acad Dermatol. 2019;81(3):765–6.
40. Sharma A, Jindal V, Singla P, Goldust M, Mhatre M. Will teledermatology be the silver lining during and after COVID-19? Dermatol Ther. 2020;33(4): e13643.
41. Grenier N, Bercovitch L, Long TP. Cyberdermatoethics II: a case-based approach to teledermatology ethics. Clin Dermatol. 2009;27(4):367–71.
42. Bickers DR, Lim HW, Margolis D, et al. The burden of skin diseases: 2004 a joint project of the American Academy of Dermatology Association and the Society for Investigative Dermatology. J Am Acad Dermatol. 2006;55(3):490–500.

Telemedicine for Inflammatory Skin Conditions

Fabio Stefano Frech, Yasmine Nousari, Ali Rajabi-Estarabadi, and Carlos Nousari

Abstract The advent of telemedicine has revolutionized healthcare delivery across various specialties, and dermatology is no exception. With the integration of technology and medical expertise, telemedicine has emerged as a powerful tool in providing remote dermatologic care. Telemedicine has the ability to break down geographical barriers, offering dermatological care to individuals who may have limited access to specialized healthcare. Rural areas, underserved communities, and regions with a shortage of dermatologists can now benefit from expert consultations through telemedicine. Patients are now able to circumvent the costs associated with transportation and time spent away from work by scheduling virtual consultations. Moreover, telemedicine allows patients to connect with dermatologists who may be in a different city or even a different country, expanding the pool of available specialists.

Keywords Inflammatory skin conditions · Telemedicine · Teledermatology · Psoriasis · Atopic dermatitis · Acne

1 Introduction

The advent of telemedicine has revolutionized healthcare delivery across various specialties, and dermatology is no exception. With the integration of technology and medical expertise, telemedicine has emerged as a powerful tool in providing remote dermatologic care. Telemedicine has the ability to break down geographical barriers, offering dermatological care to individuals who may have limited access to specialized healthcare. Rural areas, underserved communities, and regions with a shortage of dermatologists can now benefit from expert consultations through telemedicine.

F. S. Frech (✉) · Y. Nousari
Miller School of Medicine, University of Miami, Miami, FL, USA
e-mail: fabio_frech2@hotmail.com

A. Rajabi-Estarabadi · C. Nousari
Department of Dermatology, Broward Health Medical Center, Graduate Medical Center, Fort Lauderdale, FL, USA

K. Nouri (ed.), *Telemedicine and Technological Advances in Dermatology*,
https://doi.org/10.1007/978-3-031-69091-4_2

Patients are now able to circumvent the costs associated with transportation and time spent away from work by scheduling virtual consultations. Moreover, telemedicine allows patients to connect with dermatologists who may be in a different city or even a different country, expanding the pool of available specialists.

Telemedicine has streamlined the dermatological consultation process, increasing efficiency for both patients and healthcare providers. Virtual consultations enable dermatologists to review patient information, including medical histories and images, prior to the appointment, saving valuable time. Patients can upload high-quality images of their skin conditions, aiding dermatologists in making accurate diagnoses remotely. Telemedicine also facilitates rapid follow-ups, allowing patients to receive timely feedback on treatment progress without the need for an in-person visit. Consequently, telemedicine optimizes resource allocation, reducing the burden on traditional healthcare systems.

Telemedicine in dermatology has been associated with higher patient satisfaction rates [1]. The convenience of remote consultations eliminates the need for time-consuming clinic visits, minimizing waiting times and reducing anxiety for patients. Virtual appointments offer flexibility, allowing individuals to schedule consultations at their convenience, accommodating busy lifestyles. Telemedicine also empowers patients by promoting self-care and education, as they can engage in meaningful conversations with dermatologists regarding their conditions, treatment options, and preventive measures. Enhanced patient engagement and shared decision-making contribute to improved health outcomes and overall satisfaction with the care received.

While telemedicine has undeniably revolutionized dermatological care, it is not without challenges. Reliable internet connectivity and access to necessary technology can be barriers for some patients, particularly those in rural or low-income areas. Security and privacy concerns must also be addressed to safeguard patient information during virtual consultations. Dermatologists need to ensure accurate diagnoses without the advantage of physical examination, relying solely on visual cues. Additionally, some dermatological procedures, such as biopsies or surgical interventions, cannot be performed remotely. Balancing the benefits of telemedicine with the limitations it presents is crucial to ensure the delivery of comprehensive and high-quality dermatological care.

Telemedicine has had a transformative impact on dermatology, offering improved access to care, enhanced efficiency, and increased patient satisfaction. By leveraging technology, dermatologists can reach patients in remote areas, optimize resource allocation, and provide convenient and timely consultations. While challenges exist, telemedicine continues to evolve, promising to reshape the field of dermatology and improve healthcare outcomes for patients worldwide. In this chapter, we delineate the uses, advantages, and disadvantages of telemedicine for inflammatory skin conditions.

2 Types of Teledermatology

Two main forms of telemedicine exist: **store-and-forward** and **live interactive**. Store-and-forward [SAF] refers to an asynchronous type of virtual consultation that allows clinicians to make decisions based on electronically transferred patient information and photographs. In contrast, live interactive is considered a synchronous type of telehealth encounter that allows patient and clinician interaction through either voice or video communication. Given that SAF uses still photography, it allows patients to forward high-quality images to the provider and forward any relevant clinical information. This comes at little cost to the patient as well as avoiding having to coordinate or schedule a visit in person. Nonetheless, this type of telehealth is generally not reimbursable. Live interactive teledermatology allows for immediate, shared decision-making with the patient as well as allowing the physician to answer any questions on management. This technology also allows the physician to be reimbursed for their time, since it requires both patient and provider to be available at the same time generally through video conferencing. For live consultations to be achieved successfully and smoothly patients need to have a reliable internet connection. Even with a reliable connection, the image quality of these consultations is generally inferior to that of still photographic technology. This drawback may hinder the ability of dermatologists to accurately identify disease processes or monitor treatment efficacy. Therefore, a hybrid model of telehealth consultations can be implemented to limit any drawbacks of both types of teledermatology. In this combined model, patients can send medical information including high-quality images for review before any live interactive consultation. When the live interactive consultation begins, dermatologists and patients may discuss treatment strategies or make changes to current management protocols. After the live interactive telehealth visit, SAF consultations can be used to monitor patient progress and help in decision making at future visits.

Several limitations to both asynchronous and synchronous teledermatology models need to be considered, including the patients' ability to understand applications, take high-quality pictures, and reliably document pertinent changes of disease progression. Additionally, a patient's socioeconomic status may affect the likelihood of having a mobile device with a good quality camera, which may make the diagnosis as well as management through video or photography challenging. Finally, one of the biggest challenges that asynchronous visits may face is the lack of appropriate reimbursement for the time spent during these types of consults.

3 Inflammatory Skin Diseases

The role of teledermatology in treating inflammatory skin disorders is multifaceted and may be used at different stages of management. A retrospective cohort study of 286,364 patients assessing the role of telemedicine during the COVID-19 pandemic showed that the most common primary dermatologic diagnoses were inflammatory conditions [2]. The authors found that patients with inflammatory skin diseases were more likely to be evaluated and managed through telemedicine compared to patients with neoplastic disorders [2]. Thus, visual diagnosis, management, and follow-up of certain inflammatory skin conditions may be performed through teledermatology.

3.1 Acne

Acne is the most common inflammatory skin disease in the United States affecting over 85% of people in the ages of 12–25 [3]. Acne is known to have first onset and greater severity in the adolescent stages of life. However, this skin condition is not unique to adolescence and can affect adults. It has been show that about 26% of women and 12% of men in the United States experience acne in their 40s [4]. Acne is a known inflammatory skin disorder that affects the pilosebaceous unit and the specific pathophysiology is multifactorial. Increased sebum production, inflammation, infection with *Cutibacterium acnes*, and hyperkeratinization of the follicular unit have been shown to be likely factors responsible for the development of acne [4]. Given that the diagnosis of acne is clinical, both the diagnosis, management, and follow-up may be carried out using teledermatology. Ideally, a hybrid system, involving synchronous and asynchronous telemedicine, can be used. The use of SAF technology has been successfully validated and implemented in several practice models and studies. A single center, randomized controlled superiority trial of 69 patients compared mobile teledermatology in the form of SAF and regular outpatient follow-ups in the treatment of acne with isotretitinoin [5]. The patients were randomized into the teledermatology and outpatient groups in a 1:1 ratio. The teledermatology visits consisted of a mobile application that allows patients to report side effects and medical information as well as take photographs to report progress. Patients in the teledermatology group captured three pictures and entered relevant clinical information every 2 weeks. Within 24 hours the providers responded with specific instructions to either maintain or change any treatment strategy. Importantly, the baseline and the 24-week visit were conducted both in person. Using standardized tests to compare acne severity over the study period, the authors found that both groups were comparable in their satisfaction, with the SAF group reporting less adverse reactions to treatments [5]. This suggests that SAF technology is a safe and effective means of communication that allows more frequent follow-ups without the need of having in-person visits. SAF technology, however, frequently relies on patient's ability to reliably use technology and take high-quality pictures that would allow the clinician to make an accurate assessment for the management of the specific disease in question. A pilot study of 69 patients using a mobile application to take self-photographs studied the reliability of patient-take photographs for the assessment and management of acne compared to in-person visits [6]. The investigators reported that patient-taken photographs were comparable to in-person physical dermatology evaluations in the diagnosing of acne [6]. Taken together these studies suggest that not only can the management of acne be carried out with teledermatological visits but clinicians can rely on patient-taken photographs for appropriate diagnosis and treatment. Interestingly, when comparing asynchronous and synchronous visits for the management of acne with isotretinoin, about 75% of asynchronous visits were completed successfully without the need to convert to synchronous visits [7]. Likely, a hybrid model of using both synchronous and asynchronous telemedicine will be the most optimal, allowing for enough flexibility to the clinicians and patients. A retrospective study of 213 acne patients using a combination of patient-captured photographs and video visits showed that all patients reported a high level of satisfaction, especially those living at a distance [8]. When given the option for in-person visits, about 51.7% of patients opted in for live consultations suggesting a high degree of satisfaction with virtual visits [8]. Taken together these studies suggest that SAF teledermatology in combination with in-person or synchronous visits for diagnosis and long-term follow up allows patients to maintain constant communication with their dermatologists without significant interruption of their daily activities.

3.2 Hidradenitis Suppurativa

Hidradenitis Suppurativa [HS] is an inflammatory skin disease that consists of chronic and recurrent suppurativa nodules arising from apocrine glands. Affected patients generally have lesions within the folds of the skin, including axillae, groin, inframammary area, and perianal regions. It is estimated that the prevalence of HS ranges from 0.05 to 4.10% [9, 10]. Several modifiable and nonmodifiable risk factors have been elucidated and include larger body habitus, smoking, African race, and genetic predisposition. The pathogenesis of HS has been extensively studied and it has been posited to start with follicular occlusion through hyperkeratosis, leading to follicular rupture and formation of inflammatory nodules and abscesses, which ultimately with disease progression develop into chronic sinus tracts [11]. HS has been associated with significant negative implications to quality of life in patients. Therefore, prompt diagnosis and management are necessary for timely improvement of the course of the disease and to prevent exacerbation and flairs. Initial diagnosis is likely more amenable to be performed at in-person visits given that the assessment of the severity (i.e., staging) may involve inspection of areas which patients may not feel comfortable revealing during video visits or sharing through photography. Additionally, the severity of the disease might necessitate intralesional treatments at the first visit for symptom control and reduction of inflammation in the affected areas. The role of telemedicine in the management of HS has not been clearly elucidated or extensively studied. Several studies have evaluated patient satisfaction of telemedicine visits with HS patients. Ruggiero et al. performed a qualitative, question-based study on 54 HS patients undergoing management through some form of telemedicine to determine patients' feelings and concerns [12]. About 28.5% of patients reported that they prefer in-person visits compared to 22.5% of patients preferring teledermatology consults. About 49% of patients reported no preference [12]. Interestingly, a slight majority of patient [57%] reported feeling safe sharing required photos and videos through a teledermatology service [12]. In this particular study, up to 90% of respondents reported lesions in sensitive body parts [12], likely affecting the willingness of many patients to undergo examination through video or photography. Okeke et al. suggest that patients who are hesitant to show sensitive areas through video conferencing may be advised to send digital photographs prior to the video appointment [13]. This would allow patients to feel more comfortable discussing their disease progression without exposing sensitive areas during video visits. Additionally, this provides the advantage of having objective patient progress through digital images prior to the video visit, allowing clinicians to evaluate patient progress and make necessary adjustments to the plan in preparation of the upcoming video appointment. Another study investigated patient perspectives during the COVID-19 pandemic in the management of 335 HS patients. The authors found that patients with higher Hurley staging were more likely to disagree that telemedicine visits were equally effective compared to in-person visits [14]. This suggests that increased burden of disease within each patient results in lower satisfaction with teledermatology visits. More extensive disease may necessitate a higher degree of involvement and a more comprehensive treatment strategy that may not be carried out solely through telemedicine visits. Additionally, video visits may not accurately depict the severity or staging of the disease thus may result in inadequate outcomes and poorer satisfaction. Similarly, a recent study using a standardized questionnaire evaluated patient perspectives in the effectiveness of telemedicine in managing HS during the COVID-19 pandemic [15]. In this study, about 77.14% of respondents reported that teledermatology visits were not sufficient or adequate to address all patient concerns during the visit [15]. Although the role of telemedicine in the management of HS has not been extensively studied, current literature suggests that virtual appointments alone may not be adequate to treat these patients. A combination of virtual and in-person visits would likely yield the best outcomes and provide the highest satisfaction.

3.3 Atopic Dermatitis

Atopic dermatitis [AD] is a chronic, recurrent, inflammatory disease characterized by erythematous, pruritic patches most commonly located in the flexural areas of the body [16] It is estimated that it affects about 20–30% of people in developed countries, and affects 13% of children and 7% of adults in the United States [17, 18]. Atopic dermatitis is characterized by different phases: acute and chronic [or subacute]. Generally, in the acute phase patients have red, erythematous patches along the flexural areas that are open or have overlying hemorrhagic crusts caused by scratching. Chronic scratching may cause these lesions to become lichenified and hyperpigmented [16]. This hyperpigmentation may last many months and resolves with time when the underlying disease process is treated. The chronic, remitting course of the disease makes it especially challenging for patients due to the continual monitoring and treatment modifications that need to be undertaken to assure proper management. Teledermatology may provide a medium through which clinicians can follow disease progression without the limitations of in-person visits. Recently, the European Academy of Allergy and Clinical Immunology published a position stamen outlining the role of mobile or telehealth within dermatologic diseases such as AD [19]. The statement outlines that mobile teledermatology may be used to track disease progression, medication adherence, and treatment outcomes [19]. Additionally, the statement recommends the use of patient self-assessment tools for AD, such as the Patient-Oriented Scoring Atopic Dermatitis [PO-SCORAD] and the Patient Oriented Eczema Measure from Nottingham [20], as an aid for monitoring disease progression and treatment success without the necessity of in-person visits. The Atopic Dermatitis Symptom Score is another tool that has been recently validated as an effective and useful tool in the self-tracking of AD symptoms [21]. The use of these scoring systems may allow the patient to take ownership of their disease management and may aid the tailoring of the appropriate management algorithm. These tracking tools can be integrated by providing the questionnaire through mobile applications or paper surveys, allowing the clinicians to determine disease improvement more objectively. The onset of SARS-CoV-2 pandemic urged healthcare professionals to move towards different methods of delivering their services, especially the monitoring of treatment success and disease progression, including the monitoring of the safety and effectiveness of biologic therapeutics in treating atopic dermatitis [22]. A randomized clinical trial of 156 participants compared direct-access online asynchronous telehealth visits to in-person visits for the treatment of atopic dermatitis [23]. The direct-access group transmitted pictures and history of disease through an asynchronous manner allowing clinicians to provide recommendations online without the necessity of live visits. The authors showed that both the asynchronous group and regular in-person group showed equivalent improvements in atopic dermatitis clinical outcomes [23]. Another study similarly compared the efficacy of asynchronous teledermatology to in-person visits in the capacity of improving quality of life for atopic dermatitis patients [24]. To measure any improvement in quality of life, the Dermatology Life Quality Index [DLQI], Children's Dermatology Life Quality Index [CDLQI], and Short Form [SF] were used [24]. All visits for the direct-access care group were conducted asynchronously, wherein patients submitted pictures and progress as well as standardized questionnaires. The dermatologists reviewed the information and within 3 days responded with a treatment plan and recommendations. Both the in-person visit and the asynchronous direct-access care groups had equivalent improvements in quality of life scores [24]. This suggests that both atopic dermatitis can be managed and treated successfully remotely. However, it is important to note that these studies included participants in which the diagnosis of atopic dermatitis was already made and generally the first clinical visit was conducted in person. Ideally, for the purposes of diagnostic accuracy and disease severity assessment, the first visit can be conducted in person and the subsequent visits conducted remotely if feasible.

3.4 Psoriasis

Psoriasis is a chronic, immune-mediated disease that is characterized by thick erythematous plaques with overlying silvery scale that generally affects the extensor surfaces of the body [25]. There are multiple subtypes including plaque, guttate, pustular, erythrodermic, inverse, nail, and palmoplantar psoriasis—the most common of which is plaque psoriasis accounting for 80% of the cases [25]. Psoriasis has been estimated to affect 0.54–11.43% of adults and 1.37% of children in the world [26]. In the USA, it has been estimated that psoriasis affects about 7.4 million adults [27]. The management of psoriasis generally requires considerable follow up and consistent modification of treatment strategies to optimize outcomes. This characteristic lends itself well to management through telemedicine. The use of telemedicine for psoriasis has been evaluated as early as 2010. A pilot study was conducted to assess the feasibility of asynchronous teledermatology in the management of psoriasis [5]. The study involved the use of a mobile telephone application that used a 1.4 megapixel camera to take digital photos and upload relevant medical information. Patients were treated with etanercept biologic therapy and progress was assessed every 2 weeks by two teledermatologists. Progression of disease was assessed using Psoriasis Area and Severity Index [PASI] or Palmoplantar PASI [PPPASI] scores and compared to data from routine outpatient face-to-face consultations within the same timeframe. The study showed that there was concordance in PASI and PPASI assessments between the teledermatologists and in-person consultations [5]. Additionally, most of the pictures taken by patients were deemed to be at least satisfactory for analysis and decision making [5]. Interestingly, this study was conducted using a 1.4 megapixel phone camera which in modern times is considered to be of low quality given that most current phones have cameras with 48 megapixels or more. This suggests that the phone or camera type may not significantly impact decision-making during teledermatology consultations, but rather patient education will ensure that picture quality will be optimized. Another study similarly compared PASI scoring between face-to-face dermatology visits and dermatologists evaluating psoriasis patients through digital imaging [28]. The authors reported that there was moderate to good agreement in PASI scores between teledermatologists as well as good agreement between in-person encounters and teledermatologists scores [28]. The use of telemedicine has also been evaluated for the use as a monitoring tool in patients undergoing therapy with biologics [29]. The authors of the study enrolled patients that were being treated with efalizumab and etanercept for moderate-to-severe psoriasis [29]. They compared the "tele-PASI" scores to PASI scores for in-person visits. The authors reported that about 95% of the images were of sufficient quality to evaluate and perform accurate assessment of PASI scores [29]. Additionally, studies conducted during the COVID-19 pandemic due to the cessation of biologic therapy in psoriatic patients showed that there was significant adverse effects in quality-of-life and psychological status due to disease progression [30]. Therefore, the use of telemedicine as a monitoring system in patients that have limitations to in-person appointments may be used as an alternative. Additionally, studies evaluating preferences in patients undergoing biologic therapy in regards to telemedicine appointments versus physical appointments have shown that up to 48% prefer telemedicine visits, and of those who favor in-person visits report that biggest challenge with telehealth was their inability to use video-conferencing [31]. A 1:1 randomized clinical trial of 296 patients sought to evaluate the effectiveness of an online healthcare deliver model to in-person visits for the management of psoriasis [32]. Participants were enrolled to either an in-person or online group wherein patients and primary care physicians [PCP] had the ability to interact with teledermatologists through an asynchronous manner. The PCP or patient was able to contact the teledermatologists through an online platform and within 2 days recommendations were provided to PCPs by dermatologists for further management [32]. The differences in mean change of body surface area and PASI score between the two groups was − 0.27 [95% CI, − 0.85 to − 0.31] and − 0.05% [95% CI, − 1.58 to − 1.48%], respectively. This suggests that there were no differences in effectiveness between the in-person and telemedicine group in the management of psoriasis [32]. A similarly conducted randomized controlled clinical trial that evaluated the impact of online healthcare versus in-person visits in patient's functional and mental health status showed that both healthcare delivery systems were equivalent in reducing depressive symptoms and functional impairments for psoriasis patients [33]. Taken together these studies suggest that teledermatology is a feasible alternative to in-person visits that may provide equivalent outcomes in regards to managing disease progression as well as disease burden.

4 Conclusion

The integration of telemedicine into dermatology has brought about significant advancements in the provision of care for various inflammatory skin conditions. Telemedicine's ability to overcome geographical barriers, increase efficiency, and enhance patient satisfaction has been evident across different stages of patient care. Through store-and-forward and live interactive approaches, dermatologists can accurately diagnose, manage, and monitor inflammatory conditions like acne, atopic dermatitis, and psoriasis.

Despite the benefits, challenges remain, including the need for reliable technology and internet access, maintaining diagnostic accuracy without physical examination, and addressing reimbursement disparities. Striking a balance between the advantages of telemedicine and the limitations it presents is essential for delivering comprehensive and high-quality care.

As technology continues to evolve, telemedicine's role in dermatology will likely expand, contributing to improved patient outcomes and healthcare accessibility. Collaborative efforts between healthcare providers, patients, and policymakers will be crucial to address the challenges and maximize the potential of telemedicine in the management of inflammatory skin conditions. Through careful consideration and adaptation, the integration of telemedicine will likely reshape the landscape of dermatological care, breaking barriers by allowing the treatment of patients worldwide.

References

1. Santiago S, Lu J. Patient satisfaction in teledermatology: an updated review. Curr Dermatol Rep. 2023;12(1):23–6. https://doi.org/10.1007/s13671-023-00382-z.
2. He A, Ti Kim T, Nguyen KD. Utilization of teledermatology services for dermatological diagnoses during the COVID-19 pandemic. Arch Dermatol Res. 2022;315(4):1059–62. https://doi.org/10.1007/s00403-022-02438-9.
3. Mohsin N, Hernandez LE, Martin MR, Does AV, Nouri K. Acne treatment review and future perspectives. Dermatol Ther. 2022;35(9). https://doi.org/10.1111/dth.15719.
4. Zaenglein AL. Acne vulgaris. N Engl J. Med. 2018;379(14):1343–52. https://doi.org/10.1056/nejmcp1702493.
5. Frühauf J, Kröck S, Quehenberger F, et al. Mobile teledermatology helping patients control high-need acne: a randomized controlled trial. J Eur Acad Dermatol Venereol. 2015;29(5):919–24. https://doi.org/10.1111/jdv.12723.
6. Singer HM, Almazan T, Craft N, et al. Using network oriented research assistant (NORA) technology to compare digital photographic with in-person assessment of acne vulgaris. JAMA Dermatol. 2018;154(2):188. https://doi.org/10.1001/jamadermatol.2017.5141.
7. Das S, Su MY, Kvedar JC, Smith GP. Asynchronous telemedicine for isotretinoin management: a direct care pilot. J Am Acad Dermatol. 2022;(1097-6787 (Electronic)).
8. Villani A, Annunziata MC, Megna M, Scalvenzi M, Fabbrocini G. Long-term results of teledermatology for acne patients during COVID-19 pandemic. J Cosmetic Dermatol. 2022;21(4):1356–7. https://doi.org/10.1111/jocd.14805.
9. Jemec GB, Kimball AB. Hidradenitis suppurativa: epidemiology and scope of the problem. J Am Acad Dermatol. 2015;(1097-6787 (Electronic)).
10. Ingram JR, Jenkins-Jones S, Knipe DW, Morgan CLI, Cannings-John R, Piguet V. Population-based clinical practice research datalink study using algorithm modelling to identify the true burden of hidradenitis suppurativa. Br J Dermatol. 2018;178(4):917–24. https://doi.org/10.1111/bjd.16101.
11. Goldburg SR, Strober BE, Payette MJ. Hidradenitis suppurativa: epidemiology, clinical presentation, and pathogenesis. J Am Acad Dermatol. 2019;(1097-6787 (Electronic)).
12. Ruggiero AA-O, Marasca CA-O, Fabbrocini GA-O, Villani AA-OX, Martora FA-OX. Teledermatology in the management of hidradenitis suppurativa: should we improve this service? J Cosmetic Dermatol. 2022;(1473-2165 (Electronic)).
13. Okeke CA-O, Shipman WA-O, Perry JA-O, Kerns MA-OX, Okoye GA-O, Byrd AA-O. Treating hidradenitis suppurativa during the COVID-19 pandemic: teledermatology exams of sensitive body areas. J Dermatol Treat. 2020;(1471-1753 (Electronic)).
14. Price KN, Collier EK, Grogan TR, Hsiao JL, Shi VY. Hidradenitis suppurativa patient perspectives during the COVID-19 pandemic. Dermatol Online J. 2021;27(2). https://doi.org/10.5070/d3272052396.
15. Gierek M, Kitala D, Łabuś W, et al. The impact of telemedicine on patients with hidradenitis suppurativa in the COVID-19 era. Healthcare. 2023;11(10):1453. https://doi.org/10.3390/healthcare11101453.
16. Clebak KT, Helm L, Uppal P, Davis CR, Helm MF. Atopic dermatitis. (1558-299X (Electronic)).
17. Weidinger S, Novak N. Atopic dermatitis. (1474-547X (Electronic)).

18. McKenzie C, Silverberg JI. The prevalence and persistence of atopic dermatitis in urban United States children. (1534-4436 (Electronic)).
19. Matricardi PM, Dramburg S, Alvarez-Perea A, et al. The role of mobile health technologies in allergy care: an EAACI position paper. Allergy. 2020;75(2):259–72. https://doi.org/10.1111/all.13953.
20. Stalder J-F, Barbarot S, Wollenberg A, et al. Patient-oriented SCORAD (PO-SCORAD): a new self-assessment scale in atopic dermatitis validated in Europe. Allergy. 2011;66(8):1114–21. https://doi.org/10.1111/j.1398-9995.2011.02577.x.
21. Lee JY, Kim M, Yang H-K, et al. Reliability and validity of the Atopic Dermatitis Symptom Score (ADSS). Pediatr Allergy Immunol. 2018;29(3):290–5. https://doi.org/10.1111/pai.12865.
22. Napolitano M, Patruno C, Ruggiero A, Nocerino M, Fabbrocini G. Safety of dupilumab in atopic patients during COVID-19 outbreak. (1471-1753 (Electronic)).
23. Armstrong AW, Johnson MA, Lin S, Maverakis E, Fazel N, Liu F-T. Patient-centered, direct-access online care for management of atopic dermatitis. JAMA Dermatol. 2015;151(2):154. https://doi.org/10.1001/jamadermatol.2014.2299.
24. Kornmehl H, Singh S, Johnson MA, Armstrong AW. Direct-access online care for the management of atopic dermatitis: a randomized clinical trial examining patient quality of life. (1556-3669 (Electronic)).
25. Armstrong AW, Read C. Pathophysiology, clinical presentation, and treatment of psoriasis. JAMA. 2020;323(19):1945. https://doi.org/10.1001/jama.2020.4006.
26. Michalek IM, Loring B, John SM. A systematic review of worldwide epidemiology of psoriasis. J Eur Acad Dermatol Venereol. 2017;31(2):205–12. https://doi.org/10.1111/jdv.13854.
27. Rachakonda TD, Schupp CW, Armstrong AW. Psoriasis prevalence among adults in the United States. (1097-6787 (Electronic)).
28. Singh P, Soyer HP, Wu J, Salmhofer W, Gilmore S. Tele-assessment of Psoriasis Area and Severity Index: a study of the accuracy of digital image capture. Australas J Dermatol. 2011;52(4):259–63. https://doi.org/10.1111/j.1440-0960.2011.00800.x.
29. Koller S, Hofmann-Wellenhof R, Hayn D, et al. Teledermatological monitoring of psoriasis patients on biologic therapy. Acta Derm Venereol. 2011;91(6):680–5. https://doi.org/10.2340/00015555-1148.
30. Li S, Zhang S, Wu R, Su Y. COVID-19 and psoriasis: recommendation for patients on regular infliximab therapy. Dermatol Ther. 2020;33(6). https://doi.org/10.1111/dth.14472.
31. Gisondi P, Bellinato F, Piaserico S, Di Leo S, Cazzaniga S, Naldi L. Preference for telemedicine versus in-person visit among patients with psoriasis receiving biological drugs. Dermatol Ther. 2021;11(4):1333–43. https://doi.org/10.1007/s13555-021-00555-3.
32. Armstrong AW, Chambers CJ, Maverakis E, et al. Effectiveness of online vs in-person care for adults with psoriasis. JAMA Netw Open. 2018;1(6):e183062. https://doi.org/10.1001/jamanetworkopen.2018.3062.
33. Young PM, Chen AY, Ford AR, Cheng MY, Lane CJ, Armstrong AW. Effects of online care on functional and psychological outcomes in patients with psoriasis: a randomized controlled trial. (1097-6787 (Electronic)).

Telecosmetics and Lasers

Loren Elizabeth de la Caridad Hernandez, Noreen Mohsin, Daphne G. Eckembrecher, Francelia J. Eckembrecher, and Keyvan Nouri

Abstract The term telecosmetics refers to the utilization of telemedicine for the purpose of aesthetic consultations as well as post-procedure follow-up care. This modality has been utilized by both dermatologists and plastic surgeons alike and is gaining popularity given its relative ease of use and convenience. According to the American Society for Dermatologic Surgery (ASDS), in 2019 ASDS dermatologists performed over 10.3 million cosmetic treatments (Ibrahim et al. in Dermatol Surg 45:303–306, 2019 [1, 2]). Given this data, minimally invasive cosmetic procedures remain popular. As more individuals desire aesthetic alterations, in conjunction with a surge in telemedicine utilization secondary to the COVID-19 pandemic, it is inevitable that more dermatologists will implement the use of telemedicine in their practices for aesthetic consultations and post-procedure care. We will discuss the benefits and drawbacks of telehealth for aesthetic consultations and follow-up care from the perspectives of both practitioners and patients, as well as how telehealth continues to revolutionize the cosmetic dermatology industry. The latter of this chapter will focus on a review of laser technology and their applications in the field of dermatology.

Keywords Telecosmetics · Aesthetic consultations · Follow-up care · Lasers · Physical properties

L. E. de la Caridad Hernandez (✉) · N. Mohsin · D. G. Eckembrecher · F. J. Eckembrecher · K. Nouri
Dr. Phillip Frost Department of Dermatology and Cutaneous Surgery, University of Miami Miller School of Medicine, Miami, FL, USA
e-mail: loren.hernandez@med.miami.edu

K. Nouri (ed.), *Telemedicine and Technological Advances in Dermatology*,
https://doi.org/10.1007/978-3-031-69091-4_3

1 Introduction

1.1 Telemedicine Overview

There are three major divisions of telehealth: the store-and-forward method also known as asynchronous telemedicine, live telemedicine visits which are also referred to as synchronous telemedicine, and remote monitoring [3]. These three subdivisions are discussed in more detail elsewhere in this textbook but their implementation in telecosmetics will be discussed here.

In the store-and-forward method, patients can send their physician photographs, their medical history, and other information beforehand for the physician to review prior to their consultation [3]. Most aesthetic consultations begin with a questionnaire that delineates a patient's goals and desires for cosmetic treatment. This information may be collected prior to the consultation so that they can be reviewed by the clinician. They may include questions on topics that the patient wishes to learn more about, their concerns, and what procedures and/or treatments they are seeking. It should also inquire about their medical history, medications, and if they have had prior aesthetic procedures performed. The store-and-forward method may also be used for post-procedure care. Patients can take photographs of their procedure site(s) and send them to their clinician for further evaluation. If signs of infection are noted, they may then be scheduled for an in-person evaluation, advised to seek emergency medical care, and/or prescribed medication.

In synchronous telemedicine, visits occur in real-time and there is direct interaction between the physician and patient [3]. Although convenient, the webcams from laptop and/or desktop computers as well as cellphone and tablet cameras used for telemedicine often record at a shorter focal length [4]. This can result in distortion of imagery, giving the illusion of a rounder face with seemingly larger facial features. This may obscure physician's assessment of a patient and can require further in-person evaluation for an optimal aesthetic consultation. It is vital that patients, as well as physicians, optimize their virtual setup. It is important to minimize distractions and ensure that internet connectivity is stable. Lighting should be adequate so that the clinician may see the patient's facial expressions and area(s) of concern. Direct lighting may be too harsh and can cause shadows or overexposure [5]. It is ideal for patients to wear neutral, solid-colored clothing to avoid distractions. The physician should maintain eye contact and demonstrate attention to the patient's concerns, as they would in-person [6]. Akin to the distortions produced from webcams, photographs may provide a false perception of the patient.

It is important for patients to not use filters when taking photographs prior to sending for aesthetic consultations. Patients should also be advised to not wear any makeup or tinted skincare prior to both synchronous telemedicine visits and when taking photographs. Photographs should also be in-focus and of adequate magnification of the area(s) of concern. It is also important for patients to send more than one image to appropriately assess the patient's concern(s). Remote patient monitoring refers to the continuous evaluation of a patient's clinical status, usually with video monitoring or other tests and images collected remotely [3]. This method is used less often for telecosmetic consultations and is more useful for post-procedural care.

2 The Cosmetic Patient

Aesthetic consultations with patients over telehealth are akin to those done in-person. However, there are some distinguishing features between the two. Firstly, irrespective of modality, it is important to understand the cosmetic dermatological patient and their motivations behind seeking aesthetic alterations. A multicenter prospective observational study from 2018 found that the most common motivations for attaining minimally invasive cosmetic procedures were related to aesthetic appearance, such as the desire to attain a more youthful, attractive appearance [7]. They also found that oftentimes there was a psychosocial component behind their motivation in attaining cosmetic alterations, including insufficient self-confidence and social impairments [7]. The motivations behind patients seeking the services of a cosmetic dermatologist are varied and are not simply focused on vanity. Thus, it is vital for physicians to consider these complexities when interacting with patients, both over telehealth and in-person.

3 Approaching the Cosmetic Patient

When addressing the cosmetic patient, there are multiple approaches the clinician can take, and each is dependent on their own experiences and preferences. One method that has been described is the LEAP technique [8]. This is an acronym for listen, educate and empower, align and perform. Clinicians first listen to their patient's concerns, uninterrupted for 60 s. This allows physicians to listen to their concerns, further understand their perspectives, and observe their facial expressions/dynamics. Educating and empowering begins with re-stating the patient's goals and concerns in simplified, non-medical terminology, parallel to a reverse "teach-back" method. The physician may then describe the pros and cons of their desired procedures, suggest appropriate alternatives, and describe the realistic outcomes of their desired procedures and/or alternative procedures. Align refers to making treatment options alongside the patient and not making treatment decisions for them. Perform, aptly named, refers to the performance of the cosmetic procedure. Ultimately, regardless of what technique or method the physician uses when approaching the cosmetic patient, it is important to be understanding and empower patients to be an active participant in their medical care.

4 Advantages and Disadvantages of Telecosmetics

Teledermatology provides both patients and practitioners with a more convenient method to provide cosmetic consultations and follow-up care [9–11]. Granted that both the physician and patient have stable network access, a telemedicine visit can be held from any location and at any time without the need of ancillary staff. However, not all patients have stable network access, mobile devices and/or computers and are unable take part in cosmetic telehealth visits [12]. For these patients, telehealth is not feasible and in-office consultations and follow-up care are required.

The establishment of rapport between a patient and their physician is important in the practice of medicine but is especially vital in the field of cosmetic dermatology. For some physicians, it may be difficult to establish good rapport via telehealth especially if it is their first visit with a patient. Clearly, telehealth visits lack the physical interaction between patient and clinician. For example, virtual visits remove the opportunity for a physician to shake their patient's hand, provide their patient with a box of tissues when conversations become sentimental, or even place a hand on their shoulder for comfort. These interpersonal connections are difficult, if not impossible, to achieve via virtual visits. However, it is still very possible to develop rapport with patients over telemedicine, and some may even argue that virtual visits are beneficial to the patient–physician relationship given that the virtual visit is focused on the patient without extraneous distractions.

When discussing personal matters and/or sensitive topics, it is important for the physician to be empathic. This may include being friendly and warm in their demeanor and ensuring that they are receptive to a patient's concerns without showing judgement. Discussing a patient's appearance in a clinical environment may make them anxious and hesitant to express their concerns. By utilizing telehealth, a comfortable environment may allow patients to feel less anxious and more willing to discuss their goals and desires.

There are many factors that come into play when a patient chooses a practitioner for their cosmetic procedure(s). When choosing a plastic surgeon, it has been shown that board certification status and method of referral are the two most important attributes when it comes to a patient making their decision [13]. Although less important than board certification and recommendations, one cannot exclude the impacts that a practitioner's office staff and their physical office have in the selection process of a patient. By implementing telehealth visits for aesthetic consultations, these potential biases are reduced. This allows each consultation to focus on physician–patient interactions, thereby providing ample opportunities for patients to gain confidence in their care provider and ask questions.

As for post-procedure care, telephone applications and smartphone-based text communication have been used to follow-up with patients. Without the implementation of telemedicine for post-procedure care, patients would have to attend one or more in-person visits with their clinician. This poses many challenges, as patients may have to interrupt their schedule to attend these visits. One survey found that laser resurfacing patients who sent post-procedural images to their physician via their smartphone to be more convenient than in-person visits [14].

5 Advances in Telecosmetics

There is now a prevalence of dermatology telemedicine websites. Most cater to medical dermatological diseases such as rosacea and acne, but websites like Apostrophe [15], Rory [16], and Curology [17] offer dermatology consultations for aesthetic purposes as well. Patients who desire anti-aging treatment can now be connected with a dermatologist via these websites for a flat fee, have medication(s) prescribed if they are deemed an appropriate candidate, and have such medication(s) shipped to their home. Most, if not all, require an initial intake form to be completed with questions on their medical history, lifestyle, and concerns. Users are then connected with a dermatologist via phone, video, or message or a combination of the three. Some of the medications prescribed include the following: Latisse® (Bimatoprost ophthalmic solution 0.03%) for eyelash growth and topical tretinoin for facial wrinkles. With the advent of these websites, one can schedule an appointment and receive prescription medications all from the comfort of their home. One cross-sectional, secret shopper study found that the median appointment wait time to see a dermatologist was 7 days for persons with Blue Cross Blue Shield and Medicare, but 13 days for patients with Medicaid [18]. The advent of these websites allows for individuals to receive care with a physician in a timely manner, irrespective of insurance status.

6 Lasers in Dermatology

Lasers play a pivotal role in the field of dermatology. The term is an acronym—light amplification by stimulated emission of radiation [19]. They are commonly used in this field, as they have a broad variety of applications ranging from the treatment of vascular lesions to the improvement of inflammatory acne and acne scarring. This section will introduce important terminology, the mechanisms by which lasers work, and will briefly discuss some of their applications according to disease/concern being treated.

7 How Lasers Work

It is important to understand the mechanisms by which lasers function and their properties to fully understand their applications in dermatology. Einstein's quantum theory of light (1905) described what would become the foundation of laser physics:

electromagnetic radiation is composed of small packets of energy, referred to as quanta, or photons [20]. The light that can be seen by the human eye, aptly called visible light, only composes a small section of the electromagnetic spectrum. The limits are not precise and typically range from 360 to 400 nm as the lower limit and 760 and 830 nm as the upper limit [21]. Many of the lasers used in clinical dermatology fall in this portion of the spectrum as well as on the longer wavelength end. Lasers, at their most basic, have three components: a laser chamber, a lasing medium composed of one of three states of matter (solid, liquid, or gas), and a source of energy [22].

There are two types of laser energy emission: spontaneous and stimulated emission [23]. In spontaneous emission, an excited atom emits a photon. Upon the release of a photon, electrons transition from on excited state to a resting state [23]. In stimulated emission, an external source of energy increases the number of excited electrons. These excited electrons release photons that will collide with other electrons, thereby releasing more photons. If these collisions continue to occur between electrons and photons are released, laser light is produced [23].

There are also many properties of laser light that are important in the understanding of laser dynamics. The three most commonly described are as follows: laser light is monochromatic, collimated, and there is coherence [24]. Laser light's monochromacy refers to it being of one wavelength; this property is determined by the medium wherein the laser beam passes [23]. Coherence refers to a laser light's wavelength being in phase both temporally and spatially; they are correlated at different moments in time and are correlated at different points in space, lateral or longitudinal, respectively [23]. Collimation refers to the laser beams being parallel to one another, this allows for low beam divergence [23].

The light-tissue interaction describes how the laser beam produces effects in tissue [25]. For laser light to produce an effect, it needs to be absorbed by tissue [26]. Electrons vibrate at specific frequencies. When laser light interacts with atoms of the same frequency, the atom's electrons become excited and begin to vibrate. These interactions cause vibrational energy to be converted into thermal energy, and thus producing an effect in tissue. This is referred to as photothermolysis [27], and clinicians should utilize a laser of the appropriate wavelength to target the desired tissue. A laser's effect on tissue may be ablative or non-ablative. In ablative procedures, tissue is destroyed whereas in non-ablative procedures, there is only thermal injury of the tissue.

The targeted tissue can also be described in different terms—chromophores. Chromophores are the target tissues of laser light, each having a specific wavelength [28]. Water, melanin, and hemoglobin are examples of endogenous chromophores that can be targeted by laser beams. Tattoo ink is an example of an exogenous chromophore.

Laser light can also reflect and scatter [29, 30]. In reflection, the light does not enter the tissue but "bounces off" the surface. Scattering, also known as diffraction, is another property of laser light that is inversely proportional to the light beam's wavelength. When there is scattering, the laser light is dispersed over a larger area of tissue and the depth of tissue penetration is reduced [29]. Light of a shorter wavelength will penetrate the tissue more superficially due to absorption [24]. Conversely, light of a longer wavelength will penetrate the tissue deeper [24]. There is less scattering in the epidermis due to there being less extraneous tissue for the light to interact with. In contrast, there is more scattering in the dermal layer due to the presence of collagen fibers [24].

More important terms to be familiar with are the thermal relaxation time, pulse width, spot size, and surface cooling. The thermal relaxation time is the time for the target tissue to cool to half of its peak temperature after exposure to laser light [30]. It is proportional to the square of the size of the target. The pulse width, also referred to as the pulse duration, is the amount of time the tissue is exposed to energy [30]. To minimize thermal damage, the pulse width should be less than the thermal relaxation time. A laser's pulse duration may be either continuous or pulsed. When continuous, a constant beam of light is emitted which may result in non-selective tissue injury. There are two types of pulsed laser delivery, the first utilizes a mechanical shutter, also referred to as a pulsed laser, and the second utilizes a resonance chamber (pico and Q-switch lasers) [31]. When pulsed, the amount of energy transfer is dependent on the duration of time the target tissue is exposed to the laser beam. This produces more selective tissue damage. Laser beams may also be "fractionated." This form of laser delivery emits narrow sized, high-energy laser beams [32]. These beams may be either ablative or non-ablative, with ablative fractional lasers causing destruction of vertical columns of tissue and non-ablative fractional lasers causing columns of thermally injured tissue [33].

The spot size is akin to the cross-section of the laser beam [34]. A smaller spot size results in more scattering and a rapid reduction in energy provided to the tissue, as the square root of the spot size is proportional to irradiance and energy, also known as fluence [19]. For maximal penetration of the laser light to mid-dermal or deeper targets, a spot size of 7–10 mm is required [34]. However, the depth of penetration plateaus with a spot size of 10–12 mm [34].

Lasers may inadvertently target more superficial chromophores although the intention may be to target deeper chromophores. Surface cooling is used to avoid the inadvertent targeting of tissue [35, 36]. It is subdivided into three phases: pre-cooling, parallel cooling, and post-cooling. Pre-cooling of the epidermis occurs prior to the laser procedure and is most done with topical cryogen spray [36, 37]. Parallel cooling is performed at the same time as the laser is applied to tissue and is useful in laser treatments of longer pulse durations [36]. This type of surface cooling is commonly performed with a water-cooled sapphire tip. Post-cooling occurs after application of the laser and is done with the topical application of ice [36]. This can reduce pain and edema after treatment but does not attenuate tissue injury induced by the laser's application.

The intensity of a laser is greatest at the center of the beam with attenuation toward the periphery [19]. This plays a role in the clinician's practice, as they must overlap the treated areas to achieve a uniform distribution of energy [19]. There exist laser beams that are target or doughnut shaped, with the greatest intensity being at the rim of the device. These lasers are less clinically useful as the target must have a larger minimum spot size and if used, overlapping must be kept at a minimum.

Understanding these properties and terminology regarding laser use is key for the clinician in a dermatologist's practice.

7.1 *Vascular Lesions*

Oxyhemoglobin is the primary chromophore targeted when treating vascular lesions [34]. Hemoglobin has absorption peaks at blue, green, and yellow bands, 418 nm, 542 nm, and 577 nm, respectively [38]. There is also absorption at the larger end of the electromagnetic spectrum, from 700 to 1100 nm. On absorption of laser light, energy is converted to heat which is then transferred to the vessel wall. This results in coagulation and closure of the targeted vessels [39]. The potassium titanyl phosphate (KTP, 532 nm), pulsed dye laser (PDL, 585–595 nm), diode (800–810, 940 nm), alexandrite (755 nm), and neodymium-doped yttrium aluminum garnet (Nd:YAG, 532 and 1064 nm) lasers are commonly used in the treatment of vascular lesions [34]. However, it is important to consider the absorption of melanin when choosing the appropriate laser for patients. Melanin has absorption peaks that range from 300 to 600 nm. In persons with darker skin tones, it is preferred to choose lasers that target longer wavelengths to not target melanin. This can cause depigmentation of the skin in those with darker skin tones.

Intense pulsed light may also be used to treat vascular lesions and has been shown to be effective in the treatment of capillary and venous malformations, infantile hemangiomas, telangiectasias of the face, and poikiloderma of Civatte. Dermal penetration of tissue and minimization of inadvertent chromophore absorption can be accomplished with filters—these limit the wavelengths emitted by the laser.

Longer wavelength lasers, such as the LP alexandrite (755 nm), diode (800 nm), and Nd:YAG (1064 nm), are used in the treatment of deeper and/or larger vessels [40–42]. Smaller wavelength lasers, such as KTP (532 nm) and PDL (585–595 nm), are used to treat small vessels less than 1 mm in size [40, 43, 44].

7.2 *Hypertrophic Scars and Keloids*

Hypertrophic scarring and the formation of keloids are both variants of normal wound healing. In hypertrophic scarring and keloids, there is excess connective tissue deposited. They differ in that the excess tissue is restricted to the area within the original wound in hypertrophic scarring but extends beyond the area of the original wound in the case of keloids [45, 46]. There are many conventional treatments available, however, they recur even with treatment. International guidelines for the treatment of scars proposed an algorithmic approach with fractional or pulsed dye lasers (PDL, 585 nm) being the second-line for minor keloids and third-line for larger keloids or hypertrophic scars [47]. Ultimately, pulsed dye lasers (PDL, 585 nm) serve as the gold standard of laser therapy for hypertrophic scars and keloids [48].

7.3 *Pigmented Lesions*

Pigmented lesions may be subdivided into epidermal and dermal lesions with some occurring at the dermoepidermal junction. Epidermal lesions include lentigo simplex, solar lentigo, seborrheic keratoses, dermatosis papulose nigra, ephelides, café-au-lait macules, and nevus spilus [49]. Those that involve pigment deposition in both the dermis and epidermis include Becker's nevus, post-inflammatory hyperpigmentation, melasma, and nevocellular, congenital, junctional and compound melanocytic nevi [49]. Dermal lesions include nevus of Ota, nevus of Ito, Hori's nevus, and blue nevi [49]. Shorter wavelength lasers, such as pulsed-dye laser (PDL, 510 nm), QS-KTP (532 nm), QS-Nd:YAG (532 nm), or QS-ruby (694 nm), are used to treat more superficial pigmented lesions such as those that are located within the epidermis. Intermediate to long wavelength lasers, such as QS-Alexandrite (755 nm) or QS-Nd:YAG (1064 nm) are used with deeper lesions, such as those found in the dermis.

7.4 *Laser Tattoo Removal*

Tattoo ink is considered an exogenous chromophore. Depending on the color of the tattoo and skin type of the patient, the clinician will choose the most appropriate laser and wavelength for tattoo removal. Of all the pigment colors, black, dark blue, brown, and green are more responsive to laser removal than red, orange, light blue, and yellow [49]. QS lasers such as the QS-Nd:YAG (532 nm), QS-ruby (694 nm), and QS-Alexandrite (755 nm), deliver high-powered pulses that result in the destruction of tattoo ink particles [34]. Picosecond lasers of wavelengths 532, 694, 755, and 1064 nm are currently the mainstay of treatment in tattoo removal [50]. Given that their pulse duration is significantly less than the tattoo ink's thermal relaxation time, these lasers effectively destroy the targeted chromophores without the inadvertent targeting of nearby tissue [50].

7.5 *Laser Hair Removal*

The targeted chromophore in laser hair removal is melanin. Melanin is present in the hair follicular epithelium, shaft, and matrix [51, 52]. Of note, it is the melanin within the follicular stem cell that is the primary target. It is important to understand the "extended theory of selective photothermolysis," which postulates that there is selective thermal damage of non-uniformly pigmented structures in tissue [53]. This theory can be applied to laser hair removal. The melanin content is greater in the hair shaft and matrix than the actual hair follicle. Upon exposure to laser light, melanin captures and subsequently distributes energy to the surrounding structures, thereby destroying stem cells of the hair bulge and matrix. Lasers that are used for hair removal include the following: ruby laser (694 nm), Alexandrite laser (755 nm), diode laser (810 nm), Nd:YAG (1064 nm), and intense pulse light (IPL, 500–1200 nm). When choosing the appropriate laser for hair removal, one must consider the patient's skin type. The ruby [54] and Alexandrite [55] lasers are better suited for persons with Fitzpatrick skin types I–III. The diode laser is slightly more encompassing and can be used in patients with skin types I–V [56]. The Nd:YAG laser can be used in patients with skin types I–VI given less melanin absorption due to its longer wavelength [57]. IPL can be used in individuals with darker skin tones; however, it is less effective when compared to lasers [58–60].

8 Skin Resurfacing—Ablative, Non-ablative, and Fractional Resurfacing

8.1 Ablative Skin Resurfacing

Ablative skin resurfacing involves the destruction of the epidermal and superficial dermal layers of the skin. There are many indications for ablative skin resurfacing, some of which include the treatment of photoaging, wrinkles, acne scars, rhinophyma, seborrheic keratoses, and scar revisions [61]. The CO_2 (10,600 nm) and erbium: yttrium aluminum garnet (Er:YAG, 2940 nm) lasers are the two most common lasers used in ablative skin resurfacing. Water is the CO2 laser's primary chromophore; it is thought to produce desirable effects by denaturing collagen and stimulating neocollagenesis. This is useful in the treatment of atrophic acne scars and facial rhytides. The Er:YAG laser's chromophore is also water. These lasers produce less thermal energy than CO2 lasers, allowing for faster post-procedure healing but less tissue tightening [62]. Ablative skin resurfacing may produce many, prolonged side effects [63–67] such as erythema and edema, milia, acne, infections, post-inflammatory hyperpigmentation and delayed hypopigmentation.

8.2 Non-ablative Skin Resurfacing

In contrast to ablative skin resurfacing, non-ablative skin resurfacing does not damage the epidermal layer. Such devices include the following: intense pulsed light (IPL, 500–1200 nm), diode (980 and 1450 nm), Nd:YAG (1064 and 1320 nm), and erbium: glass (Er:glass, 1540 nm). The primary target for non-ablative devices is also water, akin to the lasers used in ablative skin resurfacing. As the primary chromophore is water, there is dermal remodeling and collagen heating. However, with non-ablative skin resurfacing, there is simultaneous application of epidermal cooling preventing damage of this cutaneous layer. Non-ablative skin resurfacing produces less undesirable side effects and offers patients a speedier post-operative recovery.

8.3 Fractional Resurfacing

In fractional resurfacing only a portion of the tissue is targeted—there is thermal ablation of columns of epidermal and dermal tissue [68]. These microtraumas allow for improvement of skin texture and tone as they heal [32]. Fractional resurfacing devices may be subdivided into ablative and non-ablative devices.

8.4 Lasers in Acne and Acne Scarring

Acne vulgaris is an inflammatory disorder of the pilosebaceous unit. Its etiology is multifactorial and may be due to increased follicular keratinization, androgen stimulated sebum production, colonization of follicles by *Cutibacterium acnes*, formerly known as *Propionibacterium acnes* (*P. acnes*), and inflammation [69–71]. The primary chromophore targeted in the laser treatment of acne is the porphyrin. Porphyrins are molecules with a tetrapyrrolic structure that are involved in many metabolic processes. Upon absorption of light, these porphyrins generate free radicals and reactive molecules, causing damage to tissue [34]. Porphyrins experience greatest absorption at 400 nm, this being the Soret band. Weaker absorption bands are also present between 450 and 700 nm, these are referred to as Q bands. The potassium titanyl phosphate (KTP, 532 nm), pulsed dye laser (585 and 595 nm), diode laser (1450 nm), Nd:YAG (1064 and 1320 nm), erbium-glass (Er:glass, 1540 and 1550 nm), intense pulsed light, and fractional resurfacing are used in the treatment of acne. KTP (532 nm) lasers are thought to destroy *C. acnes* via their photoactivation of porphyrins [72, 73]. When comparing the KTP (532 nm) laser to the PDL (595 nm) laser in the treatment of erythematous surgical scars, a study found that the KTP (532 nm) laser was comparable in efficacy to the PDL (595 nm) laser [74]. Pulsed dye lasers (585 and 595 nm) may be used in the treatment of inflammatory acne. One study found that one treatment of PDL therapy improved inflammatory acne after 12 weeks [75]. Another study, utilizing PDL laser therapy with a wavelength of 585 nm and pulse duration of 350 μs every 4 weeks, found that at 12 weeks non-inflammatory acne lesions decreased by 27% and the number of active lesions decreased by 57% in 25 patients [76]. Diode lasers (1450 nm) are postulated to work against inflammatory acne in part due to their effects on sebaceous glands and sebum production [77]. Another study found that sebum production was decreased, but did not find a change in facial sebum excretion rate [78]. A split-face study on 20 patients (Fitzpatrick types II–VI) found that 3 treatments with a diode (1450 nm) laser with 3–4 week intervals reduced inflammatory acne lesions [79].

Nd:YAG (1064 and 1320 nm) lasers have been shown to have thermolytic effects on sebaceous glands [80]. One double-blind, randomized controlled trial found that moderate-to-severe acne patients had a 42% decrease in the number of inflammatory lesions after 4 treatments with a 650 usec Nd:YAG (1064 nm) laser [81]. Er:glass (1540 nm) lasers are thought to work in acne secondary to their depth of tissue penetration and effects on sebaceous gland activity [80]. One randomized, split-face controlled study found that the Er:glass (1550 nm) laser, given for a total of 4 sessions with a 2-week interval, produced a statistically significant decrease in the average lesion number [82]. Intense pulsed light uses photodynamic therapy to selectively target and destroy *C. acnes* as the porphyrins produced by this bacteria absorb at 415 and 630 nm [83]. Photodynamic therapy also takes advantage of the porphyrins produced by *C. acnes*. This treatment modality involves the topical application of porphyrin precursors, such as methylaminolevulinate (MAL) or aminolevulinic acid (ALA) [84]. After the application of either medication, skin is exposed to light and after a period of time, porphyrins accumulate thereby damaging the sebaceous glands [85].

8.5 Lasers for Onychomycosis

Onychomycosis is a fungal infection of the nail unit. This condition may be caused by dermatophytes, yeasts, and saprophytic molds. The most common and effective treatment for onychomycosis is systemic antifungal therapy. However, laser treatment of these fungal infections is a newer approach as they are notoriously difficult to treat, even with conventional methods. The FDA has approved the neodymium-doped yttrium aluminum garnet (Nd:YAG, 532, 630–680, 1064, and 1120 nm) lasers, 870/930 nm combination diode laser, and the 980 nm diode laser. Ablative CO_2 lasers, photodynamic therapy, UV light, and the femtosecond infrared titanium sapphire (800 nm) laser may also be used in the treatment of onychomycosis.

8.6 Lasers for Non-melanoma Skin Cancers

Non-melanoma skin cancers (NMSC) include basal cell carcinoma (BCC), squamous cell carcinoma (SCC), and Merkel cell carcinoma (MCC) [86]. Cryosurgery, curettage with or without electrodessication, immunomodulator therapy, and surgical excision are the primary treatments for BCCs and SCCs [87]. MCC may also be treated with these modalities [88].

8.7 Lasers in Wound-Healing

Wound healing consists of three phases: the inflammatory, proliferative or granulation, and remodeling phases. The inflammatory phase is characterized by hemostasis and chemotaxis of inflammatory cells, such as mast cells, neutrophils and macrophages [89]. The proliferative phase is characterized by neovascularization, epithelization, neocollagenesis and collagen deposition, and formation of granulation tissues. The remodeling phase is characterized by reorganization and re-synthesis of the extracellular matrix as well as degradation of existing extracellular matrix [90]. It is important to note that there is overlap between these three phases. Lasers were first given consideration as treatment for wound healing when clinicians using surgical lasers found their patients to have less post-operative pain and inflammation. It has been shown, both in vitro and in vivo, that low incident doses of light can activate all three inflammatory cells involved in the inflammatory phase of wound healing [91–96]. LLLT has been shown in an in vivo animal model of incisional wounds to stimulate the production of new keratinocytes [97].

8.8 Lasers for Hair Growth and Hair Disorders

The current FDA approved treatments for hair loss are slim; topical minoxidil for both females and males, and oral finasteride for males. Other treatments, such as hair transplantation, are costly and may not be performed on all patients with hair loss as not every patient is a candidate. There are multiple forms of hair loss, such as androgenic alopecia and alopecia areata. Alopecia may also be caused by chemotherapy, named chemotherapy-induced alopecia, or from chronic trauma and/or inflammation, the latter referred to as cicatricial alopecia.

It is postulated that lasers help with hair growth via vasodilation. It has been shown that UV light induces nitric oxide (NO) release from vascular smooth muscle cells [98]. This dilation may then increase blood flow to hair follicles, thus promoting hair growth. Another mechanism involves regeneration of hair follicles secondary to wounding of tissue [99, 100]. The most common lasers used for hair growth include: low-level light therapy (LLLT, 600–700 nm), narrow-band UVB (311 nm), UVA/PUVA (320–400 nm), excimer laser (308 nm), fractionated laser (1550 nm), and ablative CO_2 lasers.

8.9 Androgenetic Alopecia

This form of hair loss is genetically predisposed and involves excessive androgens [101, 102]. In patients with androgenetic alopecia, excessive androgens activate androgen receptors, resulting in a shortened anagen phase, also referred to as the growth phase, of the hair growth cycle [103, 104].

Low-level light therapy (LLLT, 600–700 nm) is most used for androgenetic alopecia. It is thought to improve hair loss by prolonging the anagen phase, promoting reentry into the anagen phase from the telogen phase, and inhibiting transition to the catagen phase [105–107].

8.10 Alopecia Areata

Alopecia areata, an autoimmune disorder, involves non-scarring hair loss with follicular preservation [108]. It is characterized by a loss of immune privilege with CD4 and CD8 T-cell infiltration of hair bulbs [108]. Excimer (308 nm) lasers are the most studied in the treatment of alopecia areata [109–111]. However, more randomized clinical trials need to be performed to assess whether treatment with the excimer laser is superior to conventional medical treatment, as some studies have shown that the laser only causes increased diameter of the hair shaft [112, 113]. PUVA treatment is no longer commonly used given inconsistent results [114–118] and its potential for skin cancer development given cumulative UVA dose with treatment [117, 118].

8.11 Chemotherapy-Induced Alopecia

Low-level light therapy (LLLT, 600–700 nm) has been shown in rat models to induce hair regrowth. After chemotherapy administration (etoposide cyclophosphamide, or a cyclophosphamide and doxorubicin combination) and subsequent full body alopecia, it was found that rats treated with LLLT regrew their hair five days earlier than those rats treated with sham laser treatment or chemotherapy alone [119].

8.12 Cicatricial Alopecia

Cicatricial alopecia, also referred to as scarring alopecia, is hair loss wherein hair follicles are destroyed and are unable to produce quality terminal hairs [108, 120]. Examples of cicatricial alopecia include lichen planopilaris, frontal fibrosing alopecia, chronic cutaneous lupus erythematosus, central centrifugal cicatricial alopecia, and folliculitis decalvans. The use of lasers in the treatment of this subset of alopecia has not been studied in depth. However, there is some data to suggest that LLLT can help with scarring alopecia. Four patients with lichen planopilaris were treated with LLLT and showed improvement with reduction of inflammation, symptom disappearance and hair regrowth [121].

9 Conclusion

The field of dermatology is embracing telehealth more than ever and telecosmetics, the application of telehealth to aesthetic consultations and follow-up care, is increasing in popularity. It is convenient for both physicians and patients, although it may not be accessible to all patients given that stable network access is necessary for it to be undertaken successfully. Cosmetic patients may be complex, and whether undergoing consultations and/or receiving follow-up care in-person or via telehealth, it is important to understand their motivations behind wanting aesthetic procedures and how to approach them to optimize patient care. Ultimately, telehealth continues to revolutionize the dermatological industry as evident by its increased implementation in practice and the onset of various teledermatology websites. The latter of this chapter focused on lasers and provided a brief overview of their mechanism of action, important terminology and concepts, as well as their current applications within dermatology.

Key Points (3 main takeaway points)

a. Telehealth consultations are a convenient method for physicians to assess a patient's goals in respect to cosmetic procedures, discuss benefits and risks, and provide patients with follow-up care.
b. Telemedicine has been utilized by dermatologists and plastic surgeons for performing consultations and post-operative care, is now becoming more popular due to its convenience and relative ease of use.
c. Lasers play a pivotal role in dermatology and their applications are widespread, from treating vascular lesions to being used for anti-aging purposes.

Abbreviations

QS	Quality switched
YAG	Yttrium-aluminum-garnet
Nd	Neodymium
CW	Continuous-wave

References

1. Ibrahim O, Berson DS, Rohrer TE. Trends in dermatologic surgery: results of the American society for dermatologic surgery procedure and consumer surveys. Dermatol Surg. 2019;45(2):303–6. https://doi.org/10.1097/DSS.0000000000001524.
2. Surgeons ASoP. Plastic surgery statistics report. 2020.
3. Mechanic OJ, Persaud Y, Kimball AB. Telehealth systems. Treasure Island (FL): StatPearls; 2021.
4. Banks MS, Cooper EA, Piazza EA. Camera focal length and the perception of pictures. Ecol Psychol. 2014;26(1–2):30–46. https://doi.org/10.1080/10407413.2014.877284.
5. Tower JI, Lee JY, Lee YH. Screenshot photography: optimizing photo-documentation while using telehealth video platforms. Facial Plast Surg Aesthet Med. 2020;22(4):240–2. https://doi.org/10.1089/fpsam.2020.0225.

6. Onorato S, Joshi A, Schwartz AW. Lights, camera, action: optimizing virtual video visits to provide high-quality care. J Gen Intern Med. 2021;36(6):1751–4. https://doi.org/10.1007/s11606-020-06278-z.
7. Maisel A, Waldman A, Furlan K, Weil A, Sacotte K, Lazaroff JM, et al. Self-reported patient motivations for seeking cosmetic procedures. JAMA Dermatol. 2018;154(10):1167–74. https://doi.org/10.1001/jamadermatol.2018.2357.
8. Watchmaker J, Kandula P, Kaminer MS. L.E.A.P.ing into the cosmetic consult. J Cosmetic Dermatol. 2021;19(6):1499–500. https://doi.org/10.1111/jocd.13293.
9. Powell RE, Henstenburg JM, Cooper G, Hollander JE, Rising KL. Patient perceptions of telehealth primary care video visits. Ann Fam Med. 2017;15(3):225–9. https://doi.org/10.1370/afm.2095.
10. Saiyed S, Nguyen A, Singh R. Physician perspective and key satisfaction indicators with rapid telehealth adoption during the coronavirus disease 2019 pandemic. Telemed J E Health. 2021. https://doi.org/10.1089/tmj.2020.0492.
11. Kichloo A, Albosta M, Dettloff K, Wani F, El-Amir Z, Singh J, et al. Telemedicine, the current COVID-19 pandemic and the future: a narrative review and perspectives moving forward in the USA. Fam Med Community Health. 2020;8(3). https://doi.org/10.1136/fmch-2020-000530.
12. Scott Kruse C, Karem P, Shifflett K, Vegi L, Ravi K, Brooks M. Evaluating barriers to adopting telemedicine worldwide: a systematic review. J Telemed Telecare. 2018;24(1):4–12. https://doi.org/10.1177/1357633X16674087.
13. Waltzman JT, Scholz T, Evans GRD. What patients look for when choosing a plastic surgeon: an assessment of patient preference by conjoint analysis. Ann Plast Surg. 2011;66(6):643–7. https://doi.org/10.1097/SAP.0b013e3181e19eeb.
14. Chee SN, Lowe P, Lim A. Smartphone patient monitoring post-laser resurfacing. Australas J Dermatol. 2017;58(4):e216–22. https://doi.org/10.1111/ajd.12507.
15. Apostrophe. https://www.apostrophe.com. Accessed 23 Sept 2021.
16. Rory. https://www.hellorory.com. Accessed 23 Sept 2021.
17. Curology. https://curology.com. Accessed 23 Sept 2021.
18. Creadore A, Desai S, Li SJ, Lee KJ, Bui AN, Villa-Ruiz C, et al. Insurance acceptance, appointment wait time, and dermatologist access across practice types in the US. JAMA Dermatol. 2021;157(2):181–8. https://doi.org/10.1001/jamadermatol.2020.5173.
19. Carroll L, Humphreys TR. LASER-tissue interactions. Clin Dermatol. 2006;24(1):2–7. https://doi.org/10.1016/j.clindermatol.2005.10.019.
20. Bennett CL. Astrophysical observations: lensing and eclipsing Einstein's theories. Science. 2005;307(5711):879–84. https://doi.org/10.1126/science.1106444.
21. Sliney DH. What is light? The visible spectrum and beyond. Eye (London). 2016;30(2):222–9. https://doi.org/10.1038/eye.2015.252.
22. Luke AM, Mathew S, Altawash MM, Madan BM. Laser: a review with their applications in oral medicine. J Lasers Med Sci. 2019;10(4):324–9.
23. Takac S, Stojanovic S. Characteristics of laser light. Med Pregl. 1999;52(1–2):29–34.
24. Tanzi EL, Lupton JR, Alster TS. Lasers in dermatology: four decades of progress. J Am Acad Dermatol. 2003;49(1):1–31; quiz-4. https://doi.org/10.1067/mjd.2003.582.
25. Ansari MA, Mohajerani, E. Mechanisms of laser-tissue interaction: I. Optical properties of tissue. J Lasers Med Sci. 2011;2(3):119–25.
26. Dederich DN. Laser/tissue interaction. Alpha Omegan. 1991;84(4):33–6.
27. Anderson RR, Parrish JA. Selective photothermolysis: precise microsurgery by selective absorption of pulsed radiation. Science. 1983;220(4596):524–7. https://doi.org/10.1126/science.6836297.
28. Young AR. Chromophores in human skin. Phys Med Biol. 1997;42(5):789–802. https://doi.org/10.1088/0031-9155/42/5/004.
29. Dover JS, Arndt KA, Geronemus RG, et al. Illustrated cutaneous laser surgery: a practitioner's guide. Norwalk, CT: Appleton & Lange; 1990.
30. Patil UA, Dhami LD. Overview of lasers. Indian J Plast Surg. 2008;41(Suppl):S101–13.

31. Acland KM, Barlow RJ. Lasers for the dermatologist. Br J Dermatol. 2000;143(2):244–55. https://doi.org/10.1046/j.1365-2133.2000.03648.x.
32. Update on fractional laser technology. J Clin Aesthet Dermatol. 2010;3(1):42–50.
33. Ross EV, Zelickson BD. Biophysics of nonablative dermal remodeling. Semin Cutan Med Surg. 2002;21(4):251–65. https://doi.org/10.1053/sder.2002.36767.
34. Nouri K. Handbook of lasers in dermatology. Springer; 2014.
35. Zenzie HH, Altshuler GB, Smirnov MZ, Anderson RR. Evaluation of cooling methods for laser dermatology. Lasers Surg Med. 2000;26(2):130–44. https://doi.org/10.1002/(sici)1096-9101(2000)26:2%3c130::aid-lsm4%3e3.0.co;2-j.
36. Das A, Sarda A, De A. Cooling devices in laser therapy. J Cutan Aesthet Surg. 2016;9(4):215–9. https://doi.org/10.4103/0974-2077.197028.
37. Majaron B, Kimel S, Verkruysse W, Aguilar G, Pope K, Svaasand LO, et al. Cryogen spray cooling in laser dermatology: effects of ambient humidity and frost formation. Lasers Surg Med. 2001;28(5):469–76. https://doi.org/10.1002/lsm.1076.
38. Smit JM, Bauland CG, Wijnberg DS, Spauwen PH. Pulsed dye laser treatment, a review of indications and outcome based on published trials. Br J Plast Surg. 2005;58:981–7.
39. Srinivas CR, Kumaresan M. Lasers for vascular lesions: standard guidelines of care. Indian J Dermatol Venereol Leprol. 2011;77(3):349–68. https://doi.org/10.4103/0378-6323.79728.
40. Meesters AA, Pitassi LH, Campos V, Wolkerstorfer A, Dierickx CC. Transcutaneous laser treatment of leg veins. Lasers Med Sci. 2014;29(2):481–92. https://doi.org/10.1007/s10103-013-1483-2.
41. McDaniel DH, Ash K, Lord J, Newman J, Adrian RM, Zukowski M. Laser therapy of spider leg veins: clinical evaluation of a new long pulsed alexandrite laser. Dermatol Surg. 1999;25(1):52–8. https://doi.org/10.1046/j.1524-4725.1999.08117.x.
42. Kauvar AN, Lou WW. Pulsed alexandrite laser for the treatment of leg telangiectasia and reticular veins. Arch Dermatol. 2000;136(11):1371–5. https://doi.org/10.1001/archderm.136.11.1371.
43. Reichert D. Evaluation of the long-pulse dye laser for the treatment of leg telangiectasias. Dermatol Surg. 1998;24(7):737–40. https://doi.org/10.1111/j.1524-4725.1998.tb04242.x.
44. Raulin C, Weiss RA, Schonermark MP. Treatment of essential telangiectasias with an intense pulsed light source (PhotoDerm VL). Dermatol Surg. 1997;23(10):941–5; discussion 5–6. https://doi.org/10.1111/j.1524-4725.1997.tb00755.x.
45. Carswell L, Borger J. Hypertrophic scarring keloids. Treasure Island (FL): StatPearls; 2021.
46. Gauglitz GG, Korting HC, Pavicic T, Ruzicka T, Jeschke MG. Hypertrophic scarring and keloids: pathomechanisms and current and emerging treatment strategies. Mol Med. 2011;17(1–2):113–25. https://doi.org/10.2119/molmed.2009.00153.
47. Gold MH, Berman B, Clementoni MT, Gauglitz GG, Nahai F, Murcia C. Updated international clinical recommendations on scar management: part 1—evaluating the evidence. Dermatol Surg. 2014;40(8):817–24. https://doi.org/10.1111/dsu.0000000000000049.
48. Manuskiatti W, Fitzpatrick RE, Goldman MP. Energy density and numbers of treatment affect response of keloidal and hypertrophic sternotomy scars to the 585-nm flashlamp-pumped pulsed-dye laser. J Am Acad Dermatol. 2001;45(4):557–65. https://doi.org/10.1067/mjd.2001.116580.
49. Polder KD, Landau JM, Vergilis-Kalner IJ, Goldberg LH, Friedman PM, Bruce S. Laser eradication of pigmented lesions: a review. Dermatol Surg. 2011;37(5):572–95. https://doi.org/10.1111/j.1524-4725.2011.01971.x.
50. Henley JK, Zurfley F, Ramsey ML. Laser tattoo removal. Treasure Island (FL): StatPearls; 2021.
51. Lask G, Elman M, Slatkine M, Waldman A, Rozenberg Z. Laser-assisted hair removal by selective photothermolysis. Preliminary results. Dermatol Surg. 1997;23(9):737–9. https://doi.org/10.1111/j.1524-4725.1997.tb00406.x.
52. Dierickx CC. Hair removal by lasers and intense pulsed light sources. Dermatol Clin. 2002;20(1):135–46. https://doi.org/10.1016/s0733-8635(03)00052-4.

53. Altshuler GB, Anderson RR, Manstein D, Zenzie HH, Smirnov MZ. Extended theory of selective photothermolysis. Lasers Surg Med. 2001;29(5):416–32. https://doi.org/10.1002/lsm.1136.
54. Dierickx CC, Grossman MC, Farinelli WA, Anderson RR. Permanent hair removal by normal-mode ruby laser. Arch Dermatol. 1998;134(7):837–42. https://doi.org/10.1001/archderm.134.7.837.
55. Garcia C, Alamoudi H, Nakib M, Zimmo S. Alexandrite laser hair removal is safe for Fitzpatrick skin types IV–VI. Dermatol Surg. 2000;26(2):130–4. https://doi.org/10.1046/j.1524-4725.2000.99185.x.
56. Lou WW, Quintana AT, Geronemus RG, Grossman MC. Prospective study of hair reduction by diode laser (800 nm) with long-term follow-up. Dermatol Surg. 2000;26(5):428–32. https://doi.org/10.1046/j.1524-4725.2000.99260.x.
57. Chan CS, Dover JS. Nd:YAG laser hair removal in Fitzpatrick skin types IV to VI. J Drugs Dermatol. 2013;12(3):366–7.
58. Weiss RA, Weiss MA, Marwaha S, Harrington AC. Hair removal with a non-coherent filtered flashlamp intense pulsed light source. Lasers Surg Med. 1999;24(2):128–32. https://doi.org/10.1002/(sici)1096-9101(1999)24:2%3c128::aid-lsm8%3e3.0.co;2-m.
59. Tse Y. Hair removal using a pulsed-intense light source. Dermatol Clin. 1999;17(2):373–85.
60. Sadick NS, Weiss RA, Shea CR, Nagel H, Nicholson J, Prieto VG. Long-term photoepilation using a broad-spectrum intense pulsed light source. Arch Dermatol. 2000;136(11):1336–40.
61. Krupa Shankar D, Chakravarthi M, Shilpakar R. Carbon dioxide laser guidelines. J Cutan Aesthet Surg. 2009;2(2):72–80. https://doi.org/10.4103/0974-2077.58519.
62. Alster TS, Lupton JR. Erbium:YAG cutaneous laser resurfacing. Dermatol Clin. 2001;19(3):453–66. https://doi.org/10.1016/s0733-8635(05)70286-2.
63. Tanzi EL, Alster TS. Single-pass carbon dioxide versus multiple-pass Er:YAG laser skin resurfacing: a comparison of postoperative wound healing and side-effect rates. Dermatol Surg. 2003;29(1):80–4. https://doi.org/10.1046/j.1524-4725.2003.29012.x.
64. Bernstein LJ, Kauvar AN, Grossman MC, Geronemus RG. The short- and long-term side effects of carbon dioxide laser resurfacing. Dermatol Surg. 1997;23(7):519–25. https://doi.org/10.1111/j.1524-4725.1997.tb00677.x.
65. Nanni CA, Alster TS. Complications of carbon dioxide laser resurfacing. An evaluation of 500 patients. Dermatol Surg. 1998;24(3):315–20. https://doi.org/10.1111/j.1524-4725.1998.tb04161.x.
66. Sriprachya-Anunt S, Fitzpatrick RE, Goldman MP, Smith SR. Infections complicating pulsed carbon dioxide laser resurfacing for photoaged facial skin. Dermatol Surg. 1997;23(7):527–35; discussion 35–6. https://doi.org/10.1111/j.1524-4725.1997.tb00679.x.
67. Tanzi EL, Alster TS. Side effects and complications of variable-pulsed erbium:yttrium-aluminum-garnet laser skin resurfacing: extended experience with 50 patients. Plast Reconstr Surg. 2003;111(4):1524–9; discussion 30–2. https://doi.org/10.1097/01.PRS.0000049647.65948.50.
68. Alexiades-Armenakas MR, Dover JS, Arndt KA. The spectrum of laser skin resurfacing: nonablative, fractional, and ablative laser resurfacing. J Am Acad Dermatol. 2008;58(5):719–37; quiz 38–40. https://doi.org/10.1016/j.jaad.2008.01.003.
69. Tan AU, Schlosser BJ, Paller AS. A review of diagnosis and treatment of acne in adult female patients. Int J Womens Dermatol. 2018;4(2):56–71. https://doi.org/10.1016/j.ijwd.2017.10.006.
70. Toyoda M, Morohashi M. Pathogenesis of acne. Med Electron Microsc. 2001;34(1):29–40. https://doi.org/10.1007/s007950100002.
71. Bhat YJ, Latief I, Hassan I. Update on etiopathogenesis and treatment of acne. Indian J Dermatol Venereol Leprol. 2017;83(3):298–306. https://doi.org/10.4103/0378-6323.199581.
72. Sigurdsson V, Knulst AC, van Weelden H. Phototherapy of acne vulgaris with visible light. Dermatology. 1997;194(3):256–60. https://doi.org/10.1159/000246114.
73. Chilakamarthi U, Giribabu L. Photodynamic therapy: past, present and future. Chem Rec. 2017;17(8):775–802. https://doi.org/10.1002/tcr.201600121.

74. Keaney TC, Tanzi E, Alster T. Comparison of 532 nm potassium titanyl phosphate laser and 595 nm pulsed dye laser in the treatment of erythematous surgical scars: a randomized, controlled, open-label study. Dermatol Surg. 2016;42(1):70–6. https://doi.org/10.1097/DSS.0000000000000582.
75. Seaton ED, Charakida A, Mouser PE, Grace I, Clement RM, Chu AC. Pulsed-dye laser treatment for inflammatory acne vulgaris: randomised controlled trial. Lancet. 2003;362(9393):1347–52. https://doi.org/10.1016/s0140-6736(03)14629-6.
76. Harto A, Garcia-Morales I, Belmar P, Jaen P. Pulsed dye laser treatment of acne. Study of clinical efficacy and mechanism of action. Actas Dermosifiliogr. 2007;98(6):415–9.
77. Perez-Maldonado A, Runger TM, Krejci-Papa N. The 1,450-nm diode laser reduces sebum production in facial skin: a possible mode of action of its effectiveness for the treatment of acne vulgaris. Lasers Surg Med. 2007;39(2):189–92. https://doi.org/10.1002/lsm.20465.
78. Laubach HJ, Astner S, Watanabe K, Clifford J, Rius-Diaz F, Zurakowski D, et al. Effects of a 1,450 nm diode laser on facial sebum excretion. Lasers Surg Med. 2009;41(2):110–5. https://doi.org/10.1002/lsm.20672.
79. Jih MH, Friedman PM, Goldberg LH, Robles M, Glaich AS, Kimyai-Asadi A. The 1450-nm diode laser for facial inflammatory acne vulgaris: dose-response and 12-month follow-up study. J Am Acad Dermatol. 2006;55(1):80–7. https://doi.org/10.1016/j.jaad.2006.02.018.
80. Elsaie M, et al. Laser and light therapy for acne. In: Lasers in dermatology and medicine. 2011. p. 185–90.
81. Kesty K, Goldberg DJ. 650 usec 1064 nm Nd:YAG laser treatment of acne: a double-blind randomized control study. J Cosmet Dermatol. 2020;19(9):2295–300. https://doi.org/10.1111/jocd.13480.
82. Moneib H, Tawfik AA, Youssef SS, Fawzy MM. Randomized split-face controlled study to evaluate 1550-nm fractionated erbium glass laser for treatment of acne vulgaris—an image analysis evaluation. Dermatol Surg. 2014;40(11):1191–200. https://doi.org/10.1097/DSS.0000000000000167.
83. Kumaresan M, Srinivas CR. Efficacy of IPL in treatment of acne vulgaris: comparison of single- and burst-pulse mode in IPL. Indian J Dermatol. 2010;55(4):370–2. https://doi.org/10.4103/0019-5154.74550.
84. Sakamoto FH, Lopes JD, Anderson RR. Photodynamic therapy for acne vulgaris: a critical review from basics to clinical practice: part I. Acne vulgaris: when and why consider photodynamic therapy? J Am Acad Dermatol. 2010;63(2):183–93; quiz 93–4. https://doi.org/10.1016/j.jaad.2009.09.056.
85. Bissonnette R. Treatment of acne with photodynamic therapy. G Ital Dermatol Venereol. 2011;146(6):445–56.
86. Cives M, Mannavola F, Lospalluti L, Sergi MC, Cazzato G, Filoni E, et al. Non-melanoma skin cancers: biological and clinical features. Int J Mol Sci. 2020;21(15). https://doi.org/10.3390/ijms21155394.
87. Soleymani T, Abrouk M, Kelly KM. An analysis of laser therapy for the treatment of nonmelanoma skin cancer. Dermatol Surg. 2017;43(5):615–24. https://doi.org/10.1097/DSS.0000000000001048.
88. Brady M, Spiker AM. Merkel cell carcinoma of the skin. Treasure Island (FL): StatPearls; 2021.
89. Sinno H, Prakash S. Complements and the wound healing cascade: an updated review. Plast Surg Int. 2013;2013: 146764. https://doi.org/10.1155/2013/146764.
90. Gonzalez AC, Costa TF, Andrade ZA, Medrado AR. Wound healing—a literature review. An Bras Dermatol. 2016;91(5):614–20. https://doi.org/10.1590/abd1806-4841.20164741.
91. Calderhead RGKJ, Trelles MA, Ohshiro T. One mechanism behind LED phototherapy for wound healing and skin rejuvenation: key role of the mast cell. Laser Ther. 2008;17:141–8.
92. Morgan MC, Rashid RM. The effect of phototherapy on neutrophils. Int Immunopharmacol. 2009;9(4):383–8. https://doi.org/10.1016/j.intimp.2009.02.001.
93. Cauwels RG, Martens LC. Low level laser therapy in oral mucositis: a pilot study. Eur Arch Paediatr Dent. 2011;12(2):118–23. https://doi.org/10.1007/BF03262791.

94. Fahimipour F, Nouruzian M, Anvari M, Tafti MA, Yazdi M, Khosravi M, et al. Effect of low-level laser therapy on experimental wounds of hard palate mucosa in mice. Indian J Exp Biol. 2011;49(5):357–61.
95. Martu S, Amalinei C, Tatarciuc M, Rotaru M, Potarnichie O, Liliac L, et al. Healing process and laser therapy in the superficial periodontium: a histological study. Rom J Morphol Embryol. 2012;53(1):111–6.
96. Bolton PDM, Young S. The effect of polarized light on the release of growth factors from the U-973 macrophage-like cell line. Laser Ther. 1992;4:33–8.
97. Santuzzi CHBH, Pedrosa DF, Freire MO, Nogueira BV, Goncalves WL. Combined use of low level laser therapy and cyclooxygenase-2 selective inhibition on skin incisional wound reepithelialization in mice: a preclinical study. An Bras Dermatol. 2011;86:278–83.
98. Furchgott RF, Jothianandan D. Endothelium-dependent and -independent vasodilation involving cyclic GMP: relaxation induced by nitric oxide, carbon monoxide and light. Blood Vessels. 1991;28(1–3):52–61. https://doi.org/10.1159/000158843.
99. Kligman AM, Strauss JS. The formation of vellus hair follicles from human adult epidermis. J Invest Dermatol. 1956;27(1):19–23. https://doi.org/10.1038/jid.1956.71.
100. Ito M, Yang Z, Andl T, Cui C, Kim N, Millar SE, et al. Wnt-dependent de novo hair follicle regeneration in adult mouse skin after wounding. Nature. 2007;447(7142):316–20. https://doi.org/10.1038/nature05766.
101. Chan L, Cook DK. Female pattern hair loss. Aust J Gen Pract. 2018;47(7):459–64. https://doi.org/10.31128/AJGP-02-18-4498.
102. Tanaka Y, Aso T, Ono J, Hosoi R, Kaneko T. Androgenetic alopecia treatment in Asian men. J Clin Aesthet Dermatol. 2018;11(7):32–5.
103. Bienenfeld A, Azarchi S, Lo Sicco K, Marchbein S, Shapiro J, Nagler AR. Androgens in women: androgen-mediated skin disease and patient evaluation. J Am Acad Dermatol. 2019;80(6):1497–506. https://doi.org/10.1016/j.jaad.2018.08.062.
104. Sadick NS, Callender VD, Kircik LH, Kogan S. New insight into the pathophysiology of hair loss trigger a paradigm shift in the treatment approach. J Drugs Dermatol. 2017;16(11):135–40.
105. Avci P, Gupta GK, Clark J, Wikonkal N, Hamblin MR. Low-level laser (light) therapy (LLLT) for treatment of hair loss. Lasers Surg Med. 2014;46(2):144–51. https://doi.org/10.1002/lsm.22170.
106. Wikramanayake TC, Rodriguez R, Choudhary S, Mauro LM, Nouri K, Schachner LA, et al. Effects of the Lexington LaserComb on hair regrowth in the C3H/HeJ mouse model of alopecia areata. Lasers Med Sci. 2012;27(2):431–6. https://doi.org/10.1007/s10103-011-0953-7.
107. Kalia S, Lui H. Utilizing electromagnetic radiation for hair growth: a critical review of phototrichogenesis. Dermatol Clin. 2013;31(1):193–200. https://doi.org/10.1016/j.det.2012.08.018.
108. Pratt CH, King LE Jr, Messenger AG, Christiano AM, Sundberg JP. Alopecia areata. Nat Rev Dis Primers. 2017;3:17011. https://doi.org/10.1038/nrdp.2017.11.
109. Al-Mutairi N. 308-nm excimer laser for the treatment of alopecia areata in children. Pediatr Dermatol. 2009;26(5):547–50. https://doi.org/10.1111/j.1525-1470.2009.00980.x.
110. Al-Mutairi N. 308-nm excimer laser for the treatment of alopecia areata. Dermatol Surg. 2007;33(12):1483–7. https://doi.org/10.1111/j.1524-4725.2007.33320.x.
111. Gundogan C, Greve B, Raulin C. Treatment of alopecia areata with the 308-nm xenon chloride excimer laser: case report of two successful treatments with the excimer laser. Lasers Surg Med. 2004;34(2):86–90. https://doi.org/10.1002/lsm.20002.
112. Byun JWMJ, Bang CY, Shin J, Choi GS. Effectiveness of 308-nm excimer laser therapy in treating alopecia areata, determined by examining the treated sides of selected alopecic patches. Dermatology. 2015;231:70–6.
113. Mlacker S, Aldahan AS, Simmons BJ, Shah V, McNamara CA, Samarkandy S, et al. A review on laser and light-based therapies for alopecia areata. J Cosmet Laser Ther. 2017;19(2):93–9. https://doi.org/10.1080/14764172.2016.1248440.

114. Claudy AL, Gagnaire D. PUVA treatment of alopecia areata. Arch Dermatol. 1983;119(12):975–8.
115. Lassus A, Eskelinen A, Johansson E. Treatment of alopecia areata with three different PUVA modalities. Photodermatology. 1984;1(3):141–4.
116. Mitchell AJ, Douglass MC. Topical photochemotherapy for alopecia areata. J Am Acad Dermatol. 1985;12(4):644–9. https://doi.org/10.1016/s0190-9622(85)70088-6.
117. Healy ERS. PUVA treatment for alopecia areata—does it work? A retrospective review of 102 cases. Br J Dermatol. 1993;129:42–4.
118. Taylor CR, Hawk JL. PUVA treatment of alopecia areata partialis, totalis and universalis: audit of 10 years' experience at St John's Institute of Dermatology. Br J Dermatol. 1995;133(6):914–8. https://doi.org/10.1111/j.1365-2133.1995.tb06925.x.
119. Wikramanayake TC, Villasante AC, Mauro LM, Nouri K, Schachner LA, Perez CI, et al. Low-level laser treatment accelerated hair regrowth in a rat model of chemotherapy-induced alopecia (CIA). Lasers Med Sci. 2013;28(3):701–6. https://doi.org/10.1007/s10103-012-1139-7.
120. Filbrandt R, Rufaut N, Jones L, Sinclair R. Primary cicatricial alopecia: diagnosis and treatment. CMAJ. 2013;185(18):1579–85. https://doi.org/10.1503/cmaj.111570.
121. Randolph MJ, Salhi WA, Tosti A. Lichen planopilaris and low-level light therapy: four case reports and review of the literature about low-level light therapy and lichenoid dermatosis. Dermatol Ther (Heidelb). 2020;10(2):311–9. https://doi.org/10.1007/s13555-020-00359-x.

Teletrichology for Hair Disorder Consultations

Adaeze Nwosu, Mariya Miteva, and Antonella Tosti

Abstract The COVID-19 pandemic brought novel challenges to the practice of dermatology, including the remote clinical management of hair and scalp disorders. This chapter explores teledermatology for hair and scalp disorders, where we define teletrichology as the use of telecommunication platforms to interact with hair disorder patients remotely. We use the term to encompass triaging, consultations, remote imaging, and diagnoses (Randolph et al. in J Eur Acad Dermatol Venereol, 2020 [1]). The chapter assesses the nature of patient consultations and methods of evaluation of ailments in teledermatology, the benefits and challenges of teletrichology, and proposes triaging methods for efficient patient management. Finally, given that these remote consultations that arose due to the COVID-19 will likely endure and be integrated into routine practice, we offer policy and practical recommendations to improve patient outcomes.

Keywords Teletrichology · Teledermatology · Hair diseases · COVID-19 · Alopecia · Telehealth · Smartphone · Dermatoscopy

1 Overview of the Consultation

Teledermatology has been heralded for its ability to improve access to care and reduce patient inequality in the setting of global pandemics [2, 3]. This has been the case for our clinic as well, as patients from all over the country and from abroad can schedule appointments remotely. Patients love the ease of telemedicine for routine consultations and that is also true of teletrichology.

For some providers, teletrichology can be challenging in the accurate diagnosis of new patients, and an unsuitable long-term alternative to in-person practice for certain diseases, because dermatology depends heavily on visual acuity. However, in one of the authors' personal experience (AT) teletrichology presents a great opportunity

A. Nwosu · M. Miteva · A. Tosti (✉)
Dr. Phillip Frost Department of Dermatology and Cutaneous Surgery, University of Miami Miller School of Medicine, Miami, FL, USA
e-mail: ATosti@med.miami.edu

K. Nouri (ed.), *Telemedicine and Technological Advances in Dermatology*,
https://doi.org/10.1007/978-3-031-69091-4_4

not only for follow up sessions, particularly for patients with alopecia areata, and to provide accurate explanations of scalp biopsy results and therapy regimens, but also for diagnoses of complex hair disorders. For this purpose, I developed a way to obtain trichoscopic images with simple instruments [1]. Some creative strategies help patients' understanding during our remote consultations. For example, illustrative diagrams are useful to provide explanations on disease prognosis. At the University of Miami, teletrichology sessions are scheduled every 15–20 min and conducted securely via zoom. Consultations can be performed just using the desktop computer or using two devices: a mobile phone (or a tablet) for the video call and a desktop to review patient charts and complete electronic medical notes in real time. A secure portal allows patients to securely ask questions follow up questions and send images. Medications are prescribed electronically to the pharmacy of the patient's choice.

1.1 The Impact of COVID-19 on Hair Disorders

Emerging evidence suggests that COVID-19 is often associated with acute telogen effluvium [4, 5]. Although the mechanism has not been fully elucidated, it is likely that the cytokine storm that characterizes COVID-19 infection causes hairs to prematurely enter the telogen stage [6, 7]. Although COVID-19 induced Telogen Effluvium is self-limiting, it might trigger androgenetic alopecia. In 2021, Miami Dade County, where our clinic is located, had 650,000 COVID-19 cases. COVID-19 added a layer of complexity to diagnosis as patients often question whether the vaccine could be a source of recent flare ups.

1.2 Triaging

A few articles have already explored the concept of triaging to segregate patients into manageable segments based on their level of disease. In contrast to the study by Pararajasingam et al., where over 60% of their patients were triaged, we have found that less than 30% of our patients are triaged for telemedicine consultations and the choice is mostly dictated by the in-person availability of the dermatologist and/or the patient [8]. Most commonly, teletrichology cases consist of alopecia areata, androgenetic alopecia, seborrheic dermatitis, scalp pruritus, and scarring alopecia. Most patients follow-up, and even new cases are successfully managed via teletrichology. The need for face-to-face consultations arises when patients need to have further investigative trichoscopy and biopsies performed, such as in patients with an atypical presentation pattern, and in patients who are not responsive to therapy. In those instances, we would simply reschedule the patient for in-person evaluation (Fig. 1).

One potential way to improve triaging may be to ask patients to fill a pre-consultations questionnaire through an app to aid with monitoring and evaluation.

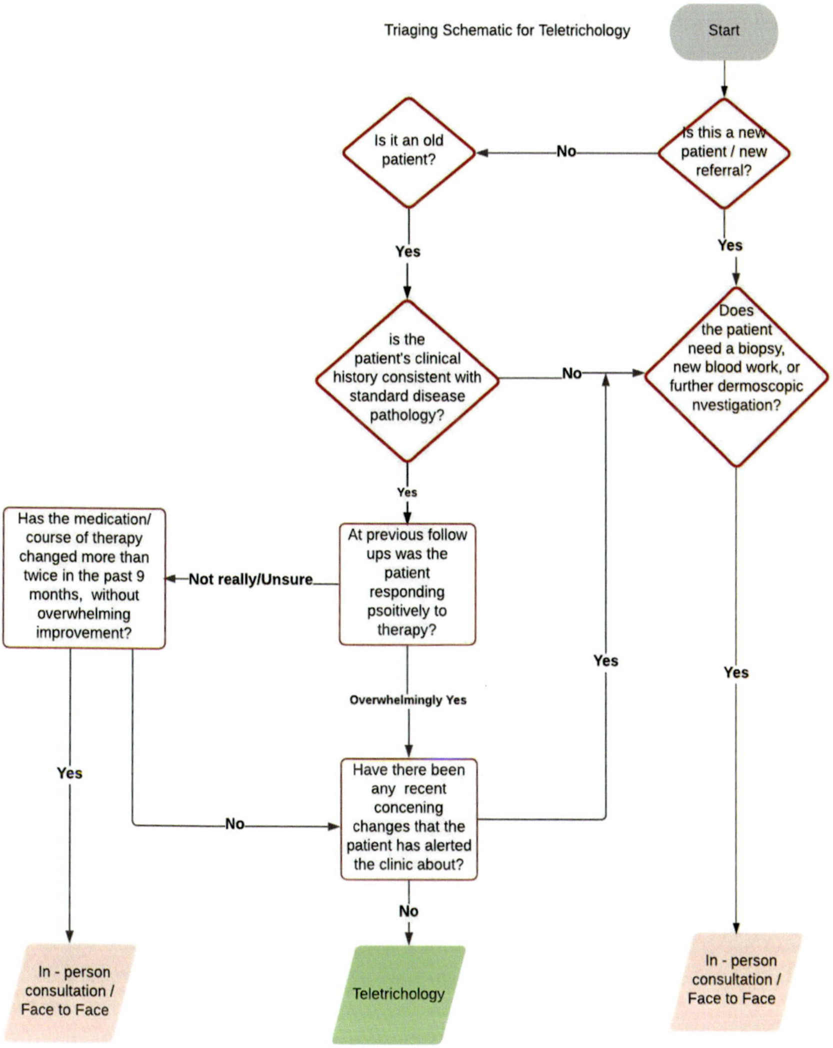

Fig. 1 Teletrichology triaging schema

Posable questions include routine patients queries that we frequently ask patients during consultations, such as new symptom development, side effects of medications, medication adherence, new lifestyle changes, and adjuvant non-prescribed therapy. The patient would upload accompanying relevant dermoscopic images, captured with a smartphone, which most, if not all our patients have. Patients can safely, take images and share with their dermatologist. Affordable and/or free applications for macrophotography are available for both Apple and Android devices (Camera +2 for apple and Camera FV-5 for android) [1]. Responses to these questions can be reviewed periodically by the nurse practitioner or a physician assistant and scaled up to the physician to alert them of any atypical or concerning changes. This may serve as a more objective and equitable way to appropriate patients who need more attention into more urgent tiers and consultation slots, while patients whose symptoms are well controlled can be placed in less urgent tiers and have their appointments moved farther out.

2 Evaluation Methods in Teletrichology

We successfully leverage existing infrastructure such as smartphones and laptops to view and evaluate the progress of hair disorders. During our telemedicine consultations, patients present their hair and scalp concerns by showcasing the relevant portion on their smartphones or laptops. Although both devices can be utilized, we recommend using laptops for patients who consult alone, as these patients more easily adjust their body's position in front of a stationery camera and in the absence of assistance from a partner. For patches, thinning and shedding that are harder to assess, such as those that present on the dorsal and occipital sides of the scalp, we recommend partner assisted consultations with a smartphone, providing the patient is comfortable. In these partner-assisted consultations, spouses or parents assist with positioning the smartphone's camera in a suitable position to evaluate the lesion. We have explored whether patients would willingly invest in a hand-held dermoscope, or hand-held mirrors to view hard to reach scalp areas, but we find patients are hesitant to invest in additional equipment (personal experience of MM). Thus far, mobile devices and laptops suffice for routine teletrichoscopy examination when there's adequate natural lighting, and assistance from a partner.

Teletrichology relies on patient participation and cooperation for a successful consultation, and evaluation of disease progression. In these instances, patients may agree to use a measuring tape to measure a lesion, participate in pull tests to assess shedding, or use a prop to part their scalp. Most patients, especially when they are in their homes, are eager to show the lesions, even without prompting. By contrast, we find patients who attend a teledermatology consultation while at work are less comfortable with using their mobile phones or laptops as a teletrichoscopy device to show scalp changes or remove a scalp prosthesis. In these cases, we recommend the patient comes in for an in-person evaluation, or to reschedule in order to be in a comfortable environment.

2.1 Teletrichology Tests

It is important to note that teletrichology may not be as sufficient for diagnosis as biopsies, and other diagnostic procedures still need to be done in-person and in a clinical setting. Evaluative tests which may be performed through teletrichology include the part test, the pull test, the tug test as well ponytail and hairline measurements [1]. The dermatologist can use a parting or "tail" comb (Fig. 6) to demonstrate to the patient how to properly part the hair at the center of the scalp. The patient replicates these actions on camera to reveal the center of the scalp. The consultant evaluates the width of the part and the density of hair to grade the severity of the disorder. The pull test is straightforward and can be used on new and follow-up patients to verify if the shedding is normal or increased. To perform the test, we show the patients how to grasp a tuft of hairs 2 cm from the scalp and gently pull with the thumb and index fingers along the hair shafts toward the distal tip. In patterned hair loss like in androgenetic alopecia, patients should pull around the affected area and normal scalp. In patchy hair loss, like alopecia areata, patients should pull form around the borders of the patch and normal hair [9]. We ask patients to repeat this in different regions of their scalp (front, sides, vertex, back). A negative pull test extracts less than five hairs and a positive pull test extracts six or more hairs from a single area [10, 11].

Other teletrichology tests include the tug test which assesses hair shaft fragility. It involves holding a few strands of hair in one hand 4–5 cm from the tip and tugging distally with thumb and index finger of the other hand. When positive, the test removes broken hair fragments. These measurements allow for follow up on conditions such as frontal fibrosing alopecia, and providers show patients how to take proper measures using a tape measure.

2.2 *Teletrichology Images*

Patients can obtain teletrichology images, by attaching a macro lens to their smartphones or by utilizing wireless, inexpensive microscopes. These technologies allow providers to see the most important diagnostic trichoscopic findings including the presence/absence of follicular openings, broken hairs, exclamation mark hairs and vellus hairs at the hairline. A wireless microscope provides higher magnifications, and can assess white dots, yellow dots, hair shaft diameters and perifollicular casts [1] (Figs. 2, 3 and 4).

2.3 *Teletrichology Props*

Given the chronic nature of hair and scalp disorders among our patients, it is important to ensure they leave consultations with a better understanding of their disease, its prognosis with therapy and without therapy, and how to manage their conditions. In teletrichology, we use props to demonstrate the pattern of disease. For example, in female patients presenting with androgenetic alopecia, we show illustrations of a Ludwig–Savin scale (Fig. 5). We find the use of illustrations particularly useful to improve therapy compliance in patients who are frustrated to learn that they would

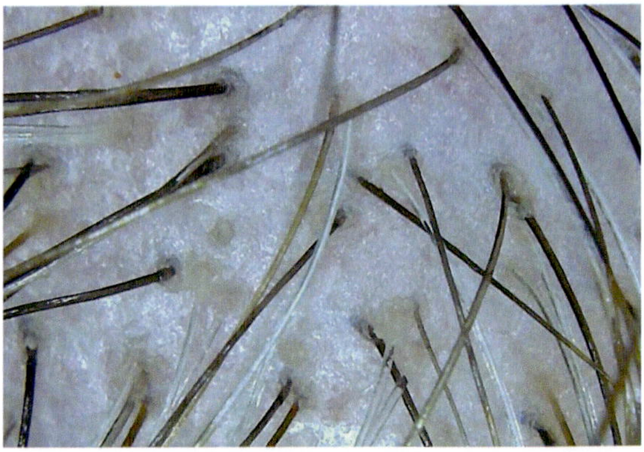

Fig. 2 Hair shaft diameter and presence of follicular openings assessed by Wi-Fi microscope at 50× magnification

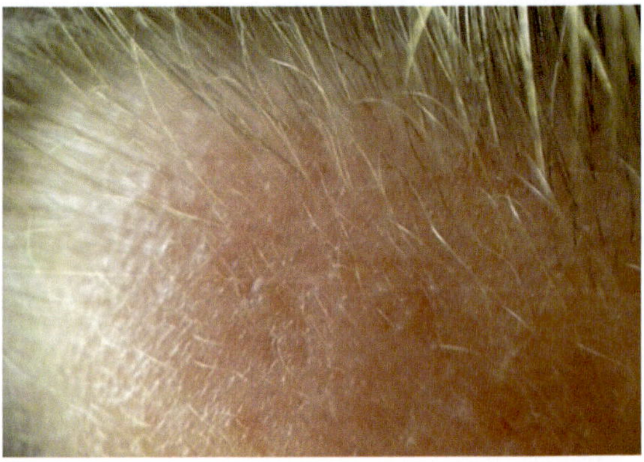

Fig. 3 Vellus hair at hairline captured by macro lens attached to smart phone at 10× magnification

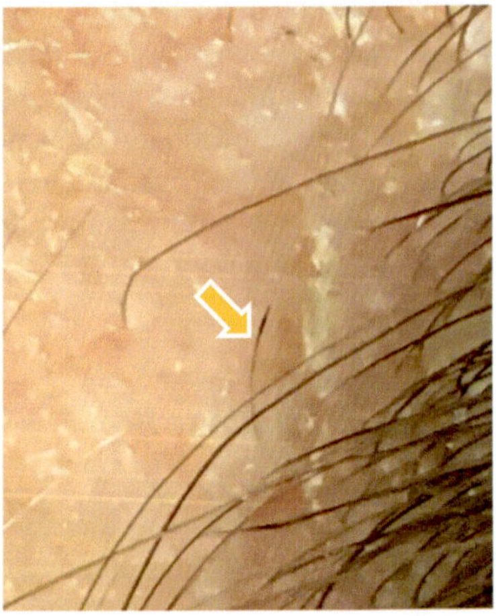

Fig. 4 Exclamation mark hair captured with smartphone

need to be on therapy for life, because of the chronic nature of their illness. For example, some patients presenting with early-stage scarring/fibrosing alopecia, may question the rationale behind a therapy that won't restore the fibrosed hair follicles and yet would be inconvenient to apply. We find once we illustrate with props how more scarring can occur without therapy, patients do become more understanding and willing to comply with medication.

While props can be useful illustrative tools, they don't replace the clinical skills required to deliver a life altering diagnosis. In these delicate circumstances, clinicians should ensure care is taken to recognize the impact of the prognosis on the patient and provide reassurance. This is done as effectively on telemedicine as it is in-person, by anticipating patient concerns, listening, quelling any unhelpful therapies patients may have read on the internet and explaining how to use treatment properly. The latter is particularly important as we find a poor response to treatment can be due to misapplication. Thus, it's important to firstly investigate how treatments are being applied before recommending alternatives. During teletrichology consultations, we ask patients use their hands to demonstrate how they apply treatments to their hair so we may correct any misapplications (Fig. 6).

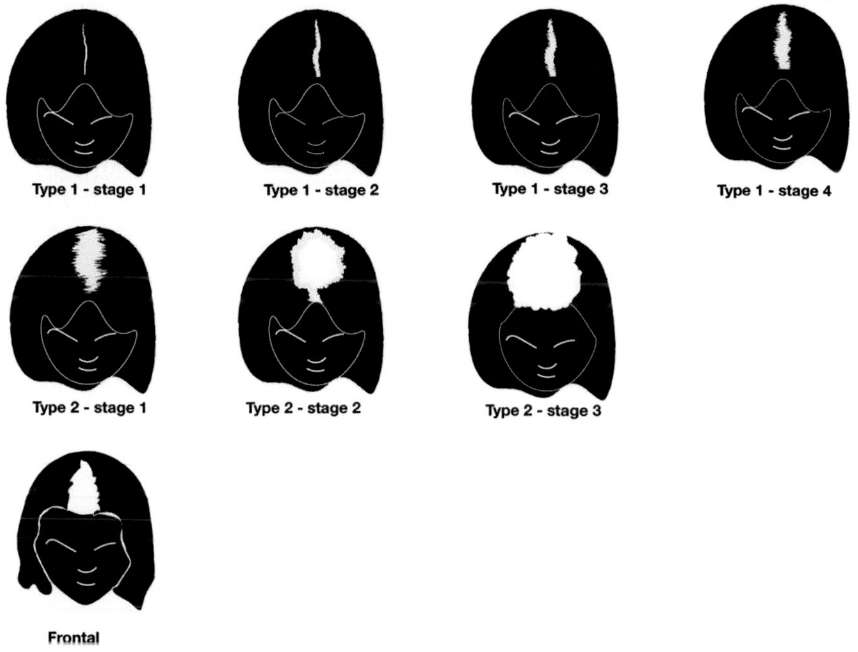

Fig. 5 Ludwig–Savin scale for female pattern baldness. Type 1 is characterized by minimal thinning, type 2 has loss of volume and widening mid-part line. Type 3 encompasses types 1 and 2 and the recession of the front line

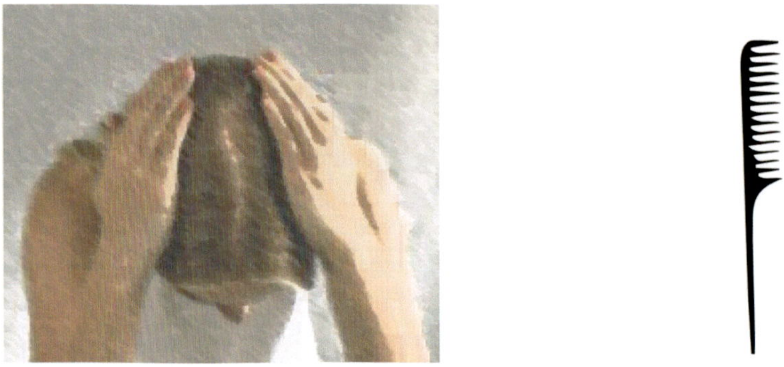

Fig. 6 Demonstration of on-screen part and a part comb used during teletrichology

2.4 Teletrichology and Patient Information

Another benefit of teletrichology is the ease and security it provides patients to share their patient information such as lab results, past medical records from other clinics and images. Patient hesitancy to share images digitally is a challenge for teledermatology, as over 50% US adults prefer to not digitally exchange health images with providers [12]. We surmount this challenge by using the screenshare tool to securely share helpful information during our teletrichology consultations. The screenshare allows dermatologist to view baseline images, captured during disease onset in real time.

3 Conclusion

In summary, teledermatology and teletrichoscopy hold significant potential to aid in the evaluation of new patients, but even more so in follow-up patients. We find it particularly useful for discussing the management plan after work up/scalp biopsies and for discussing any questions that patients may have regarding the management, side effects, prescription refills and concerns.

References

1. Randolph M, Al-alola A, Tosti A. Diagnosis of hair disorders during the COVID-19 pandemic: an introduction to teletrichoscopy. J Eur Acad Dermatol Venereol. 2020. https://doi.org/10.1111/JDV.16989
2. Zakaria A, Maurer T, Su G, Amerson E. Impact of teledermatology on the accessibility and efficiency of dermatology care in an urban safety-net hospital: a pre-post analysis. J Am Acad Dermatol. 2019;81(6):1446–52. https://doi.org/10.1016/j.jaad.2019.08.016.

3. Coustasse A, Sarkar R, Abodunde B, Metzger BJ, Slater CM. Use of teledermatology to improve dermatological access in rural areas. Telemed J E Health. 2019;25(11):1022–32. https://doi.org/10.1089/tmj.2018.0130.
4. Rivetti N, Barruscotti S. Management of telogen effluvium during the COVID-19 emergency: psychological implications. Dermatol Ther. 2020. https://doi.org/10.1111/dth.13648
5. Olds H, Liu J, Luk K, Lim HW, Ozog D, Rambhatla PV. Telogen effluvium associated with COVID-19 infection. Dermatol Ther. 2021;34(2): e14761. https://doi.org/10.1111/dth.14761.
6. Starace M, Iorizzo M, Sechi A, et al. Trichodynia and telogen effluvium in COVID-19 patients: results of an international expert opinion survey on diagnosis and management. JAAD Int. 2021;5:11–8. https://doi.org/10.1016/j.jdin.2021.07.006.
7. Malkud S. Telogen effluvium: a review. J Clin Diagn Res. 2015;9(9):WE01–3. https://doi.org/10.7860/JCDR/2015/15219.6492
8. Pararajasingam A, Lowe A, Khan W, Hancock P, Stone N. Dealing with suspended new routine general dermatology referrals during the COVID-19 pandemic: a virtual model from our local departmental experience. Clin Exp Dermatol. https://doi.org/10.1111/ced.14580
9. Tosti A, Piraccini BM. Diagnosis and treatment of hair disorders—an evidence based atlas. Oxon: Taylor and Francis; 2006, p. 10–1, 47–9.
10. Gordon KA, Tosti A. Alopecia: evaluation and treatment. Clin Cosmet Investig Dermatol. 2011;4:101–6. https://doi.org/10.2147/CCID.S10182.
11. Hillmann K, Blume-Peytavi U. Diagnosis of hair disorders. Semin Cutan Med Surg. 2009;28(1):33–8. https://doi.org/10.1016/j.sder.2008.12.005.
12. Wei G, Turner K, Hennessey K, Seminario-Vidal L. 273 Reluctance towards digital image sharing and challenges for teledermatology. J Investig Dermatol. 2021

Skin Cancer Telemedicine

Kayla D. Mashoudy, Sofia M. Perez, and Keyvan Nouri

Abstract Skin cancer treatment is an arm of dermatology that relies on accurate diagnosis and timely intervention. Teledermatology has proven useful in many stages of skin cancer care from triage to diagnosis, management, and surgical consultation. With the addition of traditional dermoscopy and store-and-forward technology, high resolution images of suspicious skin lesions can be sent to consulting dermatologists all-over for an expedited follow-up process. Both live video conference and store-and-forward telemedicine styles have assisted in narrowing the care access gap between dermatologic providers and geographically isolated patients. Teledermatology also exhibits diagnostic accuracy rates that are acceptable and, in many cases, comparable to that of face-to-face encounters, augmenting its robust clinical utility. Technologies such as artificial intelligence and reflectance confocal microscopy continue to improve image quality and the potential for increased diagnostic accuracy of virtual dermatologic care. Considering its many advantages, teledermatology serves as more of a valuable clinical tool than a comprehensive replacement for skin cancer treatment, especially for Mohs surgery and procedural interventions that must take place in-person. Nonetheless, teledermatology's role in advancing the workup of skin malignancies is gaining recognition within the dermatologic community and acquiring high approval rates amongst patients for its practicality and timely access to care.

Keywords Skin cancer · Pigmented lesions · Teledermoscopy · Cutaneous malignancy · Diagnostic accuracy · Mohs surgery · Artificial intelligence

K. D. Mashoudy (✉) · S. M. Perez · K. Nouri
Dr. Phillip Frost Department of Dermatology and Cutaneous Surgery, Miller School of Medicine, University of Miami, Miami, FL, USA
e-mail: Kmashoudy@med.miami.edu

K. Nouri (ed.), *Telemedicine and Technological Advances in Dermatology*,
https://doi.org/10.1007/978-3-031-69091-4_5

1 Introduction

Skin malignancy causes significant morbidity and mortality and is one of the most frequently diagnosed cancers in the U.S. Within this country, a man has a 1 in 37 lifetime risk and a woman has a 1 in 55 lifetime risk for developing a malignant melanoma [1]. In addition to the significant disease burden experienced by affected individuals, skin cancer generates a substantial economic burden. Estimates for treatment costs and value of life lost to society from melanoma alone vary from $8 billion per year to $15 billion per year [2]. The health and financial impacts of skin cancer are undeniably significant and increasing. It is ubiquitously known within the dermatologic community that early diagnosis and treatment of melanoma and nonmelanoma skin cancers improve patient outcomes and prognosis [3]. With the rising incidence of skin cancer cases, the demand for dermatologic care has increased in both urban and rural localities and has also increased wait time to see a specialist. Teledermatology has risen in popularity as a solution for these growing challenges and offers immediate and relatively thorough skin cancer screening for patients with poor access to health care.

Teledermatology facilitates the electronic transfer of medical information to a dermatologist for evaluation at a distance. The medical information that is utilized during a consultation may include a clinical history, clinical and/or dermoscopic images of cutaneous lesions, and self-taken photos by the patient for remote assessment. The main types of virtual consultation are store-and-forward, allowing transmission of pictures and clinical details to a medical provider for review at a later time, and live interactive, which permits real-time interaction between the patient and physician. The combination of both styles yields a hybrid consultation [4]. Although the store-and-forward consultations are generally the most effective and common type, the other formats have benefits for medically complex cases and patient education. To enhance the quality of these virtual consultations, digital photography or dermoscopic images can be added to the visit. Inclusion of both digital and mobile dermoscopic images has the potential to improve rates of diagnostic accuracy and reliability of skin examinations, especially if the images are interpreted by skilled dermatologists.

Furthermore, the role of teledermatology in the clinical steps from triage to diagnosis, management, and possible surgical intervention has been investigated in various studies. The relatively rapid time to consultation allows teledermatology to serve as a useful triage tool and may expedite the diagnosis of skin malignancy, an inherently time-sensitive matter. The process of both preoperative consultation and postoperative follow-up for Mohs surgery may also benefit from the implementation of telemedicine, promoting the resolution of patient questions and evaluation of surgical site recovery, respectively.

Prior to implementing a new health care delivery system like teledermatology, it is necessary to verify that diagnostic accuracy and thus patient care is not compromised. Although the effectiveness of teledermatology for the diagnosis of skin cancer is multifactorial, studies have shown that it has acceptable accuracy and management concordance compared with in-person clinical evaluation, especially with the addition of dermoscopic images [5] and training of non-specialty providers giving remote dermatologic care [6]. Other important considerations to acknowledge are the enhanced practicality and convenience telemedicine provides for both patients and clinicians as well as the high satisfaction rate reported by many patients. With all the advantages virtual consultation offers, the utilization and demand for teledermatology continues to increase. Technological applications to teledermatology such as reflectance confocal microscopy and artificial intelligence are continuously being updated with the potential to improve the outcomes of remote-based care. Further studies are needed to assess the safety and efficacy of making these advances permanent branches of teledermatology. Nonetheless, establishing more teledermatology networks in medically underserved areas will improve access for geographically disadvantaged patents and may significantly lower the burden of cutaneous malignancies.

2 Teledermatology Formats for Pigmented Lesions

Malignant lesions account for approximately 2.06 million dermatology visits annually [7], emphasizing the importance of skin cancer care, clinical management, and the large patient population that relies on this care. The visual component of diagnosing pigmented lesions and necessity for prompt evaluation present an ideal opportunity for the application of telemedicine to promote patient workup [8]. Telemedicine can be implemented in several ways including store-and-forward technology, live video conferencing, and a hybrid model incorporating both photographed images and live consultation. The following section will outline various methods of teledermatology as well as their benefits and disadvantages for skin cancer management.

Store-and-Forward technology is an asynchronous type of teledermatology that includes transmission of digital images from a clinician or patient to a consulting dermatologist. This method is often implemented for the diagnosis and management decision (to biopsy or not) of a suspected malignant lesion and serves as a relatively affordable, timely option for the dermatologic care of patients in medically disadvantaged areas. Specifically, store-and-forward technology has been shown to reduce long travel times and compensate for a lack of dermatologic care in rural regions of the country [9]. The telehealth process begins with a non-specialist provider or patient taking images of a lesion and electronically transferring the image, usually in JPEG format, to the consulting dermatologist via a secure database or portal. The dermatologist is then able to examine the image using Adobe Photoshop or another image processing software on a laptop, computer monitor, or tablet device. Accordingly, capturing high-quality images is essential for proper evaluation. The average image resolution of clinical photographs used for store-and-forward technology is 640 × 480 pixels [10]; increasing resolution may maximize the diagnostic capabilities of the consulting dermatologist.

Due to the limitations of image quality on diagnostic reliability, enhancing image resolution through additions like teledermoscopy can improve the virtual workup of pigmented lesions. Teledermoscopy involves archiving and web-based transferring of dermoscopic images for remote assessment [11]. This format optimizes image quality by using a dermatoscope with magnifying power rather than a mobile or digital camera and is thus associated with higher rates of diagnostic accuracy and management plan agreement [5]. as compared to telemedicine styles that don't utilize dermoscopy. Non-dermoscopic methods of capturing clinical images include using a smartphone camera or other digital devices, many of which do not require the extent of training that dermoscopy does [12]. Various devices used for photographing pigmented lesions are further discussed in ***Use of Digital photography and Dermoscopy in Teledermatology***.

Another teledermatology format is **live video conferencing**, which implements real time consultation between patients and teledermatologists. Because of its audio and video components, live interactive teledermatology requires both parties to use essential electronic equipment including a computer, video camera, and microphone. These added technological factors in combination with the increased time expenditure of the consulting dermatologist contributes to live video conferencing being a costlier teledermatology option [10]. However, this type of teledermatology is particularly useful in complex cases and management decisions requiring ample communication between the provider and patient. Live video telemedicine provides a secure digital platform for direct patient education and streamlined interactions that can improve treatment compliance and patient satisfaction [13].

Incorporating aspects of both live video and store-and-forward teledermatology yields a two-step **hybrid** telemedicine format [14].The initial stage involves electronically storing and sending images to assist the dermatologist in creating a preliminary differential. The second step integrates live video conferencing to address any doubts about the diagnosis of the lesion and patient questions as well as clarify management plans. This combined format of teledermatology is especially useful in complex cases, instances of poor initial image quality, or occasions when multiple treatment options may exist and need to be fully discussed with the patient. Hybrid and other teledermatology formats are thus beneficial for diagnosing atypical pigmented lesions and supply dermatologic care needs that are not easily met by existing health care models [15].

3 Use of Digital Photography and Dermoscopy in Teledermatology

With the rapidly changing landscape of teledermatology over the past decade, new technologies have been introduced, and workflows have been updated to include these advances in recent years. Specifically, the addition of dermoscopy and mobile dermoscopy have supplemented the teledermatology experience, offering the potential to enhance virtual skin examination. Some theoretical advantages include early detection and management, thorough skin examination, and closer inspection of skin lesions. The combination of these benefits has the potential to improve the skin cancer outcomes of teledermatology. The following section will discuss the roles and clinical utility of digital dermoscopy, mobile dermoscopy, and imaging techniques in their applications to teledermatology.

3.1 Digital Dermoscopy

In a teledermatology consultation, the touch and visualization aspects of an in-person visit are often replaced via the addition of digital photography and dermoscopic images. These photographic additions not only enhance the quality of the appointment but also supply greater diagnostic confidence and accuracy for skin lesions [4]. Dermoscopy, specifically, is the utilization of a lens-like device that enables noninvasive microscopic inspection of skin through magnifying power. In digital dermoscopy, these images are digitalized and electronically transmitted to providers. The images are initially captured with a digital dermatoscope or a digital camera configured with a dermoscopic lens and stored within a secure web-based software [16]. Stentor (currently iSite), for example, is an online picture storing and communications platform that can be used to archive and transmit dermatologic images captured with a digital camera or dermoscopic lens. One study evaluating the dermatology practice workflows of Kaiser Permanente Northern California found various advantages in using Stentor with dermoscopy. These benefits included greater probability of skin cancer detection compared with direct referral, lower probability of biopsy, fewer lesions requiring visits to the clinic, incorporation with electronic medical record (EMR), and long-term storage of images [17]. Inclusion of clinical and dermoscopic images thus has the potential to reduce healthcare costs and improve skin cancer outcomes through high diagnostic accuracy and early detection.

3.2 Mobile Dermoscopy

Many technologies, including mobile technology, are being utilized to improve the workflow of teledermatology and have the potential to enhance skin self-examination.

Mobile dermoscopy is an application of teledermoscopy that combines the photographic capabilities of mobile devices (smartphone, tablets, etc.) with their telecommunication features to capture and send clinical images of skin lesions. This technology incorporates attachable magnifying devices, mobile applications, and secure online platforms to promote a thorough skin self-examination. These images can then be transmitted directly to a clinician for remote evaluation and diagnosis [18]. The photographs can be taken directly by either the patient or a primary provider and necessitate careful inspections of skin lesions. Various algorithm-based applications can even identify features of certain malignancies, but the applications with the highest sensitivity have images interpreted by a remote dermatologist [19]. Although they can be useful for melanoma screening, smartphone applications may not be diagnostically accurate unless the image is reviewed by a skilled dermatologist and are not designed to carry out comparative analysis [20]. These points reaffirm that mobile dermoscopy serves as a supplement to regular full body skin examinations and does not suffice as a replacement. The patient may have concerning skin lesions noticeable only by a clinical examination. Improving patient instructions on types of skin lesions to capture, training patient partners for checking difficult-to-see areas, and updating algorithms to better rule out benign skin lesions at the time of photographing may improve the outcomes of this technology [18]. These and other future advances in mobile dermoscopy can increase the reliability of skin self-examinations and contribute to early detection of skin cancer.

3.3 *Imaging Techniques and Clinical Utility of Teledermoscopy*

As touched upon in the above sections, various devices are available for digital and mobile dermoscopy. These entities include dermatoscopes with built-in digital cameras, dermatoscopes that attach to smartphones or mobile devices, digital single-lens reflex cameras, Apple mobile devices, digital full frame cameras, tablets, iPods, and smartphones. There are even some all-in-one platforms that have photo capturing, data archiving, and data transmitting properties [16]. The photographs taken with digital devices can be applied to clinical environments and utilized in various ways, including teledermoscopy, sequential monitoring, and machine learning [21].

Matching the increasing popularity of telehealth in recent years, the application of teledermoscopy to virtual dermatology consultations has become very common. This technology has been particularly successful for large screening occasions and reaching rural or underserved areas that are distant from practicing dermatologists [22]. Moreover, inclusion of digital and dermoscopic photographs in teledermatology appointments has been shown to increase diagnostic accuracy with minimal changes to consultation time. This boost in reliability is important because face-to-face clinical visits tend to be more accurate than telehealth visits. Teledermoscopy's greatest strengths, however, may perhaps be in reducing healthcare costs, aiding patient triage and monitoring, and reducing the number of unnecessary referrals, surgery wait times, and "no-shows" for in-person appointments [23].

4 Teledermatology for Skin Cancer Consultation and Documentation

The management of cutaneous lesions includes multiple steps from triage and diagnosis to intervention and monitoring. Each step plays an important role in patient workup and treatment for skin malignancy, and teledermatology can help provide optimal care throughout the entire process. The following section will explore the benefits of implementing teledermatology in the triage, diagnosis, and surgical treatment of malignant lesions.

4.1 Triage

In the dermatology clinic, skin cancer triage typically involves acting on clinical suspicion and employing dermoscopy to prioritize patients based on the urgency and stage of their skin lesions. Imminent management decisions may include reassurance, biopsy, or referral to another specialist. Deciding on the best course of action is the main goal during the triage process [24], and role of telemedicine in facilitating these choices has also been evaluated in several studies.

Because the consulting dermatologist has the patient's clinical history and images digitalized and at their disposal, the store-and-forward type of teledermatology enables timely management decisions [8]. In a study conducted at the University Hospital Virgen Macarena in Spain, the average wait time to see a dermatologist in person for a concerning skin lesion was 88.62 days as compared to 12.31 days via teledermatology [8]. In addition to promptness, accuracy in management decisions is necessary to appropriately organize patients according to their needs. Shapiro et al. evaluated 49 patients with both benign and malignant lesions and reported a 100% agreement rate among clinical dermatologists and teledermatologists on the decision to biopsy a lesion [25]. Another study found a 90% agreement rate among a clinical dermatologist and 3 teledermatologists regarding the management plan of 29 patients [26]. Comparing intra-dermatologist agreement rates among three teledermatologists evaluating 168 lesions, Whited et al. reported 69–70% concordance for medical therapy plans, 64–83% concordance for clinical therapy plans, and 59–69%

concordance for diagnostic testing plans [27]. Thus, compared with traditional clinic-based dermatologic consultation, store-and-forward consultation provides relatively reliable management recommendations that may vary based on individual treatment preferences.

Additionally, live video telehealth is beneficial for process of skin cancer triage but is not regularly used for this purpose due to its multi-device dependence and fast internet speed reliance. The literature comparing live video conferencing to in-person consultation is also scarce. However, a recent study compared the management agreement (decision to biopsy or not) rates of compressed and uncompressed live video consultations to in-person consultations [28]. Of 214 patients examined, the mean proportion of cases recommended for biopsy was 0.04 for in-person consultation, 0.08 for uncompressed (higher resolution) virtual consultation, and 0.12 for compressed video virtual consultation. The higher propensity to biopsy for compressed (lower resolution) live video consultation suggests biopsy as a measure of management uncertainty and that the decision to biopsy is likely justified as a safeguard. These results highlight the importance of video quality in live video teledermatology and how this factor may influence triage decisions for skin malignancies.

4.2 Diagnosis

Pigmented lesions can be diagnosed as benign, such as seborrheic keratoses, skin tags, and lentigines, or malignant, including basal cell carcinoma, squamous cell carcinoma, and melanoma. Because malignant lesions have the potential to grow and metastasize, prompt diagnosis is essential and can be expedited using teledermatology. Furthermore, unlike dermatologic conditions like psoriasis or atopic dermatitis that bear distinct texture and clinical hallmarks, the diagnosis of cancerous lesions is largely based on visual cues. As illustrated by the ABCDE criteria of melanoma diagnosis [29], current clinical approaches to skin cancer diagnosis predominantly rely on what the lesion looks like, promoting the integration of teledermatology into dermatologic practice and the clinical workup of cutaneous malignancies due its visual nature. Dermoscopic images can also be added to teledermatology consultations to enhance the visualization of subsurface skin structures. In fact, dermoscopic features, such as black dots or hypopigmented areas, have specific histological correlates and render dermoscopy a highly sensitive and precise tool for skin cancer detection [30]. Specifically, teledermoscopy is a form of store and forward technology that transmits dermoscopic images for remote consultation [31] and supplements the telehealth experience with high-quality images [32]. Non-specialist primary care providers with access to a dermatoscope and proper training can also strengthen the reliability of their virtual dermatologic care. A recent publication [11] in conjunction with the American Telemedicine Association (ATA) outlines guidelines for the use of dermatoscopes in telemedicine. These protocols and recommendations will help create a standard of care for medical providers across all disciplines in capturing and archiving dermoscopic images for use in telemedicine and diagnosing lesions.

4.3 Treatment: Surgical Removal

After the diagnosis of cutaneous malignancy has been confirmed, common treatment options include excisional surgery or Mohs micrographic surgery (MMS). Although the actual surgical procedures take place in clinic, teledermatology can be utilized for pre-operative consultation or post-surgical follow-ups.

4.3.1 Teledermatology for Preoperative Consultation

According to a survey from the American College of Mohs Surgery, 67% of Mohs surgeons reported completing preoperative consultation with patients [33]. Consulting prior to surgery establishes an opportunity for the patient and surgeon to discuss the relative risks and benefits of the procedure. This appointment fosters patient comfort as well as acquaintanceship with the surgeon and better understanding of the surgical procedure [34]. Because this consultation is mainly informative, live video teledermatology can be implemented as a convenient and economic alternative. A retrospective analysis of Mohs surgery preoperative appointments within the Veterans Health Administration found that teledermatology consultations saved an average of 162.7 min, 144.5 miles, and $60.00 per person in average travel costs and significantly decreased consent failure rates for the surgery [35]. Teledermatology also decreased the wait time before surgery and increased the proportion of lesions treated within a 60-day period [35]. Telemedicine thus seems to be an effective modality for MMS preoperative consults and may improve the efficiency of subspecialty care.

4.3.2 Teledermatology for Post-surgical Follow Up

After a malignant lesion has been surgically removed, it is the responsibility of the surgeon to ensure that every patient properly heals. Due to the low risk of surgical site infection post Mohs surgery, [36] the primary focus of a postoperative follow-up visit is to assess scar formation, wound healing, patient satisfaction, and answer any patient questions [36]. A randomized controlled trial of 90 patients undergoing Mohs surgery reported that patients preferred to receive wound care instructions via text messages for future visits and 91% of them found the service to be "helpful" or "very helpful." [37] Thus, smartphone applications or postoperative text messaging may be beneficial in avoiding complications after dermatologic surgery and maximizing wound healing [38]. Postprocedural care and positive patient experience in the post-operative period is essential to dermatologic surgery outcomes, and telemedicine shows great potential in the domain of postoperative surveillance for promoting optimal recovery.

5 Important Considerations

Teledermatology has been well-integrated into the dermatologic community for its usefulness in increasing health care access, immediate skin cancer screening benefits, and acceptable reliability compared with face-to-face clinical assessments. Specialists and non-specialist providers alike should be familiar with the fundamental principles and circumstantial aspects of providing high quality care from a distance. The following section discusses some important considerations for providers of remote dermatologic care including accuracy rates for teledermatology diagnosis and management of cutaneous lesions, patient attitudes and potential drawbacks of virtual consultations, and new advances that are being applied to enhance teledermatology.

5.1 Reliability and Accuracy of Teledermatology Diagnosis and Management

Diagnosis and treatment recommendations made through the virtual platform of teledermatology can be rendered and accomplished remotely. The consensus of the current evidence supports and validates its diagnostic, treatment, and management reliability for skin cancers. Although teledermatology cannot fully replace the current gold standard of histopathological analysis, it yields acceptable rates of diagnostic accuracy, which continue to increase with advances in digital and dermoscopic imaging technologies. Most of the studies investigating the effectiveness of teledermatology have reported rates of accuracy to be about 75–80% in comparison with in-person clinical care and 70% in comparison with histopathological reports [39]. According to the latest Cochrane systematic review (2018) about the use of teledermatology for skin cancer, sensitivity was about 95% and specificity was about 84% across studies using photographic images for the accurate diagnosis of lesions as malignant. For individual study estimates on using only dermoscopic images or a combination of dermoscopic and clinical images, reported sensitivities were similarly high but specificities were very variable for any skin cancer [40]. The sensitivities and specificities for the various reported diagnostic thresholds of invasive melanoma or atypical intraepidermal melanocytic variants were also highly variable [40]. Another systematic review published in 2011 concluded that the levels of diagnostic accuracy and concordance of both live video teledermatology and store-and-forward dermatology were acceptable in comparison to in-person care [41].

Regarding comparing the diagnostic and management concordance between mobile dermoscopy and in-person assessment, estimates from the few studies available are generally high and range from 81 to 91% [22], but smartphone applications with algorithm-based software are currently not reliable in their diagnostic capabilities [42]. Overall, the effective use of teledermatology for the diagnosis of malignant skin lesions is multifactorial, depending on many factors such as access to high-quality images, dermoscopic analysis, specific aspects of a patient's clinical history, and the level of expertise of the teledermatologist. Results from various studies investigating the diagnostic accuracy of teledermatology for cutaneous malignancies are included in Table 1.

Although the accuracy of a clinical diagnosis for skin malignancies is important, the appropriateness of clinical management has arguably more impact on patient outcome. The decision whether to biopsy or excise a lesion, for example, may have greater implications for the criteria by which teledermatology should be assessed. Interestingly, malpractice claims for management of skin cancer via telemedicine are virtually nonexistent which could be in part due to high rates of appropriate management [43]. In a study evaluating the diagnostic and management accuracy of pigmented lesions in teledermatology, the rates of correct management plans for teledermatology were greater and/or equivalent to those of in-person dermatology for all lesions including benign lesions [44]. However, for a subgroup of malignant lesions, appropriate management via teledermatology was significantly inferior to in-person dermatology such that up to one fifth of melanomas would have been improperly managed with teledermatology [44]. Therefore, clinicians and teledermatologists should be aware of this potentially consequential limitation of teledermatology.

Acknowledging that remote dermatological care is also routinely provided by primary care providers, it is important to investigate methods to enhance diagnostic accuracy and management and reduce unnecessary referrals to the dermatology clinic. One Mayo Clinic study assessed the influence of standardized templates on the referral patterns and dermatologic knowledge of family medicine providers. Utilizing the standardized templates increased the diagnostic and management concordance by 26.2% and 33.3%, respectively [6]. This pilot study showed that improvements in primary-care based virtual dermatological care can be achieved through educational interventions. Thus, providing providers a more comprehensive protocol for teledermatology workflow is beneficial and can be further enhanced with the implementation of dermoscopy practice guidelines [11].

5.2 *Patient Satisfaction and Barriers*

In addition to its many benefits including the ability to reach geographically isolated patients and reducing unnecessary referrals from primary care providers, teledermatology is popular among patients for many reasons. For many patients who cannot drive or easily get to the dermatology clinic, teledermatology offers a relatively simple way to get access to the care they need from the comfort of their home or

Table 1 Diagnostic accuracy using teledermatology for skin malignancies

Teledermatology skin cancer diagnostic accuracy according to the literature			
Source	Population	Design	Outcome
Warshaw et al. (2015)	2152 patients: 2082 male, 70 female (mean age: 68 y)	Teledermatologist diagnosis using camera or dermoscopy taken images compared to in-person FTF dermatologist diagnosis	Primary diagnosis agreement between TD and FTF diagnosis: 45.7–75.7%
Borve et al. (2015)	772 patients: 474 female, 298 male (mean age: 54 y)	Diagnosis as malignant or benign by 3 teledermatologists using dermoscopy images and clinical information on iDoc24 app compared with histopathological diagnosis	TD benign diagnosis agreed with Histopathology benign diagnosis: 99.1% TD malignant diagnosis agreed with Histopathology malignant diagnosis: 74%
Congalton et al. (2015)	310 patients: 168 female, 142 male (mean age: 58 y)	Melanoma or non-melanoma diagnosis using MoleMapDiagnose software compared with histological diagnosis	PPV of teledermatoscopic diagnosis of melanoma and positive histology was 63%
Massone et al. (2014)	690 patients: 48 female, 642 male (mean age: 47 y)	Benign or malignant diagnosis of dermoscopic images transmitted via store-and-forward compared with histopathology diagnosis	Diagnostic agreement (as benign or malignant) between TD and histopathology: 94%
Sonet et al. (2014)	119 patients: 51 female, 68 male (mean age: 63 y)	Teledermatology diagnosis using clinical and teledermoscopy images compared with histopathologic diagnosis	TD diagnosis accuracy with clinical images: 68% (teledermatologist 1), 76% (teledermatologist 2) TD diagnosis accuracy with teledermoscopy images: 87% (teledermatologist 1), 92% (teledermatologist 2)
Van Der Heijden et al. (2013)	105 patients: 59 female, 46 male (mean age: 47 y)	Diagnosis (by 4 dermatologists) from images taken by primary care providers compared with FTF diagnosis	TD diagnostic agreement with FTF diagnosis: kappa value = 0.55–0.73 (scale 0–1: 0–0.2 slight agreement, 0.21–0.40 fair, 0.41–0.5 moderate, 0.61–0.8 substantial, 0.81–1.0 perfect agreement)

(continued)

Table 1 (continued)

Teledermatology skin cancer diagnostic accuracy according to the literature			
Source	Population	Design	Outcome
Borve et al. (2013)	62 patients: 24 female, 38 male (mean age: 64 y)	Interobserver concordance between 2 teledermoscopists and a dermatologist using dermoscopy images and clinical information on iDoc24 smartphone app and FTF diagnosis compared with histopathological diagnosis	Teledermoscopic diagnostic accuracy was 50.7% (teledermatologist 1) and 60.9% (teledermatologist 2) as compared with histopathological diagnosis FTF diagnostic accuracy was 66.7% as compared with histopathological diagnosis
Lamel et al. (2012)	86 patients: 50 female, 38 male (mean age: 45.25 y)	Diagnosis by dermatologist using pictures taken on a mobile phone compared with FTF diagnosis	Diagnostic agreement between TD and FTF diagnosis: 62%
Borve et al. (2012)	40 patients: 23 female, 17 male (mean age: 49 y)	Diagnosis by dermatologists using images taken by GP from a mobile phone camera compared with FTF diagnosis by the same dermatologists	TD diagnosis agreed with FTF diagnosis: 31/40 patients; 78%
Kroemer et al. (2011)	88 patients: 47 female, 41 male (mean age: 69 y)	Clinical image and dermoscopic image tele-evaluation by dermatologists compared with histological diagnosis	TD diagnosis of clinical images: 85% agreed with histopathology (88/104 lesions) TD diagnosis of dermoscopic images: 79% agreed with histopathology (82/104 lesions)
Boyce et al. (2011)	55 patients: 22 female, 33 male (mean age: 26 y)	Dermatologist remote diagnosis using patient-generated images taken by mobile phones compared with traditional FTF diagnosis	Exact diagnostic agreement in 116/167 analyzed lesions (69%) between remote diagnosis of patient-generated clinical images and FTF diagnosis
Warshaw et al. (2009)	542 patients: 23 female, 519 male (mean age: 66 y)	Store-and-forward teledermatology diagnosis and FTF dermatologist diagnosis compared with histopathology diagnosis	TD diagnostic agreement with histopathology diagnosis: 67% FTF diagnostic agreement with histopathology diagnosis: 81%

Published literature values reporting comparison of diagnostic accuracy or diagnostic agreement between teledermatology skin cancer diagnosis and either in-person clinical diagnosis or gold-standard histopathologic diagnosis
GP general practitioner, *FTF* face to face, *TD* teledermatology, *PPV* positive predictive value

setting of choice. Notably, Whited et al. discovered that most patients were confident in dermatologists using pictures during telemedicine visits to reach a diagnosis and viewed teledermatology consultations as more convenient than going to see a dermatologist in person [45]. In 2 studies in which patients submitted their own pictures either with or without dermoscopy, they noted being satisfied with the practicality and convenience [46] and reported willingness to pay out-of-pocket amounts for teledermatology services [47]. Additional benefits of telemedicine and teledermoscopy valued by patients include more regular skin monitoring, faster waiting times, and enhanced privacy and comfort [5].

Besides acknowledging the various advantages that teledermatology offers, it is necessary to discuss potential barriers to its use and implementation in dermatology practices. According to a database study by Fogel et al., there were no reported cases with final findings of medical malpractice resulting from inappropriate management or negligence associated with teledermatology [43]. However, there may be possible non-reported malpractice cases, such as claims that are still being processed or were settled preceding a court decision, in addition to claims that have not yet arisen due to the common legal delay after a finding of malpractice has been established [43]. Dermatologists should be mindful of the potential malpractice risk that comes with the use of telemedicine and may want to limit the scope of their virtual visits to less concerning dermatologic conditions or expedite in-person visits for patients with atypical lesions [43]. Moreover, there is always a chance of obtaining low quality clinical, dermoscopic, or patient self-captured images that can make diagnosing via teledermatology unfeasible, as well as patients skipping over concerning lesions during skin self-examination [43]. The adoption of telemedicine in Mohs Surgery can also be difficult and poses its own limitations. Incorporating telemedicine into preoperative and postoperative surgical workflow could restrict schedule flexibility for both the surgeon and the patient [48]. Another concern is the physical exam limitations of teledermatology such that certain lesion characteristics like invasion depth may be difficult to assess accurately [48]. Patient training and reception of working with new technology may also be suboptimal given the initial learning curve and that most skin cancer patients are elderly [48]. Certainly, the benefits of implementing telemedicine into the dermatologic practice workflow must be weighed against the associated challenges and should be evaluated with the unique framework of each practice in mind.

5.3 Future Directions

As the use and popularity of teledermatology continues to expand, many technologies are being applied to enhance its experience. Reflectance confocal microscopy (RCM), for example, is a noninvasive examination technique that allows for high-resolution in vivo evaluation of skin lesions and shows promise for telemedicine settings [4]. Use of RCM in research and clinical settings has been shown to render high reliability and sensitivity in diagnosing both nonpigmented and pigmented lesions, but specificity greater depends on training and skill level of the dermatologist [49]. Although there has been some integration of RCM into clinical practice, educational programs for this technique are still being developed to avoid misdiagnosis of malignant lesions in both clinical and virtual settings. The application of RCM to telemedicine learning platforms may assist in increasing the knowledge base of clinical experts as well as help to remotely connect patients to trained physicians [49].

Another technology that is being progressively used in teledermatology and has much potential in improving practice efficiency is artificial intelligence (AI). According to a meta-analysis of 70 studies, the accuracy of computer-aided diagnosis of melanoma was discovered to be comparable to that of clinical experts [50]. The reliability of AI may thus make it a complementary service in telemedicine consults by tracking lesions over time and expanding the differential diagnosis [51]. Moreover, utilizing AI as a telemedicine triage tool for patients with potentially malignant skin lesions is a convenient option to prioritize those who need expedited care [52]. In a study evaluating the application of AI in telemedicine triage and diagnosis of cutaneous lesions, Majidian et al. found no significant difference in diagnostic accuracy between a group of three dermatologists and AI using the software's first three differential diagnoses [52]. Given these findings, AI can serve as a beneficial tool in identifying lesions that require further workup and possible biopsy, especially for primary care providers or less experienced specialist providers [52]. Although AI is useful in triaging disease into broader categories, the expertise and contextual knowledge of dermatologists will always be required for meticulous diagnosis, management recommendations, and uncommon cases. Considering the rapid progression of technological developments, familiarization with the basic operations of AI along with its potential applications will be vital for practicing dermatologists and the future of the specialty.

Key Points

- Store-and-forward teledermatology and teledermoscopy facilitate the capture and electronic transmission of high-quality images, yielding diagnostic reliability of pigmented lesions as benign or malignant.
- Teledermatology expedites the dermatologic triage process for skin cancer care and significantly reduces the wait time to see a specialist.
- Most patients are satisfied with the practicality and convenience of virtual dermatologic care provided via telehealth platforms in addition to having confidence in the diagnoses given by teledermatologists.
- Technological advances in artificial intelligence and reflectance confocal microscopy are increasing telemedicine triage capacity and the potential for improved diagnostic sensitivity of both pigmented and nonpigmented lesions, respectively.

6 Conclusion

Telemedicine is emerging as a vital branch of dermatology that offers increased access to specialty providers and cost effectiveness without diminishing the quality of patient care. With the addition of equipment like mobile or digital dermoscopy, teledermatology can provide excellent skin cancer detection with fewer biopsy and nonessential dermatology clinic referrals and decreased wait times. Teledermatology can improve patient access to essential care through different telemedicine formats including store-and-forward teledermatology, live video conferencing, and the combination of both types, called a hybrid consultation. With proper dermoscopy technique training and education, primary care providers can also enhance the quality of their remote-based dermatologic care. By strategically implementing telemedicine in the triage, diagnostic workup, and management of cutaneous malignancies, screening and treatment of these lesions may be expedited through refinement of clinical workflow. Moreover, teledermatology shows great promise for boosting positive patient outcomes in the realm of preoperative and postprocedural care in Mohs micrographic surgery. Future directions of teledermatology focus on improving diagnostic accuracy through technological advances in artificial intelligence and reflectance confocal microscopy. Overall, the many advantages of teledermatology including cost efficiency, reduction of travel burden, and acceptable accuracy rates with face-to-face clinical examination in diagnosing skin cancer make it a highly utilized clinical tool within the field of dermatology.

References

1. Siegel R, Ward E, Brawley O, Jemal A. Cancer statistics, 2011: the impact of eliminating socioeconomic and racial disparities on premature cancer deaths. CA Cancer J Clin. 2011;61(4):212–36. https://doi.org/10.3322/caac.20121.
2. Federman DG, Kirsner RS, Viola KV. Skin cancer screening and primary prevention: facts and controversies. Clin Dermatol. 2013;31(6):666–70. https://doi.org/10.1016/j.clindermatol.2013.05.002.
3. Balch CM, Soong SJ, Gershenwald JE, et al. Prognostic factors analysis of 17,600 melanoma patients: validation of the American joint committee on cancer melanoma staging system. J Clin Oncol. 2001;19(16):3622–34. https://doi.org/10.1200/jco.2001.19.16.3622.
4. Walocko FM, Tejasvi T. Teledermatology applications in skin cancer diagnosis. Dermatol Clin. 2017;35(4):559–63. https://doi.org/10.1016/j.det.2017.06.002.
5. Finnane A, Dallest K, Janda M, Soyer HP. Teledermatology for the diagnosis and management of skin cancer: a systematic review. JAMA Dermatol. 2017;153(3):319–27. https://doi.org/10.1001/jamadermatol.2016.4361.
6. Cumsky HJL, Maly CJ, Costello CM, et al. Impact of standardized templates and skin cancer learning modules for teledermatology consultations. Int J Dermatol. 2019;58(12):1423–9. https://doi.org/10.1111/ijd.14437.
7. Stern RS. Dermatologists and office-based care of dermatologic disease in the 21st century. J Investig Dermatol Symp Proc. 2004;9(2):126–30. https://doi.org/10.1046/j.1087-0024.2003.09108.x.

8. Moreno-Ramirez D, Ferrandiz L, Nieto-Garcia A, et al. Store-and-forward teledermatology in skin cancer triage: experience and evaluation of 2009 teleconsultations. Arch Dermatol. 2007;143(4):479–84. https://doi.org/10.1001/archderm.143.4.479.
9. Chen TS, Goldyne ME, Mathes EFD, Frieden IJ, Gilliam AE. Pediatric teledermatology: observations based on 429 consults. J Am Acad Dermatol. 2010;62(1):61–6. https://doi.org/10.1016/j.jaad.2009.05.039.
10. Kanthraj GR. Teledermatology: its role in dermatosurgery. J Cutan Aesthet Surg. 2008;1(2):68–74. https://doi.org/10.4103/0974-2077.44162.
11. Deda LC, Goldberg RH, Jamerson TA, Lee I, Tejasvi T. Dermoscopy practice guidelines for use in telemedicine. NPJ Digit Med. 2022;5(1):55. https://doi.org/10.1038/s41746-022-00587-9.
12. Piccolo D, Ferrari A, Peris K, Diadone R, Ruggeri B, Chimenti S. Dermoscopic diagnosis by a trained clinician vs. a clinician with minimal dermoscopy training vs. computer-aided diagnosis of 341 pigmented skin lesions: a comparative study. Br J Dermatol. 2002;147(3):481–6. https://doi.org/10.1046/j.1365-2133.2002.04978.x.
13. Edison KE, Fleming DA, Nieman EL, Stine K, Chance L, Demiris G. Content and style comparison of physician communication in teledermatology and in-person visits. Telemed J e-Health. 2013;19(7):509–14. https://doi.org/10.1089/tmj.2012.0227.
14. Edison KE, Dyer JA. Teledermatology in Missouri and beyond. Mo Med. 2007;104(2):139–43.
15. Miller J, Jones E. Shaping the future of teledermatology: a literature review of patient and provider satisfaction with synchronous teledermatology during the COVID-19 pandemic. Clin Exp Dermatol. 2022. https://doi.org/10.1111/ced.15320.
16. Uppal SK, Beer J, Hadeler E, Gitlow H, Nouri K. The clinical utility of teledermoscopy in the era of telemedicine. Dermatol Ther. 2021;34(2):e14766. https://doi.org/10.1111/dth.14766.
17. Marwaha SS, Fevrier H, Alexeeff S, et al. Comparative effectiveness study of face-to-face and teledermatology workflows for diagnosing skin cancer. J Am Acad Dermatol. 2019;81(5):1099–106. https://doi.org/10.1016/j.jaad.2019.01.067.
18. Janda M, Horsham C, Vagenas D, et al. Accuracy of mobile digital teledermoscopy for skin self-examinations in adults at high risk of skin cancer: an open-label, randomised controlled trial. Lancet Digit Health. 2020;2(3):e129–37. https://doi.org/10.1016/s2589-7500(20)30001-7.
19. Wolf JA, Moreau JF, Akilov O, et al. Diagnostic inaccuracy of smartphone applications for melanoma detection. JAMA Dermatol. 2013;149(4):422–6. https://doi.org/10.1001/jamadermatol.2013.2382.
20. March J, Hand M, Grossman D. Practical application of new technologies for melanoma diagnosis: part I. Noninvasive approaches. J Am Acad Dermatol. 2015;72(6):929–41; quiz 941–2. https://doi.org/10.1016/j.jaad.2015.02.1138.
21. Bleicher B, Levine A, Markowitz O. Going digital with dermoscopy. Cutis. 2018;102(2):102–5.
22. Lee KJ, Finnane A, Soyer HP. Recent trends in teledermatology and teledermoscopy. Dermatol Pract Concept. 2018;8(3):214–23. https://doi.org/10.5826/dpc.0803a13.
23. Lee JJ, English JC 3rd. Teledermatology: a review and update. Am J Clin Dermatol. 2018;19(2):253–60. https://doi.org/10.1007/s40257-017-0317-6.
24. Jaimes N, Marghoob AA. Triage amalgamated dermoscopic algorithm. J Am Acad Dermatol. 2020;82(6):1551–2. https://doi.org/10.1016/j.jaad.2020.01.079.
25. Shapiro M, James WD, Kessler R, et al. Comparison of skin biopsy triage decisions in 49 patients with pigmented lesions and skin neoplasms: store-and-forward teledermatology vs face-to-face dermatology. Arch Dermatol. 2004;140(5):525–8. https://doi.org/10.1001/archderm.140.5.525.
26. Zelickson BD, Homan L. Teledermatology in the nursing home. Arch Dermatol. 1997;133(2):171–4.
27. Whited JD, Hall RP, Simel DL, et al. Reliability and accuracy of dermatologists' clinic-based and digital image consultations. J Am Acad Dermatol. 1999;41(5 Pt 1):693–702. https://doi.org/10.1016/s0190-9622(99)70003-4.
28. Marchell R, Locatis C, Burges G, Maisiak R, Liu WL, Ackerman M. Comparing high definition live interactive and store-and-forward consultations to in-person examinations. Telemed J e-Health. 2017;23(3):213–8. https://doi.org/10.1089/tmj.2016.0093.

29. Goldsmith SM. A unifying approach to the clinical diagnosis of melanoma including “D” for “Dark” in the ABCDE criteria. Dermatol Pract Concept. 2014;4(4):75–8. https://doi.org/10.5826/dpc.0404a16.
30. Yadav S, Vossaert KA, Kopf AW, Silverman M, Grin-Jorgensen C. Histopathologic correlates of structures seen on dermoscopy (epiluminescence microscopy). Am J Dermatopathol. 1993;15(4):297–305. https://doi.org/10.1097/00000372-199308000-00001.
31. Koelink CJ, Jonkman MF, Van Der Meer K, Van Der Heide WK. Examination of skin lesions for cancer: which clinical decision aids and tools are available in general practice? Eur J Dermatol. 2014;24(3):297–304. https://doi.org/10.1684/ejd.2014.2275.
32. Finnane A, Curiel-Lewandrowski C, Wimberley G, et al. Proposed technical guidelines for the acquisition of clinical images of skin-related conditions. JAMA Dermatol. 2017;153(5):453–7. https://doi.org/10.1001/jamadermatol.2016.6214.
33. Knackstedt TJ, Samie FH. Shared medical appointments for the preoperative consultation visit of Mohs micrographic surgery. J Am Acad Dermatol. 2015;72(2):340–4. https://doi.org/10.1016/j.jaad.2014.10.022.
34. Sharon VR, Armstrong AW, Jim On SC, Ibrahimi OA, Eisen DB. Separate-versus same-day preoperative consultation in dermatologic surgery: a patient-centered investigation in an academic practice. Dermatol Surg. 2013;39(2):240–7. https://doi.org/10.1111/dsu.12083.
35. Lee S, Dana A, Newman J. Teledermatology as a tool for preoperative consultation before Mohs micrographic surgery within the veterans health administration. Dermatol Surg. 2020;46(4):508–13. https://doi.org/10.1097/dss.0000000000002073.
36. Maragh SL, Brown MD. Prospective evaluation of surgical site infection rate among patients with Mohs micrographic surgery without the use of prophylactic antibiotics. J Am Acad Dermatol. 2008;59(2):275–8. https://doi.org/10.1016/j.jaad.2008.03.042.
37. Hawkins SD, Koch SB, Williford PM, Feldman SR, Pearce DJ. Web app- and text message-based patient education in Mohs micrographic surgery—a randomized controlled trial. Dermatol Surg. 2018;44(7):924–32. https://doi.org/10.1097/dss.0000000000001489.
38. Sohn GK, Wong DJ, Yu SS. A review of the use of telemedicine in dermatologic surgery. Dermatol Surg. 2020;46(4):501–7. https://doi.org/10.1097/dss.0000000000002230.
39. Nowell WR. Vector introduction and malaria infection on Guam. J Am Mosq Control Assoc. 1987;3(2):259–65.
40. Chuchu N, Dinnes J, Takwoingi Y, et al. Teledermatology for diagnosing skin cancer in adults. Cochrane Database Syst Rev. 2018;12(12):Cd013193. https://doi.org/10.1002/14651858.Cd013193.
41. Warshaw EM, Hillman YJ, Greer NL, et al. Teledermatology for diagnosis and management of skin conditions: a systematic review. J Am Acad Dermatol. 2011;64(4):759–72. https://doi.org/10.1016/j.jaad.2010.08.026.
42. Dascalu A, Walker BN, Oron Y, David EO. Non-melanoma skin cancer diagnosis: a comparison between dermoscopic and smartphone images by unified visual and sonification deep learning algorithms. J Cancer Res Clin Oncol. 2022;148(9):2497–505. https://doi.org/10.1007/s00432-021-03809-x.
43. Fogel AL, Lacktman NM, Kvedar JC. Skin cancer telemedicine medical malpractice risk. JAMA Dermatol. 2021;157(7):870–1. https://doi.org/10.1001/jamadermatol.2021.1475.
44. Warshaw EM, Lederle FA, Grill JP, et al. Accuracy of teledermatology for pigmented neoplasms. J Am Acad Dermatol. 2009;61(5):753–65. https://doi.org/10.1016/j.jaad.2009.04.032.
45. Whited JD, Hall RP, Foy ME, et al. Patient and clinician satisfaction with a store-and-forward teledermatology consult system. Telemed J e-Health Winter. 2004;10(4):422–31. https://doi.org/10.1089/tmj.2004.10.422.
46. Boyce Z, Gilmore S, Xu C, Soyer HP. The remote assessment of melanocytic skin lesions: a viable alternative to face-to-face consultation. Dermatology. 2011;223(3):244–50. https://doi.org/10.1159/000333363.
47. Spinks J, Janda M, Soyer HP, Whitty JA. Consumer preferences for teledermoscopy screening to detect melanoma early. J Telemed Telecare. 2016;22(1):39–46. https://doi.org/10.1177/1357633x15586701.

48. Maruthur M, Lee E, Dusza S, Nehal K, Rossi A. Pilot survey of adoption of telemedicine in mohs surgery during the COVID-19 pandemic. Dermatol Surg. 2022;48(2):187–90. https://doi.org/10.1097/dss.0000000000003352.
49. Witkowski A, Łudzik J, Soyer HP. Telediagnosis with confocal microscopy: a reality or a dream? Dermatol Clin. 2016;34(4):505–12. https://doi.org/10.1016/j.det.2016.05.013.
50. Dick V, Sinz C, Mittlböck M, Kittler H, Tschandl P. Accuracy of computer-aided diagnosis of melanoma: a meta-analysis. JAMA Dermatol. 2019;155(11):1291–9. https://doi.org/10.1001/jamadermatol.2019.1375.
51. Young AT, Xiong M, Pfau J, Keiser MJ, Wei ML. Artificial intelligence in dermatology: a primer. J Invest Dermatol. 2020;140(8):1504–12. https://doi.org/10.1016/j.jid.2020.02.026.
52. Majidian M, Tejani I, Jarmain T, Kellett L, Moy R. Artificial intelligence in the evaluation of telemedicine dermatology patients. J Drugs Dermatol. 2022;21(2):191–194. https://doi.org/10.36849/jdd.6277.

Telewound Care

Divya Chopra, Neil Seth, Noreen Mohsin, and Hadar Lev-Tov

Abstract Treatment and management of chronic wounds has a significant economic impact on healthcare and patient quality of life. As a result of the COVID-19 pandemic, an increasing amount of telehealth options are becoming available to patients. Specifically, wound care within the field of teledermatology (telewound care) is an emerging field that shows promise for improving patient health outcomes and lowering the cost of care. Patients are currently able to reach providers virtually through real-time conferencing platforms and share images and data through smart-phone applications. Imaging technologies paired with artificial intelligence and further innovations are currently in development. Despite the benefits of this technology and rapid growth of telemedicine, the implementation of telewound practices has had varied success internationally and presents its own unique set of challenges. Thus, this chapter aims to provide an overview of telewound care and to serve as a starting point for further exploration into this emerging practice. After providing a brief overview of wound care, we discuss telewound care specifically and review current available telewound options and practice. We also discuss upcoming innovations and describe the practice from a global perspective. Lastly, we highlight the benefits and discuss the challenges faced by patients, providers, and innovators involved in telewound care.

Keywords Telemedicine · Teledermatology · Telewound · Wound care · Telehealth

1 Introduction to Wound Care

Chronic wounds are defined as wounds that fail to progress through the normal healing process and heal within the expected time. The prevalence of chronic wounds is 2.21 per 1000 people with and most of the people affected are the elderly population

D. Chopra · N. Seth · N. Mohsin · H. Lev-Tov (✉)
Dr. Phillip Frost Department of Dermatology and Cutaneous Surgery, Miller School of Medicine, University of Miami, Miami, USA
e-mail: hlevtov@med.miami.edu

K. Nouri (ed.), *Telemedicine and Technological Advances in Dermatology*,
https://doi.org/10.1007/978-3-031-69091-4_6

[1, 2]. Chronic wounds are a significant economic and humanistic burden for both patients and society. Treating chronic wounds is predicted to account for 2–3% of healthcare costs in developed countries [3]. Additionally, the quality of life of people with chronic wounds is diminished to the same level as patients with chronic conditions such as cardiovascular disease and chronic obstructive pulmonary disease [4].

The most common etiologies for nonhealing wounds are pressure-induced injuries, diabetic foot ulcers, and venous leg ulcers [5]. The basic tenets of wound care aim to address the primary etiology of the wound as well as any systemic and metabolic comorbidities that would impair wound healing all combined with optimal wound care [3]. Chronic wounds require regular outpatient follow up for assessment and treatment. Standard of care varies by wound type to address the underlying pathology but often includes dressing changes tailored to each specific wound, optimization of the wound bed to avoid infection and maintenance of a healing wound bed and wound edge environment all coupled with extensive patient education. The field of wound care has made several recent developments in advanced therapies, such as advanced dressings, acellular and cellular skin substitutes, negative pressure wound therapy, platelet-rich plasma, and growth factors. Failure to implement effective wound therapeutic regimens can occur on the part of patient, the healthcare provider or the healthcare system and may have severe consequences. Without regular follow-up and proper wound care, patients are at risk for more frequent hospitalizations, wound infection, sepsis, amputation, and even death [1]. Therefore, there is a critical need to establish an effective therapeutic regimen for wound care. This can be challenged at times by various barriers such as lack of resources, lack of local experts, transportation, and other elements of healthcare delivery. Telemedicine can be used to solve some, but not all, of these barriers to wound care. Given the inherent complexity of managing chronic wounds, the added dimension of telehealth for wounds expands the access to good wound care on one hand but requires specific consideration for diagnosis and treatment which are the focus of this chapter.

2 Common Types of Chronic Wounds

2.1 Venous Leg Ulcer

Venous leg ulcers (VLUs) are the most common lower extremity ulcers. Chronic venous insufficiency (CVI) is a result of downstream blockade and/or valvular failure which can result in retrograde flow in the venous system and subsequent venous hypertension. Other causes include decreased range of motion or muscular dysfunction in the lower extremity. Clinical signs of CVI include varicose veins, edema, atrophie blanche, dyspigmentation, dermatitis and lipodermatosclerosis. Ulceration is the final stage of CVI. VLUs present as shallow ulcers with irregular borders and a granulating or fibrinous wound bed. They are commonly painful, exudative, and located on the medial aspect of the lower leg. At the core of standard care for VLU is reduction of venous hypertension via compression therapy (35–40 mm Hg), and leg elevation. Medical therapy may include the use of aspirin, pentoxifylline and horse chestnut seed extract. Various levels of evidence exist to support the use of hyperbaric oxygen therapy and tissue-based products. Surgical debridement is common practice to maintain the wound bed. Evidence also exists for the use of endovenous ablation of the great saphenous vein to improve healing time [6].

2.2 *Arterial Ulcer*

Arterial ulceration is caused by impaired perfusion of the lower limb causing ischemia and necrosis. The most common cause is progressive atherosclerosis causing large vessel disease. Other causes include vasculitis, microthrombotic disease, cryoglobulinemia and cryofibrogenemia, Raynaud's phenomenon, arteriovenous malformation, and sickle cell disease. Arterial ulcers are characterized by a "punched-out" appearance, sharply demarcated borders, and necrotic wound base. These ulcers are located on the distal portion of the lower extremity over bony prominences. Improving arterial blood flow through medical and/or surgical intervention and pain management are key to treating arterial ulcerations.

2.3 *Diabetic Foot Ulcer*

Diabetic foot ulcers (DFUs) result from peripheral neuropathy commonly with underlying arterial insufficiency. Loss of protective sensation from sensory neuropathy reduces patient's awareness of heat, excessive pressure, and physical trauma. Motor and autonomic neuropathy can lead to muscular and bony abnormalities such as Charcot's foot that create pressure points at higher risk for ulceration. Patients with diabetes should undergo frequent examination of the foot to monitor for development of DFUs. DFUs present as insensate ulcerations on pressure points that are surrounded by callus. They are often deep and should be probed with a blunt instrument to identify exposed tendon or bone which may imply the presence of osteomyelitis. Management centers around mechanical offloading with devices such as total contact cast or a removable boot. Monitoring for infection is key and exclusion of arterial disease, frequent debridement and appropriate dressing selection are common practice. Adjuvant therapies such as negative pressure wound therapy, topical growth factors, and tissue-based substitutes can be used to accelerate healing.

2.4 *Pressure Injury*

Prolonged pressure over bony prominences can cause ischemia and soft tissue necrosis due to capillary occlusion. Pressure-induced injury commonly presents in patients with reduced mobility, malnutrition and impaired sensation. Typical locations include the sacrum, ischium, and heel. Redistributing pressure through offloading techniques is key to treating active ulcerations and preventing future injury. Use of pressure redistribution devices such as specialized mattresses and cushions can be used to minimize prolonged focal compression. Nutritional support should be implemented to prevent excessive weight loss and maximize wound healing. In advanced cases, hyperbaric oxygen therapy or surgical management can be considered all combined with meticulous wound care.

2.5 *Atypical Wounds*

Atypical wounds can be loosely defined as chronic wounds with uncommon etiologies such as trauma, post-surgical wounds, DFU, VLU, arterial ulcer, or pressure ulcer. Atypical etiology should be considered in wounds that have unusual presentation or location and do not respond appropriately to standard therapies. Possible etiologies can include inflammatory processes (pyoderma gangrenosum, connective-tissue ulcers, vasculitis), infection, malignancy, and others. Management begins with thorough evaluation of risk factors (e.g. past medical history of chronic inflammatory diseases such as inflammatory bowel disease or rheumatoid arthritis), laboratory examinations including serum markers, microbiology, imaging and histopathology. Once a diagnosis is established appropriate management often leads to resolution (Table 1).

3 Teledermatology and Wound Care

Telemedicine is defined by the World Health organization as integrating modern information and communication technology to deliver health care services in conditions where distance is a critical factor [7]. This definition can probably be expanded to include other scenarios in which an in-person evaluation is less favorable such as impaired mobility or risk of infectious disease. Telemedicine was first reported to be used in dermatology in 1995 [8]. Dermatology is a largely visual field and is well suited for telemedicine. It has proven to be a reliable tool that does not sacrifice accuracy in diagnosis or treatment [9].

The COVID-19 pandemic has led to a recent boom in the field of teledermatology. Wound care, as a service that requires frequent monitoring, benefits greatly from these services. There is considerable overlap between comorbidities that would

Table 1 Diagnosis and management of most common chronic wounds

Type of wound	VLU	Arterial	DFU	Pressure injury
Risk factors	Obesity, white race, female sex, multiparity, history of DVTs	Cardiovascular disease, diabetes mellitus, male sex, smoking	Male sex, musculoskeletal deformities, peripheral vascular disease	Immobility, incontinence, poor nutrition
Clinical signs and symptoms	Pain relieved by leg elevation, edema, lipodermatosclerosis, atrophie blanche, venous dermatitis	Claudication, rest pain or pain exacerbated by leg elevation, abnormal pedal pulses, skin pallor or coolness	Neuropathy or insensate feet, xerosis or cracked skin, callus, abnormal gait	Neuropathy, skin atrophy, loss of muscle mass
Location	"Gaiter area"—medial and surface of the lower leg between the medial malleolus and lower calf	Bony prominences, distal fingertips or toes, lateral malleolus and tibial area	Foot below the ankle, usually on the plantar surface	Over bony prominences
Ulcer characteristic	Shallow, irregular borders, granulating or fibrinous base, exudative	"Punched out", deep, sharply demarcated borders, necrotic base	Deep, surrounded by callus, circular, painless or insensate	Deep, undermining borders or tunneling, macerated borders
Treatment	Compression, leg elevation, surgical management	Revascularization, pain management	Offloading of pressure by mechanical methods or surgery	Offloading of pressure, frequent repositioning, nutritional support

put patients at risk for having poor outcomes from a COVID-19 infection and for developing chronic wounds [10–12]. Additionally, patients with a greater number of these comorbidities typically have worse prognosis in each condition [13]. Additionally, people with chronic wounds are often difficult to mobilize making telemedicine a reasonable solution to maintain quality of care without compromising the patient's health. As such, this at-risk population needs to have several protective measures in place when considering their healthcare. Telemedicine has become a useful method to provide wound care and can be combined with at home nursing services for optimal care. Through the use of telemedicine for wound care (telewound hereafter), clinicians can make a diagnosis, recommend a treatment regimen, and provide assistance to home care nurses in treatment strategies [14].

4 Epidemiological Overview of Telewound Care

Globally, there is a great need for advanced treatment options and strategies for the treatment of chronic wounds. In Europe, approximately 2 million people have chronic wounds and in the United States, chronic non-healing wounds have been estimated to affect over 8 million people [15, 16]. Telewound care services serve as an additional option to standard therapies that can help alleviate this burden of disease.

The use of telewound care services has increased not only in the United States, but in other countries including Germany, France, Canada, and others [17–20]. Notably, telewound care has been adopted in France with great success demonstrating a significant reduction in the number of hospitalizations and ambulance transfers to wound healing centers [19]. However, this success has not be replicated in the United States and has been thought to be a result of increased constraints on patients and decreased access to expeditious care [20]. From a global perspective, the use of teleconsultation services has been valued highly by participants in trials involving patients healing from wounds. Furthermore, the implementation of telewound care options in developing countries located in Africa, Asia, and South America can potentially provide patients access to care that would not have had been otherwise available due to limited resources and difficulty to the proper completion of in-person visits [21].

5 Current Telewound Options and Practice

Telehealth options for wound care patients have been available since the early 2000s and resources have increased in number due to the COVID-19 pandemic. Initially, web-based communications became available for patients to share images with their providers before in-person visits and to view protocols relevant to their wounds [22]. Soon after, real-time conferencing options became available as well and hybrids merging the two mediums [23, 24]. A well-studied example of a telewound service used currently that incorporates both real-time, synchronous video conferencing and information sharing avenues is the TeleWound Practice program used by the Veteran Affairs healthcare system; recent analysis assessing the outcomes of this program highlight the importance of clear communications between team members and demonstrate a notable reduction in cost to patients [25].

Smart phone applications focused on telewound care are another option available to patients and have been increasing in popularity [26]. Smart phone applications used to measure wound size and progress became increasingly available over a decade ago and often include camera adapters that are attached externally to the smart phone [27]. However, most smart phone applications used in the field of telewound care can be accessed directly through the device. For instance, the Swift Mobile App is a mobile application currently available use with various smart phones that uses image measurement software to track the progression of wounds over time; this technology is currently used by wound centers across the globe and has been shown to reliably measure and track the progression wound healing [28]. Over time and with the influence of the pandemic, smart phone application options become increasingly available and are used more often by patients and providers [29].

6 Typical Telewound Visit

Patients completing their visits online avoid unnecessary and potentially harmful exposure to pathogens and decrease time spent commuting. The vast majority of telewound visits follow a similar structure despite variation in style and technological platforms. Prior to the first visit, patients will usually provide pertinent demographic and medical information on the phone and complete the necessary onboarding documentation through privacy protected email communications. A link to the telewound visit and pre-visit instructions will then be sent to the patient via email or SMS messaging and many clinics will call patients a day or two beforehand to confirm the appointment time and patient's availability and offer basic troubleshooting for first time users of the technology.

Before seeing the clinician via teleconferencing, patients will be expected to upload digital photos of their wound(s) to the telehealth system. Quality lighting and clear photo definition are important for the provider to properly assess the state of the wounds. Furthermore, patients can provide measurements of their wound and other information such as type of dressings used, frequency of dressing changes, wound status, etc. Many times, questions and concerns can be uploaded before seeing the clinician on the video conferencing platform.

During a typical visit, patients will first log onto a third-party telehealth web portal partnering with the wound clinic. The telehealth web portal will produce prompts notifying patients if they need to adjust their audio and video settings. It is recommended to carry out the visit in a private setting with good lighting and satisfactory internet connection. Once the teleconferencing session starts, the provider will begin the visit. Despite limited physical exam options, the clinician may ask the patient to place their wound closer to the camera or add a light source to better see the wound. However, they usually will be able to access previously uploaded photos and other media to aid in developing a management strategy. Once the visit concludes, an email communication or message will be provided with a visit summary and any important information regarding treatment plan, prescriptions, follow up and billing.

From the perspective of the provider, telewound care visits involve similar steps across various clinics and technological telehealth platforms. Notably, providers will need to sign up and provide information, such as photo of medical license or hospital ID badge, to acquire health care professional verification in the system. This may take several days to process. Once verified, the provider will be able to access the appointment information and view patient information through a privacy-secure portal. Next, a secure link will be provided that allows clinicians to join the video call and start patient visits. Most telehealth platforms have a chat message function that allows patients to share media and text communications with the provider. If video connection is poor or the visit gets interrupted, most telehealth portals will provide the patients phone number to continue the visit on the phone. Once the visit concludes, providers can schedule follow up visits through the system and respond to messages if needed.

An additional option for telewound care practice is store-and-forward telemedicine. Store-and-forward technology refers to methods that collect clinical information and send it electronically to another site for evaluation. A common application of this practice in the wound clinic involves a resident physician or nurse capturing images of a patient's wound and using a communications system to send the images to an offsite wound care physician for proper assessment and evaluation. The physician's assessment is then sent back to the clinic and communicated to the patient to update the wound care plan. This workflow greatly increases the clinical efficiency of wound care and grants patients' greater access to receiving quality care from expert physicians [30, 31].

7 Benefits of Telewound Care

The use of telemedicine in wound management has several benefits. Remote services can improve patient access to care. There is a widespread lack of physicians who specialize in wound care. Through telemedicine, these specialists can reach a larger, underserved population or patients in rural areas [14]. These specialists can also use telemedicine services to consult with other physicians to improve coordination of care [32]. Additionally, chronic wounds are common in elderly patients or patients with conditions that limit mobility. Telemedicine is a more convenient option for these patients and would increase patient participation and prevent complications [33].

Wound care by telemedicine also has a substantial economic benefit. Remote care would eliminate cost of transportation and "time costs" from lost employment or lost wages in both patients with chronic wounds and their families. Telemedicine reduces lengthy waiting times for appointments in specialized wound centers as well. More frequent and immediate follow up by telemedicine would also help prevent future complications from improper wound care such as infection, sepsis, or amputation. Managing these complications would involve costly inpatient hospitalizations and can be avoided [34].

These benefits can collectively improve quality of care and quality of life in patients with chronic wounds. Telemedicine allows for faster and better quality of care to remote or underserved populations by providing direct access to specialists. Overall, patients report satisfaction when using telemedicine services [35, 36]. Higher quality of care and decreased financial burden can improve quality of life for patients with chronic wounds [35, 37].

8 Setbacks and Barriers of Telewound Care

The use of telemedicine provides an array of benefits to patients and providers. However, successful execution of telemedicine practices on a widespread scale has not occurred due to many limitations. Telewound care practice presents with unique challenges and barriers to success. Those are added to many of the limitations of in-person medical delivery systems.

In contrast to communication through screens and electronic devices, face-to-face visits are superior in determining patients' mood, level of psychological stress, and understanding of their condition—which are all important factors in management of their wounds [38]. Furthermore, effective use of the options available requires a certain level of understanding of how to use technology and varying degrees of technical literacy. A substantial portion of patients with chronic wounds are over the age of 65 and may lack the skills to properly navigate telehealth visits and track wound progress via smart phone apps [39]. Lastly, a notable barrier to the success of the proper implementation of telewound care is a lack of resources. Smart phone technologies and visual based telewound care options often rely on the image capturing and processing abilities of the patient's phone. There are an estimated 7 billion phone subscriptions worldwide however, regarding telewound care patients with lower resolution devices are at a disadvantage compared to the newer generation of smart phones that are required to properly measure the wounds and support the "data heavy" software programs [40]. Despite these limitations and barriers, telewound care is advancing rapidly and has proved to be impactful for improving management of chronic wounds.

9 Telewound Management Considerations for Specific Wound Types

If camera quality permits, providers can perform a satisfactory visual exam of the wound to assess stage of healing and response to past treatments. However, many patients with ulcers require routine debridement procedures or graft placement to improve their wounds. Many patients also require diagnostic procedures such as wound biopsy. These treatment and diagnostic modalities are not amenable to virtual visits and require in-person care from a qualified clinician. Furthermore, providers at the wound clinic can work in tandem with home health care nurses to develop a management plan. This strategy may work for many patients, but patients with chronic non-healing wounds will likely have to come to the clinic in person to heal their wounds.

Regardless of specific wound etiology, telewound services must consider aspects of treatment that broadly apply to the field of wound care. Asking patients to describe various features of their wounds during telewound visits is crucial. Through concerted verbal communication, providers can make note of changes in odor, pain, itchiness, sensation, and other features that are less readily assessed during telewound visits due to heavy reliance on visual and verbal communication. Telewound management practices also need to emphasize patient adherence to care. Many patients receiving treatment for their wounds are prescribed compression devices and have extensive regimens consisting of multiple layers of dressings and product applications. Providers should engage in discussion with patients to assess their understanding of treatment plans and should also provide instructive feedback. Additionally, clinicians should insist on visually examining old dressings that have been removed from wounds. Removed dressings are often an important source of information and can provide clinicians an opportunity to gauge exudate quantity and character and evaluate the progress of wound healing. To improve care and efficiency, clinicians can develop a pre-visit checklist and intake form to aide with telewound management. Examples of information pertinent to wound care assessment include the date of last dressing change, the types of dressing used, changes in pain and discomfort, and amount of time per day spent wearing compression.

9.1 Venous Leg Ulcer

Management of VLU through telewound services provides several benefits. A large proportion of patients with VLU are prescribed compression devices or wraps to facilitate healing. Patients are often able to better demonstrate how they use their compression and express any difficulties or concerns when receiving care from the comfort of their own home. Additionally, VLU tend to be very exudative and infrequent care is often the case in the traditional in-person setting and may lead to poor outcomes such as infection, contact dermatitis and delayed healing. Telewound care allows more frequent visits early in the care period which will help to avoid these complications. Clinicians should consider more frequent visits initially and space out the visits as the wound improves.

9.2 Arterial Ulcer

Patients with arterial ulcers often have comorbidities that contribute to their disease. Telewound care for these patients often allows them to receive medical management for these conditions without having to set foot in the clinic. However, a crucial component of this type of wound is lack of blood flow and assessing blood flow through virtual visits remains a difficulty. Doppler ultrasound studies or in-person vascular exams are commonly used to measure blood flow to assess disease. Furthermore, treatment for these ulcers often involves reestablishing proper circulation to the ulcer site through surgical intervention, which requires the patient to travel to the hospital. Therefore, telewound visits for these patients should be limited to general wound care considerations, monitoring the wound clinically, and ensuring follow up visits with appropriate specialists are in place.

9.3 *Diabetic Foot Ulcer*

A large proportion of patients with DFU develop their ulcerations because of diabetic neuropathy and associated vascular disease. These patients often need frequent examinations to make sure that the wound has not deteriorated and that they are not developing new wounds. The convenience of telewound appointments is beneficial for patients to routinely receive care. However, providers are unable to physically probe ulcerations through virtual visits, making it difficult to screen for exposed tendon or bone and potential osteomyelitis. Mechanical overloading treatments are a mainstay for managing these wounds. During telewound visits, physicians can instruct patients on how to use removable boots and assess patient understanding of the treatment. Nevertheless, advanced therapies such as skin substitute application and total contact cast application need to be administered at the wound clinic. Providers at the wound clinic can work together with home health nurses and develop a quality treatment plan that incorporates virtual and in-person visits.

9.4 *Pressure Injury*

Patients with wounds due to pressure injury often have limited mobility and motor strength and benefit immensely from telewound care options since they often have trouble commuting to in-person visits because of their disease. For providers to properly examine patients during telehealth visits, patients will often have to change position. Having a caregiver present during the visit or adequate assistance helps immensely and is often a requirement for telewound management. Additionally, assessing nutritional support, screening for hyperbaric oxygen therapy, and setting up home health visits can easily be accomplished with virtual visits. Notably, many pressure injuries are deep and have considerable undermining. These wounds are often difficult to examine via video and patient measurements may lack the necessary precision to develop a proper treatment plan. Telewound visit also offer an ability to directly view the offloading setup at the patient's home or care facility. This advantage should be leveraged, and clinician should examine the patient's set up and make recommendations for adjustments as needed.

10 Upcoming Innovations of Telewound Care

There are several upcoming innovations in telewound care that may improve quality of care. The use of wearable medical devices that provide useful data and continuous monitoring can contribute to the quality of telewound care. For example, one promising new technology is the remote temperature monitoring (RTM) mat. Studies have shown that these RTM mats reliably detect inflammation and pre-ulcerative lesions, and especially if used once daily, allow for timely and cost-effective care [41–43]. A 2017 longitudinal study involving 129 participants showed that RTM mats detected 97% of nonacute plantar diabetic foot ulcers with a lead time of 37 days on average [44]. Another study showed similar findings, even when participants had partial foot amputations [45]. Thus, RTM mats could improve patient outcomes and decrease healthcare resource utilization if used routinely in patients who are predisposed to developing wounds. Going beyond the daily RTM mat monitoring, some companies are designing shoes, insoles, and temperature-monitoring socks that will allow for real-time monitoring, although these technologies are still under development [46–48].

In addition to remote patient monitoring, artificial intelligence (AI) technology relevant to telewound care has developed rapidly in recent years. AI integrated into smartphone applications has the potential to help better monitor wound sizes, which would be a valuable tool in remotely caring for patients [40]. Currently, AI in dermatology is still in its infancy, although this area is rapidly progressing. As technology solutions become more readily available, considerations should be made to their smooth integration into the existing platforms and hardware (i.e. phones and computers). This will help to avoid decreased quality care due to excessive technological complications. Additionally, added monitoring by wearable devices and other adjunct datapoints has not been shown to improve the overall quality of care and healing rates. Therefore, a strict risk and benefit analysis should be continuously employed by healthcare systems and other practitioners to understand if more information is actually useful or only impedes care without adding real value.

11 Conclusion/Discussion

Caring for chronic wounds represents a large economic and humanistic burden to society. Treatment involves regular examination of the wound with dressing changes tailored to the individual and debridement or microbial assessment as needed. The underlying cause of the wound (prolonged pressure, vascular status, metabolic abnormalities, etc.) should be addressed, as well.

Telewound has been practiced for over two decades but has become of particular interest due to the COVID-19 pandemic. The implementation of telewound has been easier through widespread access to appropriate technology such as smartphones and computers with audiovisual capability. Patients can communicate with their physicians and other caretakers in three ways: (1) store and forward, (2) synchronous telemedicine, and (3) a hybrid of the previous two.

Telewound has expanded rapidly recently; however, it should be integrated as a long-term option for patients with chronic wounds. It can improve quality and consistency of care, especially for patients of limited mobility and access to wound care specialists. Unfortunately, full wound care cannot be provided solely through telemedicine. Physical assessment of the wound and procedures such as debridement, culture and application of tissue-based products are best done in a clinical setting. Additionally, while a vast population has access to necessary technology, some do not have the technological literacy or access for an adequate consultation. Rapid technological advancements may be the answer to these critical issues, but these recent developments may take years before they can be fully implemented. In summary, telewound has become an essential component of care and is "here to stay." The wise wound clinician can find ways to incorporate these capabilities into their practice and by being cognizant of the appropriate care that can be given over telewound visit will elevate their practice and improve their patients' care.

References

1. Sen CK. Human wound and its Burden: updated 2020 compendium of estimates. Adv Wound Care (New Rochelle). 2021;10(5):281–92. https://doi.org/10.1089/wound.2021.0026.
2. Martinengo L, Olsson M, Bajpai R, et al. Prevalence of chronic wounds in the general population: systematic review and meta-analysis of observational studies. Ann Epidemiol. 2019;29:8–15. https://doi.org/10.1016/j.annepidem.2018.10.005.
3. Frykberg RG, Banks J. Challenges in the treatment of chronic wounds. Adv Wound Care (New Rochelle). 2015;4(9):560–82. https://doi.org/10.1089/wound.2015.0635.
4. Olsson M, Järbrink K, Divakar U, et al. The humanistic and economic burden of chronic wounds: a systematic review. Wound Repair Regen. 2019;27(1):114–25. https://doi.org/10.1111/wrr.12683.
5. Kirsner RS, Romanelli M. Use of advanced technologies across the wound care spectrum: prologue. Int Wound J. 2016;13(S3):5–7. https://doi.org/10.1111/iwj.12633.
6. Vivas A, Lev-Tov H, Kirsner RS. Venous leg ulcers. Ann Int Med. 2016;165(3):ITC17–32. https://doi.org/10.7326/AITC201608020.
7. World Health Organization. Telemedicine: opportunities and developments in member states. Report on the second global survey on eHealth. World Health Organization; 2010.
8. Tensen E, van der Heijden JP, Jaspers MWM, Witkamp L. Two decades of teledermatology: current status and integration in national healthcare systems. Curr Dermatol Rep. 2016;5(2):96–104. https://doi.org/10.1007/s13671-016-0136-7.
9. Whited JDMDMHS. Teledermatology. Med Clin North Am. 2015;99(6):1365–79. https://doi.org/10.1016/j.mcna.2015.07.005.
10. Jockenhöfer F, et al. Aetiology, comorbidities and cofactors of chronic leg ulcers: retrospective evaluation of 1000 patients from 10 specialised dermatological wound care centers in Germany: aetiology, comorbidities and cofactors of chronic leg ulcers. Int Wound J. 2016;13(5):821–8.

11. Raeder K, et al. Prevalence and risk factors of chronic wounds in nursing homes in Germany. Int Wound J. 2020;17(5):1128–34.
12. Ko JY, et al. Risk factors for coronavirus disease 2019 (COVID-19)-associated hospitalization: COVID-19-associated hospitalization surveillance network and behavioral risk factor surveillance system. Clin Infect Dis. 2021;72(11):E695–703.
13. Oropallo A. COVID-19: issues related to wound care and telehealth management. In: Eidt JF, Mills JL, editors. UpToDate; 2020.
14. Chanussot-Deprez C, Contreras-Ruiz J. Telemedicine in wound care: a review. Adv Skin Wound Care. 2013;26(2):78–82. https://doi.org/10.1097/01.ASW.0000426717.59326.5f.
15. Graves N, Phillips C, Harding K. A narrative review of the epidemiology and economics of chronic wounds. Br J Dermatol. 2021. https://doi.org/10.1111/bjd.20692.
16. Sen CK. Human wound and its Burden: updated 2020 compendium of estimates. Adv Wound Care. 2021;10(5):281–92.
17. Rees RS, Bashshur N. The effects of telewound management on use of service and financial outcomes. Telemed J e-Health. 2007;13(6):663–74. https://doi.org/10.1089/tmj.2007.9971. PMID: 18069917.
18. Schlager JG, Kendziora B, Patzak L, Kupf S, Rothenberger C, Fiocco Z, French LE, Reinholz M, Hartmann D. Impact of COVID-19 on wound care in Germany. Int Wound J. 2021;18(4):536–42. https://doi.org/10.1111/iwj.13553. Epub 7 Feb 2021. PMID: 33554436; PMCID: PMC8014846.
19. Sood A, Granick MS, Trial C, Lano J, Palmier S, Ribal E, Téot L. The role of telemedicine in wound care: a review and analysis of a database of 5,795 patients from a mobile wound-healing center in Languedoc-Roussillon, France. Plast Reconstr Surg. 2016;138(3S):248S–56S. https://doi.org/10.1097/PRS.0000000000002702.
20. Mufti A, Sachdeva M, Maliyar K, Sibbald RG. COVID-19 and wound care: a Canadian perspective. JAAD Int. 2020;1(2):79–80. https://doi.org/10.1016/j.jdin.2020.05.003.
21. Le Goff-Pronost M, Mourgeon B, Blanchère J, Teot L, Benateau H, Dompmartin A. Real-world clinical evaluation and costs of telemedicine for chronic wound management. Int J Technol Assess Health Care. 2018;34(6):567–75. https://doi.org/10.1017/S0266462318000685.
22. Rees R, Bashshur N. The effects of telewound management on use of service and financial outcomes. Telemed J e-Health Off J Am Telemed Assoc. 2008;13:663–74. https://doi.org/10.1089/tmj.2007.9971.
23. Chittoria RK. Telemedicine for wound management. Indian J Plast Surg. 2012;45(2):412–7.
24. Santamaria N, Kapp S. Telewound care—providing remote wound assessment and treatment in the home care setting: current status and future directions. Smart Homecare Technol Telehealth. 2013;1:35–41. https://doi.org/10.2147/SHTT.S34353.
25. Etingen B, Patrianakos J, Wirth M, Hogan TP, Smith BM, Tarlov E, Stroupe KT, Kartje R, Weaver FM. Telewound practice within the veterans health administration: protocol for a mixed methods program evaluation. JMIR Res Protoc 2020;9(7):e20139. https://doi.org/10.2196/20139.
26. Wang SC, Au Y, Ramirez-GarciaLuna JL, Lee L, Berry GK. The promise of smartphone applications in the remote monitoring of postsurgical wounds: a literature review. Adv Skin Wound Care. 2020;33(9):489–96. https://doi.org/10.1097/01.ASW.0000694136.29135.02. PMID: 32810062.
27. Chakraborty C, Gupta B, Ghosh SK. Identification of chronic wound status under telewound network through smartphone. In: Information Resources Management Association (ed.) Human-computer interaction: concepts, methodologies, tools, and applications. IGI Global. 2016; 991–1007. https://doi.org/10.4018/978-1-4666-8789-9.ch046.
28. Wang SC, Anderson J, Evans R, Woo K, Beland B, Sasseville D, Moreau L. Point-of-care wound visioning technology: reproducibility and accuracy of a wound measurement app. PLoS ONE. 2017;12(8):e0183139. https://doi.org/10.1371/journal.pone.0183139.
29. Iyengar K, Upadhyaya GK, Vaishya R, Jain V. COVID-19 and applications of smartphone technology in the current pandemic. Diab Metab Syndr. 2020;14(5):733–7. https://doi.org/10.1016/j.dsx.2020.05.033.

30. Dobry A, Begaj T, Mengistu K, Sinha S, Droms R, Dunlap R, Wu D, Adhami K, Stavert R. Implementation and impact of a store-and-forward teledermatology platform in an urban academic safety-net health care system. Telemed J e-Health. 2021;27(3):308–15. https://doi.org/10.1089/tmj.2020.0069. Epub 9 Jun 2020. PMID: 32522105.
31. Nelson CA, Takeshita J, Wanat KA, Bream KD, Holmes JH, Koenig HC, Roth RR, Vuppalapati A, James WD, Kovarik CL. Impact of store-and-forward (SAF) teledermatology on outpatient dermatologic care: a prospective study in an underserved urban primary care setting. J Am Acad Dermatol. 2016;74(3):484–90.e1. https://doi.org/10.1016/j.jaad.2015.09.058. Epub 8 Dec 2015. PMID: 26679528.
32. Joshua SJ, Sydney AS, Seth AS. Telemedicine broadening access to care for complex cases. J Surg Res. 2017;220:164–70.
33. Ratliff CR, Shifflett R, Howell A, Kennedy C. Telehealth for wound management during the COVID-19 pandemic: case studies. J Wound Ostomy Continence Nurs. 2020;47(5):445–9. https://doi.org/10.1097/WON.0000000000000692.
34. Dávalos ME, French MT, Burdick AE, Simmons SC. Economic evaluation of telemedicine: review of the literature and research guidelines for benefit-cost analysis. Telemed J e-Health. 2009;15(10):933–48. https://doi.org/10.1089/tmj.2009.0067.
35. Hofmann-Wellenhof R, Salmhofer W, Binder B, Okcu A, Kerl H, Soyer HP. Feasibility and acceptance of telemedicine for wound care in patients with chronic leg ulcers. J Telemed Telecare. 2006;12(1_suppl):15–17. https://doi.org/10.1258/135763306777978407.
36. Edward H, Howard G, Keyvan N. Definitions, survey methods, and findings of patient satisfaction studies in teledermatology: a systematic review. Arch Dermatol Res. 2021;313(4):205–15.
37. Salmhofer W, Hofmann-Wellenhof R, Gabler G, et al. Wound teleconsultation in patients with chronic leg ulcers. Dermatology (Basel). 2005;210(3):211–7. https://doi.org/10.1159/000083512.
38. Currell R, Urquhart C, Wainwright P, Lewis R. Telemedicine versus face to face patient care: effects on professional practice and health care outcomes. Cochrane Database Syst Rev. 2000;2:CD002098. https://doi.org/10.1002/14651858.CD002098. Update in: Cochrane Database Syst Rev. 2015;9:CD002098. PMID: 10796678.
39. Carlin A. Wound care in older adults. Br J Commun Nurs. 2018;23(Suppl 12):S18–22. https://doi.org/10.12968/bjcn.2018.23.Sup12.S18. PMID: 30521355.
40. Okita AL, Molina Tinoco LJ, Patatas OH, Guerreiro A, Criado PR, Gabbi TV, Ferreira PS, Neto CF. Use of smartphones in telemedicine: comparative study between standard and teledermatological evaluation of high-complex care hospital inpatients. Telemed J e-Health. 2016;22(9):755–60. https://doi.org/10.1089/tmj.2015.0086. Epub 9 Mar 2016. PMID: 26959500.
41. Lavery LA, Petersen BJ, Linders DR, Bloom JD, Rothenberg GM, Armstrong DG. Unilateral remote temperature monitoring to predict future ulceration for the diabetic foot in remission. BMJ Open Diabetes Res Care. 2019;7(1):e000696.
42. Killeen AL, Brock KM, Dancho JF, Walters JL. Remote temperature monitoring in patients with visual impairment due to diabetes mellitus: a proposed improvement to current standard of care for prevention of diabetic foot ulcers. J Diabetes Sci Technol. 2020;14(1):37–45.
43. Frykberg RG, Gordon IL, Reyzelman AM, Cazzell SM, Fitzgerald RH, Rothenberg GM, Bloom JD, Petersen BJ, Linders DR, Nouvong A, Najafi B. Feasibility and efficacy of a smart mat technology to predict development of diabetic plantar ulcers. Diabetes Care. 2017;40(7):973–80. https://doi.org/10.2337/dc16-2294.
44. Gordon IL, Rothenberg GM, Lepow BD, Petersen BJ, Linders DR, Bloom JD, Armstrong DG. Accuracy of a foot temperature monitoring mat for predicting diabetic foot ulcers in patients with recent wounds or partial foot amputation. Diabetes Res Clin Pract. 2020;161:108074.
45. Najafi B, Ron E, Enriquez A, Marin I, Razjouyan J, Armstrong DG. Smarter sole survival: will neuropathic patients at high risk for ulceration use a smart insole-based foot protection system? J Diabetes Sci Technol. 2017;11(4):702–13.
46. Reyzelman AM, Koelewyn K, Murphy M, Shen X, Yu E, Pillai R, Ma R, et al. Continuous temperature-monitoring socks for home use in patients with diabetes: observational study. J Med Internet Res. 2018;20(12):e12460.

47. Bus SA, Waaijman R, Nollet F. New monitoring technology to objectively assess adherence to prescribed footwear and assistive devices during ambulatory activity. Arch Phys Med Rehabil. 2012;93(11):2075–9.
48. Kuziemsky C, Maeder AJ, John O, Gogia SB, Basu A, Meher S, Ito M. Role of artificial intelligence within the telehealth domain. Yearb Med Inform. 2019;28(1):35–40.

Teledermatological Surgery

Soraya Azzawi and Keyvan Nouri

Abstract Telesurgery is broad field encompassing the remote performance of procedures, consultation with other physicians and mentorship of trainees. The astronomical pace of advancements in robotic surgical systems have enabled life-saving patient care. Although teledermatologic surgery is still an evolving field, the utilization of telehealth technologies in preoperative evaluation and intraoperative consultation has proven beneficial.

Keywords Teledermatological surgery · Dermatologic surgery · Skin neoplasms · Telepathology · Mohs surgery

1 Introduction

Diligent preparation underlies the success of any venture, particularly one as vital as surgery. On September 7th 2001, Dr. Jacques Marescaux and his team prepared for a laparoscopic cholecystectomy [1]. While cholecystectomies are generally considered standard procedures, the Lindbergh operation was commemorated in the annals of history for how it was performed— across 3860 miles between New York, USA and Strasbourg, France [1]. As the world's first telesurgery, the Lindbergh operation utilized asynchronous transfer mode (ATM) telecommunications to conduct a transatlantic robot-assisted procedure [1]. The surgery and postoperative course proceeded without complication, demonstrating that telesurgery could safely and reliably be performed in situations where traditional surgery is not feasible.

As the evolving surgical workforce shortage [2–10] continues to deprive patients of optimal treatment, the development of telesurgery becomes even more critical. Over the last decade, the United States population grew by 10.1%, representing 96.8 million people [11], while the number of general surgeons graduating residency has remained relatively stagnant across the last 30 years [8]. This alarming

S. Azzawi (✉) · K. Nouri
Dr. Phillip Frost Department of Dermatology and Cutaneous Surgery, Miller School of Medicine, University of Miami, Miami, USA
e-mail: soraya.azzawi@jhsmiami.org

K. Nouri (ed.), *Telemedicine and Technological Advances in Dermatology*,
https://doi.org/10.1007/978-3-031-69091-4_7

undersupply traverses surgical specialties; one study predicted that the number of practicing cardiothoracic surgeons will fall 21% by 2025 [12]. The dearth of specialized surgical care has profound consequences on morbidity and mortality [13–15], and thereby embodies an area for innovation.

2 Nomenclature

Telesurgery is a broad term that refers to utilization of robotic intermediaries to perform a procedure from a remote location. In contrast to other forms of telemedicine, telesurgery is contingent on the ability to execute tasks synchronously, or in real-time, from a remote location. By contrast, telepresence encompasses the audio and visual connection to a remote surgical field. A surgeon utilizing telepresence can oversee, but lacks the capacity to directly manipulate, the operating theater. Traditional nomenclature designates the surgeon console as the "master" domain, which employs a human system interface (HSI) to guide the surgical robot, referred to as the "slave" domain [16–19]. HSI provide audio and visual information through haptic devices, headphones and a video console. Surgical robots ae outfitted with a 3D camera and microphone, with newer models containing more dependable tactile sensors. Teleconsulting, in which two seasoned surgeons collaborate on a complex case, and telementoring, whereby an expert surgeon advises another surgeon through an unfamiliar procedure, are related benefits of telesurgery [20, 21].

Key Points

- Telesurgery can be conducted synchronously or asynchronously and utilizes a surgeon console that guides the surgical robot through a human system interface.

3 History of Technologic Development

Numerous advances in telesurgery can be attributed to the groundwork laid by the Defense Advanced Research Agency (DAPRA) and the National Aeronautics and Space Administration (NASA), who have invested significant resources into devising solutions for healthcare delivery in challenging locations [22, 23]. These ventures have led to the commercialization of several robotic surgical systems.

The first robotic surgical system approved by the US Food and Drug Administration (FDA) was the Automated Endoscopic System for Optimal Positioning (AESOP) in 1994 [24, 25]. Developed by Computer Motion, Inc. (Goleta, CA), the AESOP assisted in procedures by holding and manipulating an endoscope as directed by a surgeon. AESOP was subsequently integrated into the ZEUS platform, which became FDA approved in October 2001 achieved worldwide fame for successfully enabling the first transatlantic surgery in 2001 [26]. ZEUS' success was rivaled by the da Vinci surgical system, a product of Intuitive Surgical Inc. (Mountain View, CA) approved by the FDA in July 2000 [24, 25, 27]. After the two companies merged in 2003, AESOP and ZEUS would be largely replaced by the Da Vinci Surgical System, which involves a surgeon operating a console to guide the interactive robotic arms. Additional features of this system include three-dimensional vision, tremor elimination and wristed instrumentation [24, 25, 27, 28]. Intuitive Surgical Systems Inc. (Davis, CA) has also generated commercially available systems, including the NeuroMate stereotactic robot, with predominantly neurosurgical applications, and ROBODOC, which assists in precision bone machining during orthopedic procedures [16, 29]. When contrasted with traditional laproscopy, robot assisted laparoscopic procedures improve patient outcomes by reducing hemorrhage, hospitalization time and conversion to open surgery [30, 31].

Building on these advancements, the United States Army's Telemedicine and Advanced Technology Research Center (TATRC), NASA and the University of Cincinnati combined their expertise to investigate the potential of robotic surgical systems through NASA's Extreme Environment Mission Operations (NEEMO) program. These experiments were conducted by surgical researchers and physician astronauts in a laboratory located 60 ft underwater known as the Aquarius Habitat. The NEEMO12 mission featured M7 Telerobotic surgical system, provided by Stanford Research International Robotics (SRI), and the RAVEN robotic surgical system, developed by the University of Washington. Both these systems were successfully operated by surgeons in distant geographic locations [32]. In addition to experiments conducted in the Aquarius habitat, the M7 system has also been trialed in simulated zero gravity [32, 33]. The utility of robotic surgical systems in extreme, desolate environments is an active area of investigation.

In 2011, Shenai and colleagues developed the virtual interactive presence and augmented reality (VIPAR) platform for remote surgical assistance utilizing a standard internet connection [34, 35]. The novelty of the VIPAR system lies in its sophisticated connectivity between local and remote participants. Each station has a binocular videoscope demonstrating not only the shared surgical field, but also the perspectives of both the local and remote surgeons. Augmented reality mingles digital and virtual renderings with the surgical field. The remote surgeon is able to identify critical anatomy and demonstrate operative techniques synchronously, enhancing communication and collaboration between surgical teams. Beyond its use with the binocular videoscope, VIPAR has been further adapted to other audiovisual platforms, including Google Glass and the iPad [36]. Candidate procedures for VIPAR include endoscopic, endovascular and microsurgical cases, all of which are predicated on video capture.

A breakthrough achievement within robotic surgical systems was the development of haptic feedback, which facilitates tactile feedback [37–39]. While traditional robotic surgical systems relied exclusively on transmission of video information, the advent of haptic feedback allows surgical operators to sense suture tension and tissue consistency, minimizing suture tearing and tissue injury. Telelap Alf-x (SOFAR S.p.A., ALF-X Surgical Robotics Department, Trezzano Rosa, Milan, Italy), which debuted in 2015, first demonstrated haptic feedback technology in the context of surgery [40]. The additional tactile information afforded by haptic feedback decreased the mean duration of cholecystectomy by one hour. Eye-tracking technology within Telelap Alf-x are an added safety feature that detects when a surgeon's gaze is not directed to the screen, and accordingly ceases motions of the robotic arms. Implementing reusable components adds to the cost-efficiency of Telelap Alf-x, in contrast to many other robotic surgical systems. Recently, an MRI-guided telesurgery system is exploring the production of haptic feedback through pneumatic pressure [41].

Key Points

- Accelerating technologic advances, including haptic feedback technology and eye-tracking, are helping improve the feasibility, safety and efficiency of telesurgery.

4 Advantages of Telesurgery

4.1 Bridging Disparities

Geographic or circumstantial constraints have a determinative role in shaping patient outcomes. In both domestic and international spheres, inequalities in the provision of surgical and perioperative care have been well documented. Survival of non-small cell lung cancer, for example, has been correlated to geographic area and is at least partially dictated by disparities in access to surgical care [42]. Superseding these obstacles, telesurgery has the remarkable ability to connect underserved populations with the care they require.

Locations as remote as Antarctica have benefited from telesurgery. In an unforgiving environment where the slightest delay in evaluation can be detrimental, telecommunication has played an instrumental role. Utilizing the International Telecommunications Satellite (INTELSAT) system, orthopedic and other surgical specialists in Japan could consult on patients partaking in the Japanese Antarctic Research Expedition. Another study established a telerobotic surgical service between St. Joseph's Hospital in Hamilton and North Bay General Hospital, a rural hospital located in Ontario, Canada [43]. At the time of publication, this system resulted in 21 successful telerobotic laparoscopic surgeries collaboratively performed by the two surgical teams. These included fundoplications, sigmoid resections, right hemicolectomies, inguinal hernia repairs and anterior resection. It bears mention that there was a transient disturbance in signal transmission during the first colectomy; however, the telerobotic surgeon immediately shifted to the alternative telecommunication line with an interruption of less than 1 s, and continued without further incident. All operations proceeded without serious complications, and none of the procedures were converted to open surgeries. Furthermore, there was no difference in length of stay between patients who received the telerobotic laparoscopic procedures at the rural hospital, and those who received the equivalent procedure in the academic hospital.

Telesurgery has demonstrated utility in sites of military conflict. Orthopedic telemedicine consultations for soldiers serving in Afghanistan, Iraq and Navy Afloats resulted in decreased aeromedical evacuation frequency, costs and time to treatment [44].

Yet another relevant demographic for telesurgery is patients within correctional facilities. The evolving telemedicine network between the Virginia Commonwealth University Health System and the Department of Corrections showed the efficacy of telemedicine consultation for general surgery and postoperative care [45]. Out of the 55 consultations completed during the year of the study, 49% led to surgeries.

4.2 Surgical Collaboration and Telementoring

Capacity-building, whether through consultation or pedagogy, constitutes a vital part of addressing the global undersupply of surgeons. Conventionally, surgical education has been conducted through on-site, interactive training. The finite amount of experienced surgeons, who tend to cluster in metropolitan areas, translates to a tacit exclusion of many rural and international trainees from optimal surgical training. The resources and time necessary to commute to locations with surgical experts can be prohibitive, compounding the gap in access to surgical care [46].

As technology continues to advance, telesurgery is better able to facilitate collaboration on complex cases between distant surgical teams, interweaving the global surgical community. This shared expertise can be life-changing for patients. Even cases as intricate as operative fetoscopy, which merges endoscopy and ultrasound technology to correct birth defects in utero, has been accomplished via telesurgery. At present, operative fetoscopy is limited to very few experienced facilities around the world. Consultation between a team in Tampa, Florida and Santiago, Chile enabled a telesurgical fetoscopy for an acardiac twin, leading to the delivery of a healthy infant at 37.5 weeks [47].

Emphasizing the scarcity of surgical expertise, this particular study draws attention to some of major forces fueling the workforce shortage. The disparity of access to surgical care is magnified by narrow opportunities for trainees around the world to acquire surgical skills. Capitalizing on technological innovation to swiftly disseminated surgical proficiency could ameliorate the geographically-based differences in patient outcomes. Telementoring has been validated as an efficacious and economic approach to imparting surgical knowledge [48–50]. One review exploring the outcomes and educational benefits of surgical telementoring found that the most common telementored operations consisted of laparoscopic cholecystectomy, endovascular treatment of aortic aneurysm, laparoscopic colectomy and nephrectomies [51]. Out of 433 total telementored procedures, only 5% were converted to open surgery. Furthermore, there was a fairly low complication rate at approximately 5%. Reported complications included bile collection, conversion to open surgery, iliac artery rupture, liver bleeding, postoperative ileus, serosa tears, trocar port bleeding and wound infection. The response from surgical mentees has been overwhelmingly positive [46, 52–59]. Cited benefits included acquisition of surgical maneuvers, increased familiarity in identifying critical anatomy and enhanced confidence in surgical performance.

A groundbreaking collaboration between facilities in Ho Chi Minh City, Vietnam and Birmingham, Alabama highlighted the utility of VIPAR in facilitating the training of local neurosurgeons [36]. Local and remote surgical teams successfully jointly performed 15 endoscopic third ventriculostomy with choroid plexus coagulation surgeries without serious complications. Of these patients, 80% remain remained free of a ventricular shunt at follow-up. Contrast this to outcomes prior to the introduction of VIPAR, which included grave complications such as severe intraventricular bleeding necessitating an external ventricular drain, postoperative cerebrospinal fluid leak, subdural hematoma and death due to basilar artery injury and hemorrhage.

Despite benign intentions, both the efficacy and morality of medical voluntourism have come under greater scrutiny [60, 61]. International medical missions face a significant challenge in ensuring sustainability. Capacity building in underdeveloped countries is hindered by limits placed on their trainees who embark on rotations abroad. Furthermore, practices learned abroad are governed by the availability of resources, and therefore may not be directly applicable to systems in their home country. Given the highly technical nature of surgical skillsets, interactive pedagogy through telesurgery offers an appealing solution to the impending global surgery crisis.

4.3 Enhancement of Operator Accuracy

Telesurgery utilizing robotic surgical systems can improve surgical performance [62]. Laproscopy and microsurgery both involve image magnification, which can intensify a surgeon's baseline tremor and the frequency of purposeless movements [1, 63, 64]. The natural consequence of this arrangement is that the surgeon slows the operation to ensure precise execution of surgical choreography. Although this may transiently correct these issues, ultimately, the prolonged operative time and the surgeon's stagnant posture contribute to exhaustion, aggravating any underlying purposeless movements. The evolution of accelerometer technology has been shown to mitigate the effects of physiologic tremor on surgical performance, although efficacy can be limited by lag time, drift, noise and gravity [65–68]. Robotic systems have been used to negate physiologic tremor during vitroretinal microsurgery, and have demonstrated efficacy in sutured coronary artery bypass anastomoses in plastic models [15, 69–71]. Telesurgical robotic systems can also bypass ergonomic constraints, providing enhanced dexterity and flexibility when wielding instruments.

Key Points

- Telesurgery carries a myriad of applications, including improving health equity, fostering educational and research collaboration between remote locations and enhancing technical proficiency.

5 Challenges to Adoption of Telesurgery

5.1 Latency

The distance over which telesurgery can be conducted is limited by communication latency, defined as the lag time from initiation of movement by the remote surgeon until execution by the surgical robot and recapitulation of this movement on video feedback [72]. Without fiber-optic lines, surgeons operating remotely can contend with latency times ranging from 500 to 900 ms [73–76]. Studies have found a significant deterioration in accuracy and user experience with increasing latency, with one analysis characterizing the threshold as low as 105 ms of artificial latency [77–84]. This poses a substantial hurdle to the safe clinical translation of telesurgery. Communication latency can lead to surgeon disorientation and fatigue, prolonged intraoperative time and compromised patient outcomes [83, 85].

5.2 Cost

The monumental successes of telesurgery have long been haunted by the colossal expenses associated with the system [86]. Operation Lindbergh, the quintessential procedure in telesurgery, exceeded 1 million euros in cost [15]. Beyond the cost of acquisition, realistic integration of a robotic surgical system into a medical facility requires an investment in training of personnel, swift and reliable data transmission with a backup system and maintenance of robotic system with annual service contracts [87].

5.3 Ethical and Legal Considerations

The dizzying acceleration of innovation within the field of telesurgery has outpaced the development of ethical and legal frameworks. A major concern in the performance of any surgery is patient safety and liability. In the event of a prolonged disturbance of data transition or equipment failure, what entity is responsible—the remote surgeon, the facility housing the patient or the scientists who engineered the robotic surgical system? Telesurgical procedures conducted across geographically distant locations raises questions about conflicts of jurisdiction.

Given reported incidences of theft of data from cloud technology, patient privacy remains a key issue in the successful implementation of telesurgery. When obtaining informed consent, patients must be made aware of a variety of risks, including breaches of confidentiality and equipment failure. Caution must be taken with respect to the storage and transmission of patient data [88, 89].

Key Points

- Despite its numerous benefits, telesurgery mis mired in several challenges, including the technologic limitations, the substantial cost of equipment and continuously evolving legal frameworks.

6 Applications to Teledermatologic Surgery

Surgical skills are a are an integral element of the practice of dermatology. Furthermore, dermatology-focused surgical training has a substantial impact on patient outcomes with respect to the management of skin neoplasms. Although not recommended by current guidelines, up to 10% of basal cell carcinomas (BCCs) are excised by general practitioners, which may partially be explained by the dearth of dermatologists in underserved areas [90]. In a set of 277 BCC excisions, only 42.7% of the excisions performed by general practitioners achieved adequate excision margins, compared to 72% of the excisions performed by consultant dermatologists [91]. Other studies have similarly echoed a significant difference in BCC excision and diagnosis between general practitioners and dermatologists [92, 93], highlighting the value of dermatologic surgery the need for enhanced access to specialized dermatologic care.

6.1 Preoperative Evaluation

Preoperative care has proven an ideal juncture at which to implement telehealth technologies [94, 95]. Teledermatologic assessment prior to surgery has been demonstrated as a feasible and cost-effective method for preoperative to consult, resulting in an equivalent percentage of treated cancers and significantly reduced consult failure rates [94]. Historically, teledermatologic evaluation has been constrained by the visual quality of the images or video conferencing modality provided; however, the introduction of teledermoscopy can overcome this hurdle [96].

In a study assessing the utility of store-and-forward dermatologic consultation, clinical information and 2 digital images were provided to the consultant dermatologist [97]. It bears mention that the study excluded lesions thought to require significant reconstruction through flaps or grafts. After a report including suspected diagnosis, preoperative instructions and a surgery date was forwarded to the consulting physician, the patient would present to the dermatologic surgeon for examination on the day of surgery. Unless any contraindications to surgery were identified, the patient was then immediately operated on.

This model resulted in a remarkable decrease in time to surgical procedure, from mean interval of 60.57 days through the conventional referral system to just 26.20 days through the teledermatology consultation system [97]. A plethora of other studies have reaffirmed this finding, with teleconsultation patients consistently receiving intervention earlier than their counterparts in the traditional referral process [98–102].

Interestingly, the teledermatology consultation system devised by Ferrandiz and colleagues also achieved a lower rate of on-the-day surgery cancellation (2.99%) when compared to the conventional referral system (8.85%) [97]. Of the patients in the teledermatology cohort who did cancel, two of these cases were attributed to clinical evolution resulting in surgical contraindication, while the remaining two failed to present for surgery. Teleconsulting resulted in high diagnostic accuracy, with a diagnostic kappa concordance of $\kappa = 0.86$ (95% CI, 0.83–0.89) when contrasted with histopathologic diagnosis. Highlighting the reliability of teledermatologic preoperative consultation, this study demonstrated robust agreement between the planned and perfomed surgical approach $\kappa = 0.75$ (95% CI, 0.71–0.79). Discrepancy with regards to surgical technique can be attributed to the performance of direct suture in cases where local graft had been planned through teleconsultation.

The value of teledermatology in preoperative evaluation is perhaps best recapitulated through the convenience afforded to patients. By enabling the dermatologic surgeon to plan treatment (surgical technique, type of anesthesia, outpatient vs. inpatient surgery), teleconsultation spares patients the time and costs of unnecessary face-to-face visits. This is of the utmost importance to patients with physical limitations or disability, financial hardship, remote geographic location or residency in living facilities for whom transportation is logistically challenging.

6.2 Telepathologic Intraoperative Consultation

Given the highly visual nature of pathology, telemedicine naturally lends itself to this service. The diagnostic accuracy and efficiency of telepathology have been validated throughout the literature, leading to the exploration of its use in teledermatology [103–106].

One of the key benefits of Mohs surgery, minimal tissue sacrifice when excising a neoplasm, is contingent on intraoperative evaluation of frozen sections to secure tumor-free margins. A spectrum of technologic advancements has enabled this process to be successfully adapted to telemedicine [107–110]. Dynamic telepathology utilizes live transmission to convey histopathologic images to a remote pathologist. Methods used include motorized microscopes in addition to commercially available digital cameras poised at the microscope eyepiece followed by videoconferencing using iChat AV (Apple Computer Inc., Cupertino, CA) [107–110]. In this context, telepathology has yielded high diagnostic accuracy when contrasted to conventional light microscopy [107–110]. Furthermore, telepathology has proven cost-effective; utilizing consumer-grade products, McKenna and Florell demonstrated complete agreement between telepathology and Mohs frozen section diagnosis during intraoperative consultation [110]. Beyond assessing tumor margins, telepathology consultations enabled the resolution of diagnostic conundrums such as confirming of tumor type when distinct from the original biopsy diagnosis or discerning similarly-appearing benign and malignant epithelial proliferations (for instance, trichoblastoma, pilar sheath acanthoma and basal cell carcinoma) [107–110]. Remote consultation also provided valuable prognostic information.

Integrating dynamic telepathology into Mohs surgery allows greater diagnostic clarity, sparing patients from unnecessary excision of benign neoplasms or overly-aggressive excision when margin assessment is complicated by an unrelated inflammatory infiltrate. In malignant cases, telepathology facilitates swift tumor excision. Fostering collaboration between dermatologists and pathologists can thus optimize patient outcomes while also lending credence to excision when confronted with nonspecific findings.

Despite these benefits, extensive use of telepathology has traditionally hindered by the cost of the necessary equipment; however, this is anticipated to be less of a barrier as technology advances. While the dynamic telepathology arrangement of McKenna and Florrell in 2007 cost $1250, in 2019 Kantor and colleagues implemented a consumer-grade plastic binocular adapter attached to a smartphone to transmit histopathologic images and videos, an approach which cost less than $150 [110, 111].

Beyond the expense of the requisite equipment, legal burdens have also complicated widespread use of telepathology. Many current, billing frameworks do not take into account intraoperative telepathology consultation; because reimbursement for Mohs surgery depends on the Mohs surgeon performing surgery as well as evaluating frozen sections, the consultant dermatopathologist is not compensated for their efforts [10]. Buoyed by a growing body of literature attesting to the benefits of telemedicine, proposed legislature reforms may help broaden insurance coverage to include intraoperative telepathology consultation in the future.

Additional factors complicating the use of telepathology including ensuring encryption of patient identifying information, a lack of standardized protocols for results reporting and division of responsibility for malpractice. In McKenna and Florell's study, for example, results were discussed between the Mohs surgeon and dermatopathologist, but the name of the dermatopathologist was not included in the operative report.

6.3 Telesurgical Intraoperative Consultation

Intraoperative surgical consultation presents another avenue for telehealth innovation, although its current use within teledermatologic surgery remains limited.

To date, the literature evaluating the utility of telemedicine to intraoperative dermatologic surgery has focused predominantly on Smartglasses (Google Glass, Google Inc, Mountain View, CA), a voice-activated instrument that enables hands-free image and video capture capability [113–115]. Because the monitor attaches above the field of vision, the dermatologic surgeon can document preoperative visits, consults or surgery [114]. Fitting a pair of Smartglasses with a 5 megapixel 720p HD camera, Hamann and colleagues demonstrated the wide-ranging applications of this technology at Loma Linda University, where the departments of Dermatology and Otolaryngology and Head and Neck Surgery collaboratively manage the caseload for reconstruction of Mohs surgery defects [113]. Using store-and-forward telehealth, dermatologic surgeons performing Mohs micrographic surgery on patients could capture and transmit complex defects or anticipated challenging reconstructions to Plastic Surgery or Otolaryngology and Head and Neck Surgery colleagues for triage and consultation [113]. The videoconferencing feature of the Smartglasses also permits live consultation. Consultant surgeons in remote locations can visualize the operative field, lend their expertise in closure approach or provide referrals when necessary [98, 113]. Intraoperative telesurgical consultation also presents a unique educational opportunity for residents or fellows scrubbed into a case. The remote video streaming functionality has also been used to arrange a live surgery observation course at a private practice for residents from a local academic institution. Future directions may include incorporating patient vital signs onto the monitor for observation during surgery as well as the addition of loupes [98].

Evoking other concerns with telemedicine as a whole, preserving patient privacy when transmitting information during an intraoperative consult remains a top priority.

6.4 Postoperative Follow Up

Perioperative education has been shown to reduce complication rates, diminish pre- and postoperative anxiety, enhance medication compliance and improve patient satisfaction [116, 117]. As electronic medical records continue to evolve, many program are starting to incorporate web portals that enable communication and image transfer [98]. Particularly for uncomplicated cases, this facilitates remote perioperative education and postoperative follow up that alleviates the financial and logistic burdens of travel from patients.

One randomized controlled trial assessed four different modalities of postoperative wound care instructions: videos with text messages, videos-only, text messages-only or a control group using only pamphlets [118]. While knowledge scores were relatively similar between groups, patient rated the instructional video and text messages as "very helpful" when compared with the pamphlet. Patient preference also favored text message instructions rather than the pamphlet.

Similar approaches have been used in the cosmetic branch of dermatology. Smartphone monitoring following laser resurfacing was found to efficient and convenient alternative to face-to-face appointments for both patients and dermatologists [119].

The Plastic Surgery literature is replete with evidence of the applications of telemedicine during postoperative follow up. Text messaging has been used to transmit postoperative images, enabling remote monitoring of the postprocedural course. Of 57 patients who were subject to a smartphone-based postoperative protocol utilizing text messaging, 96.2% reported improved quality of postoperative experience [120]. This protocol also enabled the early detection of complications in 3 cases, in addition to prompt management prior to the scheduled face-to-face follow up. Similarly, smartphone applications have been used for surveillance of free flap outcomes, leading to prompt diagnosis of flap compromised and overall increased flap survival [121, 122].

Smartphone-based postoperative surveillance regimens could benefit both dermatologic surgeons and patients by facilitating prompt recognition of complications, optimizing flap or graft survival and improving patient experience.

Key Points

- Teledermatologic surgery holds immense promise by reducing the logistic and financial burden of transportation on patients, cultivating interdisciplinary cooperation and improving recognition of postoperative complications.

7 Conclusions

Since the first transatlantic operation, telesugery has progressed from a mythical venture into a feasible and efficacious treatment modality. Emerging as a creative response to the undersupply of the global surgical workforce, telesurgery mitigates disparities in access to surgical care. Providing meaningful capacity-building in resource-scarce areas makes telesurgery a more sustainable intervention than transient medical missions. Robotic surgical systems can also improve surgeon accuracy by canceling physiologic tremor and circumventing the positioning constraints of traditional surgeon. Despite the exciting technologic advances, widespread use of telesurgery is still limited by communication latency, exorbitant costs and ethical and legal quagmires.

Key Concepts

- The rapid evolution of telecommunications technology and robotics have helped democratize the field of medicine, enabling specialized healthcare delivery to remote geographic locations andmarginalized populations.
- Hurdles to widespread implementation of telemedicine in the realm of surgery include the cost of equipment, ligstics of installation and maintenance of

equipment, nebulous legal infrastructure, malpractice accountability and privacy concerns.

- Ideal paradigms in which teledermatologic surgery has been deployed include preoperative consultation, intraoperative consultation, postoperative surveillance, surgical education and mentorship. Further intraoperative utility, as well as applications in laser and cosmetic dermatology, are ripe for further investigation.

References

1. Marescaux J, Leroy J, Rubino F, et al. Transcontinental robot-assisted remote telesurgery: feasibility and potential applications. Ann Surg. 2002;235(4):487–92. https://doi.org/10.1097/00000658-200204000-00005.
2. Cobey JC. The surgeon shortage: constructive participation during health reform. J Am Coll Surg 2010;211:568 (Letter).
3. Cofer JB, Burns RP. The developing crisis in the national gen-eral surgery workforce. J Am Coll Surg. 2008;206:790–7.
4. Cohn SM, Price MA, Villarreal CL. Trauma and surgical critical care workforce in the United States: a severe surgeon shortage appears imminent. J Am Coll Surg. 2009;209:446–52.
5. Polk HC Jr, Vitale DS, Qadan M. The very busy urban sur-geon: another face of the evermore obvious shortage of gen-eral surgeons. J Am Coll Surg. 2009;209:144–7.
6. Sanchez M, Sariego J. The general surgeon shortage: causes, consequences, and solutions. South Med. 2009;J102:291–4.
7. Satiani B, Williams TE, Go MR. Predicted shortage of vas-cular surgeons in the United States: population and workload analysis. J Vasc Surg. 2009;50:946–52.
8. Sheldon GF, Ricketts TC, Charles A, King J, Fraher EP, Meyer A. The global health workforce shortage: role of surgeons and other providers. Adv Surg. 2008;42:63–85.
9. Voelker R. Experts say projected surgeon shortage a "looming crisis" for patient care. JAMA. 2009;302:1520–1.
10. Williams TE Jr, Sun B, Ross P Jr, Thomas AM. A formidable task: Population analysis predicts a deficit of 2000 cardiotho-racic surgeons by 2030. J Thorac Cardiovasc Surg. 2010;139:835–41.
11. https://www.census.gov/library/stories/2021/08/united-states-adult-population-grew-faster-than-nations-total-population-from-2010-to-2020.html.
12. Grover A, et al. Circulation. 2009;120(6):488–94.
13. Sanchez M, Sariego J. The general surgeon shortage: causes, consequences, and solutions. South Med J. 2009;102(3):291–4. https://doi.org/10.1097/SMJ.0b013e31818c96ac. PMID: 19204642.
14. Lynge DC, Larson EH. Workforce issues in rural surgery. Surg Clin North Am. 2009;89(6):1285–91, vii. https://doi.org/10.1016/j.suc.2009.07.003. PMID: 19944809.
15. Sheldon GF. Access to care and the surgeon shortage: American surgical association forum. Ann Surg. 2010;252(4):582–90. https://doi.org/10.1097/SLA.0b013e3181f886b6. PMID: 20881763.
16. Lum MJH, Friedman DCW, Sankaranarayanan G, et al. The RAVEN: design and validation of a telesurgery system. Int J Robot Res. 2009;28(9):1183–97.
17. Tozal ME, Wang Y, Al-Shaer E, et al. On secure and resilient telesurgery communications over unreliable networks. In: Proceedings of the IEEE conference on computer communications workshops (INFOCOM WKSHPS), Shanghai, China, 10–15 Apr 2011. New York: IEEE; 2011. pp. 714–9.
18. Iqbal S, Farooq S, Shahzad K, Malik AW, Hamayun MM, Hasan O. SecureSurgiNET: a framework for ensuring security in telesurgery. Int J Distrib Sens Netw. 2019.

19. Gupta R, Tanwar S, Tyagi S, Kumar N. Tactile-internet-based telesurgery system for healthcare 4.0: an architecture, research challenges, and future directions. IEEE Netw. 2019;33(6):22–9. https://doi.org/10.1109/MNET.001.1900063.
20. Cheriff AD, Schulam PG, Docimo SG, Moore RG, Kavoussi LR. Telesurgical consultation. J Urol. 1996;156(4):1391–3. Erratum in: 1997;158(4):1530. PMID: 8808879.
21. Wagner A, Millesi W, Watzinger F, Truppe M, Rasse M, Enislidis G, Kermer C, Ewers R. Clinical experience with interactive teleconsultation and teleassistance in craniomaxillofacial surgical procedures. J Oral Maxillofac Surg. 1999;57(12):1413–8. https://doi.org/10.1016/s0278-2391(99)90722-x. PMID: 10596661.
22. Lendvay TS, Hannaford B, Satava RM. Future of robotic surgery. Cancer J. 2013;19(2):109–19. https://doi.org/10.1097/PPO.0b013e31828bf822.
23. George EI, Brand TC, LaPorta A, Marescaux J, Satava RM. Origins of robotic surgery: from skepticism to standard of care. JSLS. 2018;22(4):e2018.00039. https://doi.org/10.4293/JSLS.2018.00039.
24. Takacs A, Nagy DA, Rudas IJ, Haidegger T. Origins of surgical robotics rom space to the operating room. Acta Polytech Hung. 2016.
25. Doarn C, Latifi R. Telementoring and teleproctoring in trauma and emergency care. Curr Trauma Rep. 2016;13(1):13–30.
26. Jacobs LK, Shayani V, Sackier JM. Determination of the learning curve of the AESOP robot. Surg Endosc. 1997;11(1):54–5. https://doi.org/10.1007/s004649900294. PMID: 8994989.
27. Ghodoussi M, Butner SE, Wang Y. Robotic surgery—the transatlantic case. Proc IEEE Int Conf Robot Autom. 2002;2:1882–8. https://doi.org/10.1109/ROBOT.2002.1014815.
28. Guthart G, Salisbury JK Jr. The intuitive telesurgery system: overview and application. Proc IEEE Int Conf Robot Autom. 2000;1:618–21.
29. Sugano N. Computer-assisted orthopaedic surgery and robotic surgery in total hip arthroplasty. Clin Orthop Surg. 2013;5(1):1–9. https://doi.org/10.4055/cios.2013.5.1.1.
30. Lim P, Kang E, Park DH. A comparative detail analysis of the learning curve and surgical outcome for robotic hysterectomy with lymphadenectomy versus laparoscopic hysterectomy with lymphadenectomy in treatment of endometrial cancer: a case-matched controlled study of the first one hundred twenty two patients. Gynecol Oncol. 2011;120:413–8.
31. Holloway RW, Patel SD, Ahmad S. Robotic surgery in gynecology. Scand J Surg. 2009;98(2):96–109.
32. Doarn CR, Anvari M, Low T, Broderick TJ. Evaluation of teleoperated surgical robots in an enclosed undersea environment. Telemed J e-Health. 2009;15(4):325–35.
33. Hannaford B, Friedman D, King H, Lum M, Rosen J, Sankaranarayanan G. Evaluation of RAVEN surgical telerobot during the NASA extreme environment mission operations (NEEMO) 12 mission. University of Washington Electrical Engineering Department Technical Report; 2009.
34. Shenai MB, Dillavou M, Shum C, Ross D, Tubbs RS, Shih A, Guthrie BL. Virtual interactive presence and augmented reality (VIPAR) for remote surgical assistance. Neurosurgery. 2011;68(1 Suppl Operative):200–7. Discussion 207. https://doi.org/10.1227/NEU.0b013e3182077efd. PMID: 21304333.
35. Shenai MB, Tubbs RS, Guthrie BL, Cohen-Gadol AA. Virtual interactive presence for real-time, long-distance surgical collaboration during complex microsurgical procedures. J Neurosurg. 2014;121(2):277–84. https://doi.org/10.3171/2014.4.JNS131805. Epub 6 Jun 2014. PMID: 24905563.
36. Davis MC, Can DD, Pindrik J, Rocque BG, Johnston JM. Virtual interactive presence in global surgical education: international collaboration through augmented reality. World Neurosurg. 2016;86:103–11. https://doi.org/10.1016/j.wneu.2015.08.053. Epub 3 Sept 2015. PMID: 26342783; PMCID: PMC5476961.
37. Stark M, Benhidjeb T, Gidaro S, Morales ER. The future of telesurgery: a universal system with haptic sensation. J Turk Ger Gynecol Assoc. 2012;13(1):74–76. Published 1 Mar 2012. https://doi.org/10.5152/jtgga.2012.05.

38. Stark M, Morales ER, Gidaro S. Telesurgery is promising but still need proof through prospective comparative studies. J Gynecol Oncol. 2012;23(2):134–5. https://doi.org/10.3802/jgo.2012.23.2.134.
39. Stark M, Pomati S, D'Ambrosio A, Giraudi F, Gidaro S. A new telesurgical platform–preliminary clinical results. Minim Invasive Ther Allied Technol. 2015;24(1):31–6. https://doi.org/10.3109/13645706.2014.1003945. PMID: 25627435.
40. Gidaro S, Buscarini M, Ruiz E, Stark M, Labruzzo A. Telelap Alf-X: a novel telesurgical system for the 21st century. Surg Technol Int. 2012;22:20–5 PMID: 23225591.
41. Su H, Shang W, Li G, Patel N, Fischer GS. An MRI-guided telesurgery system using a Fabry-Perot interferometry force sensor and a pneumatic haptic device. Ann Biomed Eng. 2017;45(8):1917–1928. https://doi.org/10.1007/s10439-017-1839-z. Epub 26 Apr 2017. PMID: 28447178; PMCID: PMC5529224.
42. Osuoha CA, Callahan KE, Ponce CP, Pinheiro PS. Disparities in lung cancer survival and receipt of surgical treatment. Lung Cancer. 2018;122:54–9. https://doi.org/10.1016/j.lungcan.2018.05.022. Epub 23 May 2018. PMID: 30032845.
43. Anvari M, McKinley C, Stein H. Establishment of the world's first telerobotic remote surgical service: for provision of advanced laparoscopic surgery in a rural community. Ann Surg. 2005;241(3):460–4. https://doi.org/10.1097/01.sla.0000154456.69815.ee.
44. Waterman BR, Laughlin MD, Belmont PJ Jr, Schoenfeld AJ, Pallis MP. Enhanced casualty care from a global military orthopaedic teleconsultation program. Injury. 2014;45(11):1736–40. https://doi.org/10.1016/j.injury.2014.03.012. Epub 28 Mar 2014. PMID: 24810665.
45. Lavrentyev V, Seay A, Rafiq A, Justis D, Merrell RC. A surgical telemedicine clinic in a correctional setting. Telemed J e-Health. 2008;14(4):385–8. https://doi.org/10.1089/tmj.2007.0061. PMID: 18570570.
46. Huang EY, Knight S, Guetter CR, Davis CH, Moller M, Slama E, Crandall M. Telemedicine and telementoring in the surgical specialties: a narrative review. Am J Surg. 2019;218(4):760–6. https://doi.org/10.1016/j.amjsurg.2019.07.018. Epub 18 July 2019. PMID: 31350010.
47. Quintero RA, Muñoz H, Pommer R, Diaz C, Bornick PW, Allen MH. Operative fetoscopy via telesurgery. Ultrasound Obstet Gynecol. 2002;20(4):390–1. https://doi.org/10.1046/j.1469-0705.2002.00809.x. PMID: 12383324.
48. Sebajang H, Trudeau P, Dougall A, Hegge S, McKinley C, Anvari M. The role of telementoring and telerobotic assistance in the provision of laparoscopic colorectal surgery in rural areas. Surg Endosc. 2006;20(9):1389–93. https://doi.org/10.1007/s00464-005-0260-0. Epub 3 Jul 2006. PMID: 16823656.
49. Singh S, Sharma V, Patel P, Anuragi G, Sharma RG. Telementoring: an overview and our preliminary experience in the setting up of a cost-effective telementoring facility. Indian J Surg. 2016;78(1):70–3. https://doi.org/10.1007/s12262-015-1429-y. Epub 11 Jan 2016. PMID: 27186048; PMCID: PMC4848219.
50. Ereso AQ, Garcia P, Tseng E, Gauger G, Kim H, Dua MM, Victorino GP, Guy TS. Live transference of surgical subspecialty skills using telerobotic proctoring to remote general surgeons. J Am Coll Surg. 2010;211(3):400–11. https://doi.org/10.1016/j.jamcollsurg.2010.05.014. PMID: 20800198.
51. Augestad KM, Bellika JG, Budrionis A, Chomutare T, Lindsetmo RO, Patel H, Delaney C, Mobile Medical Mentor (M3) Project. Surgical telementoring in knowledge translation—clinical outcomes and educational benefits: a comprehensive review. Surg Innov. 2013;20(3):273–81. https://doi.org/10.1177/1553350612465793. Epub 30 Oct 2012. PMID: 23117447.
52. Ponce BA, Jennings JK, Clay TB, May MB, Huisingh C, Sheppard ED. Telementoring: use of augmented reality in orthopaedic education: AAOS exhibit selection. J Bone Joint Surg Am. 2014;96(10):e84. https://doi.org/10.2106/JBJS.M.00928. PMID: 24875036.
53. Challacombe B, Kandaswamy R, Dasgupta P, Mamode N. Telementoring facilitates independent hand-assisted laparoscopic living donor nephrectomy. Transplant Proc. 2005;37(2):613–6. https://doi.org/10.1016/j.transproceed.2005.01.065. PMID: 15848474.

54. Fuertes-Guiró F, Vitali-Erion E, Rodriguez-Franco A. A program of telementoring in laparoscopic bariatric surgery. Minim Invasive Ther Allied Technol. 2016;25(1):8–14. https://doi.org/10.3109/13645706.2015.1083446. Epub 11 Sept 2015. PMID: 26360307.
55. Agarwal R, Levinson AW, Allaf M, Makarov D, Nason A, Su LM. The RoboConsultant: telementoring and remote presence in the operating room during minimally invasive urologic surgeries using a novel mobile robotic interface. Urology. 2007;70(5):970–4. https://doi.org/10.1016/j.urology.2007.09.053. PMID: 18068456.
56. Agrawal R, Mishra SK, Mishra A, Chand G, Agarwal G, Agarwal A, Verma AK. Role of telemedicine technology in endocrine surgery knowledge sharing. Telemed J e-Health. 2014;20(9):868–74. https://doi.org/10.1089/tmj.2013.0164. Epub 31 July 2014. PMID: 25078673.
57. Janetschek G, Bartsch G, Kavoussi LR. Transcontinental interactive laparoscopic telesurgery between the United States and Europe. J Urol. 1998;160(4):1413 PMID: 9751366.
58. Micali S, Virgili G, Vannozzi E, Grassi N, Jarrett TW, Bauer JJ, Vespasiani G, Kavoussi LR. Feasibility of telementoring between Baltimore (USA) and Rome (Italy): the first five cases. J Endourol. 2000;14(6):493–6. https://doi.org/10.1089/end.2000.14.493. PMID: 10954305.
59. Lee BR, Caddedu JA, Janetschek G, Schulam P, Docimo SG, Moore RG, Partin AW, Kavoussi LR. International surgical telementoring: our initial experience. Stud Health Technol Inform. 1998;50:41–7 PMID: 10180584.
60. Dupuis CC. Humanitarian missions in the third world: a polite dissent. Plast Reconstr Surg. 2004;113(1):433–5. https://doi.org/10.1097/01.PRS.0000097680.73556.A3. PMID: 14707671.
61. Maki J, Qualls M, White B, Kleefield S, Crone R. Health impact assessment and short-term medical missions: a methods study to evaluate quality of care. BMC Health Serv Res. 2008;2(8):121. https://doi.org/10.1186/1472-6963-8-121.PMID:18518997; PMCID:PMC2464597.
62. Cazac C, Radu G. Telesurgery—an efficient interdisciplinary approach used to improve the health care system. J Med Life. 2014;7:137–41.
63. Cuschieri A, Szabo Z. Philosophy and set up. In: Cuschieri A, Szabo Z, editors. Tissue approximation in endoscopic surgery. Oxford: Isis Medical Media; 1995. pp. 68–81.
64. Soper NJ, Hunter JG. Suturing and knot tying in laparoscopy. Surg Clin North Am. 1992;72:1139–52.
65. Ghorbanian A, Zareinejad M, Rezaei SM, Sheikhzadeh H, Baghestan K. A novel control architecture for physiological tremor compensation in teleoperated systems. Int J Med Robotics Comput Assist Surg. 2013;9:280–97. https://doi.org/10.1002/rcs.1436.
66. Veluvolu KC, Ang WT. Estimation of physiological tremor from accelerometers for real-time applications. Sensors (Basel). 2011;11:3020–36. https://doi.org/10.3390/s110303020.
67. Gonzalez JG, Heredia EA, Rahman T, Barner KE, Arce GR. Optimal digital filtering for tremor suppression. IEEE Trans Biomed Eng. 2000;47:664–73.
68. Zhang J, Chu F. Real-time modeling and prediction of physiological hand tremor. In: Proceedings of IEEE international conference on acoustics, speech, and signal processing, vol. 5, Philadelphia, PA, USA, 18–23 Mar 2005, pp. 645–648.
69. Gomez-Blanco M, Riviere CN, Khosla PK. Intraoperative tremor monitoring for vitreoretinal microsurgery. Stud Health Technol Inform. 2000;70: 99–101.
70. Riviere CN, Jensen PS. A study of instrument motion in retinal microsurgery. Abstract presented at 21st annual conference of IEEE engineering in medicine and biology society, 26 June 2000, Chicago.
71. Garcia-Ruiz A, Smedira NG, Loop FD, et al. Robotic surgical instruments for dexterity enhancement in thoracoscopic coronary artery bypass graft. J Laparoendosc Adv Surg Tech A. 1997;7:277–83.
72. Haidegger T, Sándor J, Benyó Z. Surgery in space: the future of robotic telesurgery. Surg Endosc. 2011;25(3):681–90. https://doi.org/10.1007/s00464-010-1243-3. Epub 22 July 2010. PMID: 20652320.

73. Rayman R, Croome K, Galbraith N, et al. Robotic telesurgery: a real-world comparison of ground- and satellite-based internet performance. Int J Med Robot. 2007;3(2):111–6.
74. Nguan CY, Morady R, Wang C, et al. Robotic pyeloplasty using internet protocol and satellite network-based telesurgery. Int J Med Robot. 2008;4(1):10–4.
75. Arata J, Takahashi H, Pitakwatchara P, et al. A remote surgery experiment between Japan and Thailand over Internet using a low latency CODEC system. In: IEEE international conference on robotics and automation, 2007. pp. 953–959.
76. Sterbis JR, Hanly EJ, Herman BC, et al. Transcontinental telesurgical nephrectomy using the da Vinci robot in a porcine model. Urology. 2008;71(5):971–3.
77. Fabrizio MD, Lee BR, Chan DY, Stoianovici D, Jarrett TW, Yang C, Kavoussi LR. Effect of time delay on surgical performance during telesurgical manipulation. J Endourol. 2000;14(2):133–8. https://doi.org/10.1089/end.2000.14.133. PMID: 10772504.
78. Kim T, Zimmerman PM, Wade MJ, Weiss CA 3rd. The effect of delayed visual feedback on telerobotic surgery. Surg Endosc. 2005;19(5):683–6. https://doi.org/10.1007/s00464-004-8926-6. Epub 23 Mar 2005. PMID: 15776211.
79. Anvari M, Broderick T, Stein H, Chapman T, Ghodoussi M, Birch DW, McKinley C, Trudeau P, Dutta S, Goldsmith CH. The impact of latency on surgical precision and task completion during robotic-assisted remote telepresence surgery. Comput Aided Surg. 2005;10(2):93–9. https://doi.org/10.3109/10929080500228654. PMID: 16298920.
80. Rayman R, Croome K, Galbraith N, McClure R, Morady R, Peterson S, Smith S, Subotic V, Van Wynsberghe A, Primak S. Long-distance robotic telesurgery: a feasibility study for care in remote environments. Int J Med Robot. 2006;2(3):216–24. https://doi.org/10.1002/rcs.99. PMID: 17520635.
81. Perez M, Quiaios F, Andrivon P, Husson D, Dufaut M, Felblinger J, Hubert J. Paradigms and experimental set-up for the determination of the acceptable delay in telesurgery. Annu Int Conf IEEE Eng Med Biol Soc. 2007;2007:453–6. https://doi.org/10.1109/IEMBS.2007.4352321. PMID: 18001987.
82. Lum MJ, Rosen J, King H, Friedman DC, Lendvay TS, Wright AS, Sinanan MN, Hannaford B. Teleoperation in surgical robotics–network latency effects on surgical performance. Annu Int Conf IEEE Eng Med Biol Soc. 2009;2009:6860–3. https://doi.org/10.1109/IEMBS.2009.5333120. PMID: 19964184.
83. Xu S, Perez M, Yang K, Perrenot C, Felblinger J, Hubert J. Determination of the latency effects on surgical performance and the acceptable latency levels in telesurgery using the dV-Trainer(®) simulator. Surg Endosc. 2014;28(9):2569–76. https://doi.org/10.1007/s00464-014-3504-z. Epub 27 Mar 2014. PMID: 24671353.
84. Perez M, Xu S, Chauhan S, Tanaka A, Simpson K, Abdul-Muhsin H, Smith R. Impact of delay on telesurgical performance: study on the robotic simulator dV-trainer. Int J Comput Assist Radiol Surg. 2016;11(4):581–7. https://doi.org/10.1007/s11548-015-1306-y. Epub 8 Oct 2015. PMID: 26450105.
85. Kumcu A, Vermeulen L, Elprama SA, Duysburgh P, Platiša L, Van Nieuwenhove Y, Van De Winkel N, Jacobs A, Van Looy J, Philips W. Effect of video lag on laparoscopic surgery: correlation between performance and usability at low latencies. Int J Med Robot. 2017;13(2). https://doi.org/10.1002/rcs.1758. Epub 3 July 2016. PMID: 27373237.
86. Brower V. The cutting edge in surgery. Telesurgery has been shown to be feasible—now it has to be made economically viable. EMBO Rep. 2002;3(4):300–1. https://doi.org/10.1093/embo-reports/kvf083.
87. Gkegkes ID, Mamais IA, Iavazzo C. Robotics in general surgery: a systematic cost assessment. J Minim Access Surg. 2017;13(4):243–55. https://doi.org/10.4103/0972-9941.195565.
88. Klein CA. Cloudy confidentiality: clinical and legal implications of cloud computing in health care. J Am Acad Psychiatry Law. 2011;39:571–8.
89. Lee DWH, Tong KW, Lai PBS. Telehealth practice in surgery: ethical and medico-legal considerations. Surg Pract. 2021;25(1):42–6. https://doi.org/10.1111/1744-1633.12479.
90. Holme SA, Malinovszky K, Roberts DL. Changing trends in non-melanoma skin cancer in South Wales, 1988–98. Br J Dermatol. 2000;143(6):1224–9. https://doi.org/10.1046/j.1365-2133.2000.03892.x. PMID: 11122025.

91. Dabrera G, Wakeel R. Is the adequacy of excision of basal cell carcinoma related to operator experience? Clin Exp Dermatol. 2007;32:103–4.
92. Murchie P, Delaney EK, Thompson WD, Lee AJ. Excising basal cell carcinomas: comparing the performance of general practitioners, hospital skin specialists and other hospital specialists. Clin Exp Dermatol. 2008;33(5):565–71. https://doi.org/10.1111/j.1365-2230.2008.02710.x. Epub 18 Mar 2008. PMID: 18355357.
93. Talbot S, Hitchcock B. Incomplete primary excision of cutaneous basal and squamous cell carcinomas in the Bay of Plenty. N Z Med J. 2004;117(1192):U848 PMID: 15107870.
94. Lee S, Dana A, Newman J. Teledermatology as a tool for preoperative consultation before Mohs micrographic surgery within the veterans health administration. Dermatol Surg. 2020;46(4):508–13. https://doi.org/10.1097/DSS.0000000000002073. PMID: 31403533.
95. Kanthraj GR. Teledermatology: its role in dermatosurgery. J Cutan Aesthet Surg. 2008;1(2):68–74. https://doi.org/10.4103/0974-2077.44162.PMID:20300347;PMCID:PMC2840907.
96. Di Stefani A, Zalaudek I, Argenziano G, Chimenti S, Soyer HP. Feasibility of a two-step teledermatologic approach for the management of patients with multiple pigmented skin lesions. Dermatol Surg. 2007;33(6):686–92. https://doi.org/10.1111/j.1524-4725.2007.33144.x. PMID: 17550445.
97. Ferrandiz L, Moreno-Ramirez D, Nieto-Garcia A, Carrasco R, Moreno-Alvarez P, Galdeano R, Bidegain E, Rios-Martin JJ, Camacho FM. Teledermatology-based presurgical management for nonmelanoma skin cancer: a pilot study. Dermatol Surg. 2007;33(9):1092–8. https://doi.org/10.1111/j.1524-4725.2007.33223.x. PMID: 17760600.
98. Sohn GK, Wong DJ, Yu SS. A review of the use of telemedicine in dermatologic surgery. Dermatol Surg. 2020;46(4):501–7. https://doi.org/10.1097/DSS.0000000000002230. PMID: 31688234.
99. Moreno-Ramirez D, Ferrandiz L, Bernal AP, et al. Teledermatology as a filtering system in pigmented lesion clinics. J Telemed Telecare. 2005;11:298–303.
100. Whited JD, Hall RP, Foy ME, et al. Teledermatology's impact on time to intervention among referrals to a dermatology consult service. Telemed J e-Health. 2002;8:313–21.
101. Whited JD, Datta S, Hall RP, et al. An economic analysis of a store-and-forward teledermatology consult system. Telemed J e-Health. 2003;9:351–60.
102. Krupinski E, Barker G, Rodriguez G, et al. Telemedicine versus in-person dermatology referrals: an analysis of case complexity. Telemed J. 2002;8:143–7.
103. Massone C, Soyer HP, Lozzi GP, Di Stefani A, et al. Feasibility and diagnostic agreement in teledermatopathology using a virtual slide system. Hum Pathol. 2007;38:546–54.
104. Leinweber B, Massone C, Kodama K, Kaddu S, et al. Teledermatopathology: a controlled study about diagnostic validity and technical requirements for digital transmission. Am J Dermatopathol. 2006;28:413–6.
105. Piccolo D, Soyer HP, Burgdorf W, Talamini R, et al. Concordance between telepathologic diagnosis and conventional histopathologic diagnosis: a multiobserver store-and-forward study on 20 skin specimens. Arch Dermatol. 2002;138:53–8.
106. Berman B, Elgart GW, Burdick AE. Dermatopathology via a still-image telemedicine system: diagnostic concordance with direct microscopy. Telemed J. 1997;3:27–32.
107. Nehal KS, Busam KJ, Halpern AC. Use of dynamic telepathology in Mohs surgery: a feasibility study. Dermatol Surg. 2002;28:422–6.
108. Chandra S, Elliott T, Vinciullo C. Telepathology as an aid in Mohs micrographic surgery. Dermatol Surg. 2004;30:945–7.
109. Sukal SA, Busam KJ, Nehal KS. Clinical application of dynamic telepathology in Mohs surgery. Dermatol Surg. 2005;31:1700–3.
110. McKenna JK, Florell SR. Cost-effective dynamic telepathology in the Mohs surgery laboratory utilizing iChat AV videoconferencing software. Dermatol Surg. 2007;33:62–8.
111. Kantor J. An effective, low-cost technique for photograph and video capture, wireless transmission, and quality assurance assessments for dermatopathology, anatomic pathology, and Mohs micrographic surgery. J Am Acad Dermatol. 2019;80:e69–70.

112. Giambrone D, Rao BK, Esfahani A, Rao S. Obstacles hindering the mainstream practice of teledermatopathology. J Am Acad Dermatol. 2014;71:772–80.
113. Kantor J. Application of Google glass to Mohs micrographic surgery: a pilot study in 120 patients. Dermatol Surg. 2015;41(2):288–9. https://doi.org/10.1097/DSS.0000000000000268. PMID: 25627633.
114. Niamtu J. Google glass: dermatologic and cosmetic surgery applications. Dermatol Surg. 2014;40:1150–2. https://doi.org/10.1097/01.DSS.0000452655.37260.c5.
115. Hamann D, Mortensen WS, Hamann CR, Smith A, Martino B, Dameff C, Tully J, Kim J, Torres A. Experiences in adoption of teledermatology in Mohs micrographic surgery: using smartglasses for intraoperative consultation and defect triage. Surg Innov. 2014;21(6):653–4. https://doi.org/10.1177/1553350614552735. PMID: 25389145.
116. Johansson K, Nuutila L, Virtanen H, Salanterä S, et al. Preoperative education for orthopaedic patients: systematic review. J Adv Nurs. 2005;50:212–23.
117. Hathaway D. Effect of preoperative instruction on postoperative outcomes: a meta-analysis. Nurs Res. 1986;35:269–75.
118. Hawkins SD, Koch SB, Williford PM, Feldman SR, Pearce DJ. Web app- and text message-based patient education in Mohs micrographic surgery—a randomized controlled trial. Dermatol Surg. 2018;44(7):924–32. https://doi.org/10.1097/DSS.0000000000001489. PMID: 29406486.
119. Chee SN, Lowe P, Lim A. Smartphone patient monitoring post-laser resurfacing. Australas J Dermatol. 2017;58(4):e216–22. https://doi.org/10.1111/ajd.12507. Epub 10 Jun 2016. PMID: 27282697.
120. Pozza ED, D'Souza GF, DeLeonibus A, Fabiani B, et al. Patient satisfaction with an early smartphone-based cosmetic surgery postoperative follow-up. Aesthet Surg J. 2017;38:101–9.
121. Engel H, Huang JJ, Tsao CK, Lin CY, et al. Remote real-time monitoring of free flaps via smartphone photography and 3G wireless Internet: a prospective study evidencing diagnostic accuracy. Microsurgery. 2011;31:589–95.
122. Kiranantawat K, Sitpahul N, Taeprasartsit P, Constantinides J, et al. The first smartphone application for microsurgery monitoring: SilpaRamanitor. Plast Reconstr Surg. 2014;134:130–9.

Teledermatopathology

Samantha Ouellette, Phillippe Hans Jean-Pierre, Shelley Uppal, and Babar K. Rao

Abstract Teledermatopathology involves the real-time or static (store-and-forward) transmission of microscopic images to a remote pathologist or dermatopathologist. Teledermatopathology allows for specimens to be expertly analyzed by pathologists all over the country, increasing access to specialist care in underserved regions and countries. Studies have shown that diagnostic accuracy with utilizing teledermatopathology is comparable to that of glass microscopy. Teledermatopathology can lead to improvements in clinical workflow and efficacy, as well as increased job satisfaction and schedule flexibility for specialists. It also facilitates collaboration between pathologists and dermatologists, and serves as a resource for educational and research purposes. Nonetheless, widespread implementation of teledermatopathology is limited by several factors, including variation in image quality of digital slides, costs associated with implementation and maintenance of teledermatopathology services, and hesitancy among specialists. Furthermore, legal considerations, such as licensure and regulations, have also been frequently cited as obstacles. Despite these challenges, dermatology and pathology are increasingly becoming more digitized, especially with emphasis on remote care in the setting of the recent COVID-19 pandemic.

Keywords Teledermatopathology · Pathology · Telemedicine

S. Ouellette (✉)
Department of Dermatology, Rutgers Robert Wood Johnson Medical School, 1 Robert Wood Johnson Place, New Brunswick, NJ 08901, USA
e-mail: sjo55@rwjms.rutgers.edu

P. H. Jean-Pierre
Miller School of Medicine, University of Miami, Miami, FL, USA

S. Uppal
Albany Medical College, Albany, NY, USA

B. K. Rao
Department of Dermatology, Weill Cornell Medicine, New York, NY 10065, USA

K. Nouri (ed.), *Telemedicine and Technological Advances in Dermatology*,
https://doi.org/10.1007/978-3-031-69091-4_8

1 Introduction

Teledermatopathology can utilize dynamic real-time transmission of images or the static store-and-forward model involving the digital transmission of microscopic images taken by a dermatologist and transmitted to remote pathologists or dermatopathologists [1]. With advancements in broadband technology in the digital age, telemedicine has become one of the most important strides in the modern era of medicine, allowing for long-distance patient-to-provider and provider-to-provider clinical interactions [1]. Given the inherent visual nature of histological specimen analysis in dermatopathology, telemedicine lends itself particularly well to dermatopathology, as there are many cutaneous conditions that can be diagnosed, monitored, and treated remotely [1]. During the height of the global COVID-19 pandemic, demand for telepathology has dramatically increased and is expected to continue seeing increased usage beyond the pandemic [1]. Teledermatopathology allows for collected specimens to be expertly and efficiently analyzed by dermatopathologists all over the country, and therefore, has the potential to increase access to care in remote communities that have a shortage of dermatopathologists. Given that skin cancer is the most diagnosed malignancy domestically and globally, and that early detection of cancerous lesions typically correlates with an improved prognosis, implementation of teledermatopathology can greatly improve prognosis and health outcomes. This section will discuss some of the different modalities through which teledermatopathology can be accomplished: store-and-forward technology, whole slide imaging, real-time imaging (dynamic), hybrid, and robotic.

1.1 Store-and-Forward Telepathology

First introduced in 1985, store-and-forward (static) telemedicine was the first iteration of telepathology introduced. Store-and-forward telepathology involves the automatic generation of an image derived from a histological glass slide through a light microscope integrated with a camera, which creates a digital image based on the specimen of interest [2]. The image generated can be of different optical objectives [2]. Images can then be securely shared between colleagues who can view the digital slides on their computer, as opposed to a conventional light microscope [2]. The era of telepathology marks a significant change in the field of pathology (including dermatopathology), as previously histological specimens could only be manipulated and viewed one person at a time, which was impractical and expensive. Store-and-forward technology remains the least expensive modality of teledermatopathology [2]. One notable drawback of store-and-forward usage, however, is the potential for inadequately sampling of a histological specimen. However, this risk can be mitigated by having an experienced and knowledgeable photographer handle specimen collection and digital image creation [3]. Store-and-forward telepathology is also limited to only one field of view, in contrast to whole-slide imaging (WSI), and thus WSI is preferred modality over store-and-forward telepathology [4].

1.2 Whole-Slide Imaging (WSI)

Early efforts to introduce whole-slide imaging (WSI) began in the late 1990s by Ferreira at the University of Maryland Institute for Advanced Computer Studies and Joel Saltz from John Hopkins University, where the first software program was designed to support WSI [4]. It is a newer modality for teledermatopathology and has tremendously improved since its original inception [5]. WSI works by using a robotic microscope and computer software program to simultaneously capture and stitch individual static images of a histological slide [4]. This results in a digital image of much higher resolution than static technology, allowing the receiving pathologist to effectively manipulate the image with different optical resolutions and make annotations [4]. WSI is often used in a hybrid model in conjunction with either real-time (dynamic) telepathology or robotic microscopy, modalities that allow the receiving pathologist to optimize magnification levels and visualize areas of interest within a histological specimen [6]. The live teledermatopathology sessions include the interactive control of microscope by a remote presenter and a viewing pathologist, allowing slides to be viewed in their entirety at different magnification levels and for the viewing pathologist to direct the remote operator to areas of specific interest within the sample [6]. The main disadvantage of WSI is that it requires highly sophisticated equipment to generate higher resolution images, and higher storage and bandwidth requirements to transmit images [5]. As a result, the economic investment of WSI is greater than that of store-and-forward technology [5]. Because of the increased costs, accessibility of WSI is limited to wealthier countries and academic institutions [5]. Nonetheless, WSI is in high demand and further research will likely increase efficiency, decrease cost, and improve accessibility in the future [6].

1.3 Real-Time (Dynamic) Teledermatopathology

Real-time (dynamic) teledermatopathology involves the interactive control of a microscope by a remote presenter and a viewing pathologist, allowing slides to be viewed in their entirety at different magnification levels [6]. This modality can also effectively prevent inadequate sampling, as the viewing pathologist can preemptively direct the remote operator to areas of specific interest within the histological sample [6]. Similar to real-time teledermatopathology, robotic teledermatopathology gives control of the microscope stage, objectives, and focus to the receiving pathologist while transmitting a live dynamic image feed. However, pathologists are given direct control of these features, eliminating the need to dictate verbal orders to a host photographer [3]. Like with real-time teledermatopathology, inadequate sampling is a non-issue in robotic teledermatopathology, as the pathologist themselves control the sampling of histological specimen [3].

2 Advantages of Teledermatopathology

Teledermatopathology allows for the interdisciplinary collaboration between general pathologists and dermatopathologists, which can help reduce interpretive errors and their associated healthcare costs [7]. Errors in the diagnosis of biopsy specimens can lead to treatment delay, which is especially critical in cases of melanoma, where prognosis is largely determined by time of detection and early intervention. A study conducted in 2012 by Ho et al. showed that general pathologists analyzing melanomas had a false negative and positive interpretive error rate of 0.21% and 0.23%, respectively [8]. False negative diagnoses led to melanomas progressing to more advanced stages and subsequently to more costly and invasive treatments. False positive diagnoses, similarly, led to unnecessary treatment and psychological distress for patients [8]. The treatment of false negative and positive diagnoses, furthermore, lead to a total incremental annual cost of approximately $144,756 [8]. Teledermatopathology leads to increased diagnostic accuracy, improved patient outcomes, and reduced costs by improving access to dermatopathologists, particularly in situations with equivocal, complex cases, [7, 8].

Another significant advantage of teledermatopathology is its diagnostic accuracy compared to direct glass microscopy in evaluating skin lesions. Numerous studies have found no significant diagnostic discordance between teledermatopathology and glass microscopy in the assessment of melanocytic, non-melanocytic, and inflammatory diagnoses [9, 10]. Furthermore, studies using static images acquired through smartphones and microscope adapters have high diagnostic compared to conventional glass slide review [9]. Availability of digital slides also helps with the development of image analysis software or neural networks as part of artificial intelligence (AI) to help improve diagnostic accuracy [11, 12]. While this technology is unlikely to completely replace physicians, it can help assist in monitoring lesions or draw focus to regions of particular interest [11].

As a whole, telepathology is a cost-effective modality for both the provider and the patient [13]. Telepathology circumvents costs associated with transporting and shipping glass slides between sites, restructuring personnel, storing glass slides, and optimizing resources such as laboratories and microscopes [13, 14]. While many facilities implementing telepathology are required by law to store glass slides, the costs can be minimized by storing slides in more remote, inexpensive locations [14]. Patients seen via teledermatology also have shorter distances to travel and spend less time overall attending to the appointment compared with patients seen in-person. According to earlier studies, the profitability of telepathology is dependent on factors such as the distance between sites and service level of activity [15]. More recent studies carried out at a two large academic centers calculated a projected 5-year savings of $18 million and $1.3 million respectively following implementation of digital pathology systems [8, 14]. Further studies are required to elucidate the costs and benefits of teledermatopathology in the clinical setting.

Utilization of telepathology has also been shown to lead to improvements in clinical workflow and efficiency. Pathologists have on-demand access to all of a patient's digital slides, allowing for ease of slide retrieval and comparison [14]. One study showed that digital pathology has the potential to increase a pathologist's efficiency by at least 13% [16]. This finding was attributed to time saved on mundane tasks including searching for and retrieving prior cases, error correction, transporting cases, organizing cases, and accessing new cases [16]. In one study, the quickest diagnosis for a digital consultation was only 18 min after data submission, compared to approximately 5–10 days with conventional consultation using glass sides [17]. In addition, digital pathology allows for distribution of workload among a network of pathologists regardless of their geographic location [8]. Finally, since digital pathology decouples pathologists from the histology laboratory and conventional microscopes, it will also facilitate centralization of pathology services, reduce the number of facilities needed, and promote more efficient lab staffing models [8].

Additionally, the use of digital pathology has been shown to increase satisfaction and confer schedule flexibility for pathologists [14, 18]. 80% of general and dermatopathologists reported that the use of digital pathology improved their clinical sign-out experience, and was quicker and more convenient than conventional glass sides [17]. The ability to access slides from any location also increases satisfaction by avoiding the need for pathologists to travel to or reside in remote regions [18]. With more flexibility in a pathologist's day-to-day schedule, there is more time to incorporate other academic and professional activities as well as personal activities that can reduce physician burn-out.

A base of digital slides is also beneficial for fellows, residents, and medical students as a resource for educational material and an archive for research cases. Pathologists can easily organize digital slides into folders for teaching and research purposes, or multidisciplinary team meetings [11]. Currently available software program also now allow for slide annotation and report creation [11]. Digital pathology has become an integral component of dermatology residency curricula in the United States, as the American Board of Dermatology (ABD) has increasingly incorporated digital pathology images into medical licensing exams [19]. It is no surprise that digital pathology has far-reaching implications for dermatology on an international level. In a study by Yeung et al., an international virtual grand rounds curriculum was successfully piloted with teledermatopathology images from Kabul, Afghanistan with the goal of increasing exposure to socioeconomic, cross-cultural, and ethical issues that influence global skin health [20].

Importantly, teledermatopathology allows access to dermatopathologists in rural and underserved areas both in the United States and internationally. This is especially important as the incidence of skin cancer has been increasing in the context of a shortage of dermatopathologists [21]. Approximately half of all trained pathologists currently reside in the United States, where they serve less than 5% of the global population [22]. In resource-limited settings, remote review of difficult cases via teledermatopathology can increase the likelihood of definitive diagnosis and guide appropriate treatment of patients with serious dermatologic diseases. A two-year study at a dermatology clinic in sub-Saharan Africa revealed that teledermatopathology consultation allowed for correct diagnosis in 300 clinically equivocal cases [23]. In nearly 1/3 of cases, the histologic diagnosis was not considered in the clinical differential [23]. Similarly, a study carried out at an academic teaching hospital in Kabul, Afghanistan, showed that static image SAF teledermatopathology in resource-limited settings improves the diagnostic outcomes in a clinically significant way [24]. Final diagnosis from teledermatopathology consultation differed from the most likely clinical diagnosis in 34.7% of cases [24].

3 Limitations of Teledermatopathology

One of the limitations of teledermatopathology is the variation in image quality of digital slides.

Commercially available slide scanning systems scan conventional glass slides at a high magnification ($\times$ 20 or $\times$ 40) and at multiple focal planes in depth to generate a digital slide [25]. The size of a whole slide image (WSI) is dependent on the objective lens magnification of the scanner, the size and number of individual pixels within the digital camera's sensor, and the size and number of individual pixels within the monitor [25]. When digital images are compared with viewing images from microscope, the cellular features can vary in size, ultimately altering what the pathologist visualizes [26]. Some studies have assessed digital image quality by calculating the concordance rate between teledermatopathology and conventional glass slide assessment [27, 28]. Concordance rates between 73 and 100% have been cited in literature [27, 29–31]. Nonetheless, comparison of concordance rates is difficult as other factors such as pathologist experience, case complexity, and sample size can impact diagnosis [7, 32]. Despite the variation in range of reported concordance rates, most studies agree that the image quality of digital slides is sufficient for diagnosis [11, 27–31]. Use of digital slides, however, is limited in discerning inflammatory cell microscopic features on digital slides [28, 33]. Other histopathologic features that are difficult to assess on digital slides include melanocytic dysplasia, parakeratosis, Civatte bodies, epidermal melanin, and microorganisms on Gram and other special stains [28, 29, 33]. Possible reasons for difficulty identifying these specific features include lower resolution, distortion of color, and inconsistent image quality due to human operator error [28, 29].

Another disadvantage of teledermatopathology is the cost associated with more widespread implementation. A whole-slide scanner costs between $50,000 and $300,000 depending on slide capacity, as more expensive whole-slide scanners are able to read several hundred slides at a time [34]. While an image viewer is typically included with whole-slide scanners, additional features are also available which can lead to a higher cost [34]. Examples of these include more advanced image viewing tools, image management platforms, and image analysis software [34]. Furthermore, the need to obtain larger amounts of storage, carry out routine maintenance and technical support, train staff and pathologists, and employ personnel to operate the device also add to the cost of maintaining a whole-slide scanning system [34]. The costs associated with maintenance and operation may be difficult to incur, especially for smaller labs [35]. While cost–benefit analyses conducted at large academic centers have shown projected savings in the long-term with implementation of whole-slide scanning, data for smaller labs is lacking as cost–benefit analyses have yet to be conducted [35].

Legal considerations, such as licensure and regulations, have also been frequently cited as obstacles to teledermatopathology [7]. Licensure requirements depend on factors such as degree of diagnosis (primary versus secondary) and the geographic location of sending and receiving sites [36]. For primary diagnoses, pathologists are required to have a medical license to practice where the biopsy is taken and where the pathologist physically resides [36]. For secondary diagnoses, however, pathologists are only required to have a license in the state where they practicing medicine [36]. Giambrone et al. reported that, as of 2014, 40 states, Washington DC, and Puerto Rico all required out-of-state physicians to obtain a full state medical license in dermatopathology or pathology to use teledermatopathology for primary diagnoses [37]. However, with the onset of the COVID-19 pandemic, many states have waived certain telemedicine licensure requirements, but it is unclear how long these waivers will remain active [38]. Internationally, specific regulations are even more unclear as there is no outlined framework for incorporating telemedicine into the clinical setting [36]. Furthermore, physicians are advised to confirm licensure requirements prior to practicing teledermatopathology to avoid legal repercussions, such as civil or criminal charges [36, 39].

In addition to licensure concerns, lack of regulatory approval by the U.S. Food and Drug Administration (FDA) has also been a barrier towards implementing teledermatopathology [11, 40]. Initially, the FDA stated that they considered whole slide scanners to be a class III medical device, the highest risk classification intended for new technologies [40]. Therefore, to be approved and marketed as a primary diagnostic medical device, whole slide scanners need to undergo "pre-market approval" consisting of rigorous clinical trials to confirm validity and safety in human subjects [40]. In addition, whole slide scanners are required to be reviewed by a third party to correct for interobserver differences [11]. Recently, the Digital Pathology Association negotiated with the FDA and began urging manufacturers to submit de novo applications to obtain class II classification, a moderate risk category with a less rigorous approval process [41]. Certain manufacturers, as a result, have been able to market their products as primary diagnostic medical devices. As the FDA is a highly influential regulatory body, lack of FDA approval is a considerable deterrent for physicians investing in these medical devices [11].

Despite reporting increased satisfaction and schedule flexibility with use of digital pathology, pathologists also express hesitancy with adopting telepathology for clinical practice [7, 11]. A survey of 207 pathologists in the U.S. showed that less than 50% of pathologists utilized whole slide imaging [42]. In this study, the authors attributed limited use of digital pathology to FDA regulations and perception that use of digital pathology is too slow for clinical practice [42]. However, studies on digital versus glass slide diagnostic time have reported conflicting results. One study reported that glass slides were read 22.15% faster and used 23% lower objective magnification on average compared to digital slides [28]. Another study by Vodovnik et al., however, showed that diagnostic time in digital pathology can be shorter than traditional microscopy in the routine diagnostic setting, with efficient and stable network speeds, fully integrated laboratory information management systems (LIMS), better ergonomics, and a larger viewing field [43]. A pathologist's experience using digital pathology also influences diagnostic time, and with increasing experience, pathologists will likely analyze digital slides faster than glass slides [33]. Another important factor that may contribute to physician hesitancy with digital pathology implementation includes lack of experience with digital slides, as conventional microscopy has been the norm for making accurate diagnoses [44]. Due to the nature of technology, technical and network issues are obstacles that can arise during image upload and sharing [45].

4 Future Directions

Despite challenges that still exist with teledermatopathology, pathology is increasingly becoming more digitized, as it increases work productivity and job satisfaction. Teledermatopathology also serves a vital role as an important resource for education and research, with the latter including the ongoing development of image analysis software to aid clinicians with diagnosing and treating skin lesions. With each of the advantages conferred by telepathology, the overall goal is to continue to improve patient care. With advancements in technology, changes in regulation, and emphasis placed on telemedicine due to the COVID-19 pandemic, teledermatopathology will continue to grow as an entity in the field of dermatology.

Keypoints

- Teledermatopathology involves real-time or static transmission of microscopic images taken by a dermatologist and transmitted to remote pathologists or dermatopathologists.
- The diagnostic accuracy of teledermatopathology is comparable to that of glass microscopy.
- With the disparity in access to dermatopathologists, increasing incidence of skin cancer, and emphasis placed on telemedicine due to the COVID-19 pandemic, teledermatopathology will continue to grow as an entity in the field of dermatology.

Conflicts of Interest Ms. Ouelette, Mr. Jean-Pierre, Dr. Uppal, and Dr. Rao have no conflicts of interest to declare.

References

1. Giambrone DRB, Esfahani A, Rao S. Obstacles hindering the mainstream practice of teledermatopathology. J Am Acad Dermatol. 2014;71(4):772–80. https://doi.org/10.1016/j.jaad.2014.04.043.
2. Weinstein RS, Graham AR, Richter LC, et al. Overview of telepathology, virtual microscopy, and whole slide imaging: prospects for the future. Hum Pathol. 2009;40(8):1057–69.
3. Dietz RL, Hartman DJ, Pantanowitz L. Systematic review of the use of telepathology during intraoperative consultation. Am J Clin Pathol. 2020;153(2):198–209.
4. Hanna MG, Parwani A, Sirintrapun SJ. Whole slide imaging: technology and applications. Adv Anat Pathol. 2020;27(4):251–9.
5. Saco A, Bombi JA, Garcia A, Ramírez J, Ordi J. Current status of whole-slide imaging in education. Pathobiology. 2016;83(2–3):79–88.
6. Riedl EAM, Alvarez D, Margaritescu I, Gottlieb GJ. A study assessing the feasibility and diagnostic accuracy of real-time teledermatopathology. Dermatol Pract Concept. 2012;2(2):2. https://doi.org/10.5826/dpc.0202a02.In.
7. Saleh J. Practice of teledermatopathology: a systematic review. Am J Dermatopathol. 2018;40(9):667–70.
8. Ho J, Ahlers SM, Stratman C, et al. Can digital pathology result in cost savings? A financial projection for digital pathology implementation at a large integrated health care organization. J Pathol Inform. 2014;5(1):33.
9. Wolner ZJ, Brahmbhatt M, Stoff BK. Teledermatopathology: a Review. Curr Dermatol Rep. 2020;9(2):123–30.
10. Massone C, Peter Soyer H, Lozzi GP, et al. Feasibility and diagnostic agreement in teledermatopathology using a virtual slide system. Hum Pathol. 2007;38(4):546–54.
11. Griffin J, Treanor D. Digital pathology in clinical use: where are we now and what is holding us back? Histopathology. 2017;70(1):134–45.
12. Pantanowitz L, Valenstein PN, Evans AJ, et al. Review of the current state of whole slide imaging in pathology. J Pathol Inform. 2011;2:36.
13. Meyer J, Paré G. Telepathology impacts and implementation challenges: a scoping review. Arch Pathol Lab Med. 2015;139(12):1550–7.
14. Hanna MG, Reuter VE, Samboy J, et al. Implementation of digital pathology offers clinical and operational increase in efficiency and cost savings. Arch Pathol Lab Med. 2019;143(12):1545–55.
15. Loane MA, Bloomer SE, Corbett R, et al. Patient cost-benefit analysis of teledermatology measured in a randomized control trial. J Telemed Telecare. 1999;5(Suppl 1):S1–3.
16. Stratman C Drogowski L, Ho J. Digital pathology in the clinical workflow: a time and motion study. Abstract presented at: Pathology Visions, Oct 2010, San Diego, CA.
17. Nakayama I, Matsumura T, Kamataki A, et al. Development of a teledermatopathology consultation system using virtual slides. Diagn Pathol. 2012;7:177.
18. Farahani N, Riben M, Evans AJ, Pantanowitz L. International telepathology: promises and pitfalls. Pathobiology. 2016;83(2–3):121–6.
19. Shahriari N, Grant-Kels J, Murphy MJ. Dermatopathology education in the era of modern technology. J Cutan Pathol. 2017;44(9):763–71.
20. Yeung H, Sargen MR, Luk KM, et al. Teledermatology and teledermatopathology as educational tools for international dermatology: a virtual grand rounds pilot curriculum. Int J Dermatol. 2018;57(11):1358–62.
21. De Logu F, Ugolini F, Maio V, et al. Recognition of cutaneous melanoma on digitized histopathological slides via artificial intelligence algorithm. Front Oncol. 2020;10:1559.
22. Weinstein RS, Graham AR, Lian F, et al. Reconciliation of diverse telepathology system designs. Historic issues and implications for emerging markets and new applications. APMIS. 2012;120(4):256–75.
23. Micheletti RG, Steele KT, Kovarik CL. Robotic teledermatopathology from an African dermatology clinic. J Am Acad Dermatol. 2014;70(5):952–4.

24. Ismail A, McMichael JR, Stoff BK. Utility of international store-and-forward teledermatopathology among a cohort of mostly female patients at a tertiary referral center in Afghanistan. Int J Womens Dermatol. 2018;4(2):83–6.
25. Vyas N, Markow M, Prieto-Granada C, et al. Comparing whole slide digital images versus traditional glass slides in the detection of common microscopic features seen in dermatitis. J Pathol Inform. 2016;7(1):30.
26. Sellaro T, Filkins R, Hoffman C, et al. Relationship between magnification and resolution in digital pathology systems. J Pathol Inform. 2013;4(1):21.
27. Al Habeeb A, Evans A, Ghazarian D. Virtual microscopy using whole-slide imaging as an enabler for teledermatopathology: a paired consultant validation study. J Pathol Inform. 2012;3:2.
28. Vyas NS, Markow M, Prieto-Granada C, et al. Comparing whole slide digital images versus traditional glass slides in the detection of common microscopic features seen in dermatitis. J Pathol Inform. 2016;7:30.
29. Lee JJ, Jedrych J, Pantanowitz L, Ho J. Validation of digital pathology for primary histopathological diagnosis of routine. Inflamm Dermatopathol Cases Am J Dermatopathol. 2018;40(1):17–23.
30. Shah KK, Lehman JS, Gibson LE, Lohse CM, Comfere NI, Wieland CN. Validation of diagnostic accuracy with whole-slide imaging compared with glass slide review in dermatopathology. J Am Acad Dermatol. 2016;75(6):1229–37.
31. Leinweber B, Massone C, Kodama K, et al. Teledermatopathology: a controlled study about diagnostic validity and technical requirements for digital transmission. Am J Dermatopathol. 2006;28(5):413–6.
32. Fertig RM, Sangueza O, Gaudi S, Gamret AC, Cervantes J, Jukic DM. Whole slide imaging. Am J Dermatopathol. 2018;40(12):938–9.
33. Velez N, Jukic D, Ho J. Evaluation of 2 whole-slide imaging applications in dermatopathology. Hum Pathol. 2008;39(9):1341–9.
34. Digital Pathology FAQ. Digital Pathology Association. https://digitalpathologyassociation.org/faq. Published 2020. Accessed 1 Oct 2021.
35. Kumar N, Gupta R, Gupta S. Whole slide imaging (WSI) in pathology: current perspectives and future directions. J Digit Imaging. 2020;33(4):1034–40.
36. Cornish TC, McClintock DS. Medicolegal and regulatory aspects of whole slide imaging-based telepathology. Diagn Histopathol. 2014;20(12):475–81.
37. Giambrone D, Rao BK, Esfahani A, Rao S. Obstacles hindering the mainstream practice of teledermatopathology. J Am Acad Dermatol. 2014;71(4):772–80.
38. U.S. States and territories modifying requirements for telehealth in response to COVID-19. Federation of State Medical Boards. https://www.fsmb.org/siteassets/advocacy/pdf/states-waiving-licensure-requirements-for-telehealth-in-response-to-covid-19.pdf. Published 2021. Accessed 5 Oct 2021.
39. Marsch AF, Feinberg JS. State restrictions on the interstate practice of dermatopathology are unconstitutional: the tissue is the issue. J Cutan Pathol. 2015;42(10):669–73.
40. Parwani AV, Hassell L, Glassy E, Pantanowitz L. Regulatory barriers surrounding the use of whole slide imaging in the United States of America. J Pathol Inform. 2014;5(1):38.
41. Ward M. Recommends whole slide imaging manufacturers submit De Novo applications to the FDA for primary diagnosis in the United States. Digital Pathology Association. https://www.prweb.com/releases/2016/01/prweb13163307.htm. Published 2016. Accessed 7 Oct 2021.
42. Onega T, Reisch LM, Frederick PD, et al. Use of digital whole slide imaging in dermatopathology. J Digit Imaging. 2016;29(2):243–53.
43. Vodovnik A. Diagnostic time in digital pathology: a comparative study on 400 cases. J Pathol Inform. 2016;7:4.

44. Evans AJ, Salama ME, Henricks WH, Pantanowitz L. Implementation of whole slide imaging for clinical purposes: issues to consider from the perspective of early adopters. Arch Pathol Lab Med. 2017;141(7):944–59.
45. Pantanowitz L, McHugh J, Cable W, Zhao C, Parwani AV. Imaging file management to support international telepathology. J Pathol Inform. 2015;6:17.

Optimizing Care with Teledermatology

Daphne G. Eckembrecher, Francelia J. Eckembrecher, Sofia M. Perez, Shrey Patel, Zoe Tsoukas, and Keyvan Nouri

Abstract Teledermatology can be implemented for use across a wide variety of dermatologic conditions with the goal of decreasing patient wait times, travel times, exposure to hospital and clinical environments, and the financial burden of dermatologic care on both patients and clinics. The field of dermatology is especially fit for telemedicine because of the visual nature of the dermatologic assessment. As the utilization of teledermatology is on the rise and has the potential to play an essential role in patient care, it is vital to ensure that all patients are receiving optimal virtual treatment continually. Teledermatology visits have the capability to function as effectively as their in-person equivalents if the proper measures and strategies are implemented. Steps can be taken by both the patient and the physician to optimize the efficiency and quality of care that patients receive. These optimization strategies can be implemented before, during, and after patient visits. They include perfecting workflow, technology used for meetings, room setup, security software, organization, and both patient and physician responsibilities before and after visits. These methods are outlined within this chapter and will ensure that both the patient's and physician's time is maximally utilized while optimizing for the patient's understanding and satisfaction.

Keywords Teledermatology · Telemedicine · Optimizing care · Live virtual visits · Patient education

D. G. Eckembrecher (✉) · F. J. Eckembrecher · S. M. Perez · S. Patel · K. Nouri
Dr. Phillip Frost Department of Dermatology and Cutaneous Surgery, Miller School of Medicine, University of Miami, Miami, FL, USA
e-mail: daphne.eckembrecher@gmail.com

Z. Tsoukas
Brown University, Providence, RI, USA

K. Nouri (ed.), *Telemedicine and Technological Advances in Dermatology*,
https://doi.org/10.1007/978-3-031-69091-4_9

1 Introduction

Dermatology is a visual specialty making it well suited for telemedicine [1]. The primary aim of teledermatology is to improve dermatology treatment quality in terms of access to care, timely diagnosis and management, and overall patient quality of life [2]. Teledermatology allows patients the opportunity to receive care with avoidance of exposure to a clinical environment and in the convenience of their home, reduces travel time, wait time, and cost, greatly increasing accessibility [3]. If managed correctly, teledermatology has the ability to function with the same degree of success as in-person visits and uphold high patient satisfaction ratings [4]. It also allows the opportunity to establish interpersonal connections between patients and healthcare providers despite physical distance [5].

Throughout the COVID-19 pandemic, teledermatology implementation rates rose significantly and continue to rise. Since the re-opening of many clinics to in-person visits, analyses of various workflows combining both teledermatology and in-person appointments have been done in order to optimize patient care. One such analysis has shown an effective workflow made up of initiation of a telemedicine appointment by a nurse or medical assistant while the physician consults with an in-person patient [4]. Once the in-person appointment has finished, the telehealth patient is prepped and ready for consultation with the physician. During the virtual appointment, the clinic staff have the opportunity to clean and prep the previously used patient room in preparation for the following in-person patient visit so that it is ready when the physician ends the telehealth appointment. This workflow cycle alternating between back to back in-person and telehealth appointments optimizes both the time of the dermatologist as well as the patient while also increasing the number of patients able to be seen in one day.

Workflows such as this prove the utility that teledermatology, either alone or in conjunction with in-person care, can have on the enhancement of patient care. As the use of teledermatology continues to rise and be implemented into clinic workflows, we hope that this chapter will provide the necessary guidelines that can be implemented before, during, and after telemedicine visits in order to maximally optimize dermatology patient care.

2 Preparing for Meeting

As with in-person patient appointments, preparation begins long before the moment that the patient is sitting in front of the physician. Patient chart review by the physician is recommended before every teledermatology visit in addition to certain telemedicine-specific preparations. This section explores the steps both physicians and patients can take prior to a teledermatology appointment to optimize the appointment flow and patient outcome.

2.1 Physician

Prior to the virtual meeting with the patient, the physician should ensure that they have access to a phone, desktop computer, or laptop in a private area, depending on the technological model being utilized. Teledermatology can take different forms including hybrid (image exchange with phone or video call), synchronous (live phone or video call), and asynchronous (photo exchange) care [3]. The physician should ensure that the software program that they will be utilizing during the session is up-to-date, and that the audio and video work properly. It is also critical that there is high-quality network signal and Wi-Fi so that the session can progress as smoothly as possible.

It is important that the physician has set up security elements and software to ensure that the patient's imaging, data, and personal information is protected. Some of these elements include storage and network security, data encryption, and audit trails. This will limit legal risk and also improve the patient's trust and perception of telemedicine [6].

Prior to the appointment, the physician should also ensure that the room setup is appropriate for the virtual meeting. This includes being in a quiet, private area with adequate positioning. The physician should consider being positioned in a room that has ample lighting either with a ring light or in front of a window [7]. The camera used during the session should be placed at eye level and have high-quality resolution so that the patient has a clear view of the physician.

Moreover, if indicated for the meeting, the physician should ensure that the patient's previous results are uploaded. This includes any previous lab work, histopathology results, or consultation results from other physicians. All previous data and patient history should be looked over by the physician prior to the start of the meeting [8]. This will make the appointment run more smoothly as it ensures the physician is not spending vital appointment time on uploading or interpreting results. Finally, it may be helpful to conduct a brief check in call with the patient shortly before the start of the meeting to ensure that the patient will be ready at the scheduled time of the meeting and that they are not having any issues with the software. Also, the nurse and medical staff should obtain patient consent to be treated prior to initiating virtual meeting [9].

2.2 Patient

To prepare for the virtual meeting, similar to the steps a physician takes, the patient should ensure that they have access to a desk computer or to a laptop. Patients should also make sure that the audio and camera are functioning properly. They should also verify that they have access to the portal and to the software program they will be using to attend the virtual appointment. Additionally, the patient should verify that they are connected to a high-quality network signal and Wi-Fi.

For the meeting the patient should take steps similar to the physician in regard to room set-up. The patient should be in a quiet, private room and should be positioned in front of the camera . The patients should also have ample lighting in front of a ring light or in front of a window [7]. The camera should be placed at eye level and should have high-resolution so that the physician has a clear view of the patient. If the patient is older than 60 years old, the patient should be encouraged to have a second person during the visit.

At least a week prior to the meeting, the patient should upload pictures and documentation to the portal. This includes any images or videos of skin lesions, rashes, burns, blisters, or any area of concern that the patient wishes to discuss during their dermatology consultation. Additionally, when capturing these images, the patient should try to best maximize the quality to make the interpretation as easy as possible for the physician. Methods to improve picture quality can include taking the image at a well lit angle, minimizing distracting backgrounds, and ensuring the camera is focused on the area of concern. Uploading images prior to the scheduled appointment time will allow the physician to review all information and maximize the appointment time as much as possible.

3 During Meeting

Although there has been no significant difference reported in the length of teledermatology consultations as compared to in-person appointments, there are steps that the physician can take to optimize the time spent with a patient during a virtual teledermatology visit [10]. These steps include ensuring patient charts and all relevant information has been reviewed prior to the meeting, in addition to steps that can be taken during the meeting itself that aid in maximizing the short time available during each teledermatology consultation. This section will outline the ways to optimize both patient and physician time during a teledermatology appointment.

One way proven to optimize time during a teledermatology visit is conveying the physician's expectations and patient responsibilities at the very beginning of the visit [7]. These responsibilities may include removing an article of clothing covering a region of the skin that is of concern or having an additional person present to point out any skin lesions. Outlining expectations as such at the beginning of the visit reduces time spent explaining a specific task to a patient without context at different times throughout the visit [7]. Along with outlining the expectations and visit flow, it is essential that if a visit is being recorded (although uncommon), that the physician informs the patient of this, and that consent is granted for the recording [11].

It is additionally important for the physician to communicate details regarding how the patient's images will be used during the visit and what security measures have been taken to protect the privacy of the patient [12]. Although teledermatology has been in use since 1999, the practice is new to many patients and therefore causes concern regarding information privacy and protection of personal information [13]. Not only does assurance of privacy by the physician put the patient at ease but it also aids in building a trusting physician–patient relationship.

The quality of physician–patient communication is crucial in patient satisfaction and outcomes related to treatment compliance. Aside from its virtual aspect, teledermatology communication between physician and patient should be identical to the communication style practiced during in-person appointments and consultations. This includes small talk, verbal clinical assessment, patient education , as well as providing ample opportunities for addressing patient questions and concerns. Maintaining eye contact by looking through the video camera also helps to create a comfortable environment for the patient- despite the virtual nature of the visit [14]. Including these aspects along with an interaction style comparable to that of an in-person visit ensures patient understanding and treatment compliance at rates equal to those seen in face to face appointments [15].

4 After Meeting

Continuity of care is essential for both quality of care and for patient welfare [9]. In regard to optimizing the teledermatology process, after a virtual consultation there are actions that both the physician and patient can take to ensure complete care and follow-up has been established. For the physician, these responsibilities include thoroughly checking out the patient and ensuring that all storage of medical records and images are secure in the patient chart. For the patient, responsibilities include reviewing their visit summary and following up in-person or virtually if any questions or concerns arise. The following physician and patient sections will expand upon the details of each of these responsibilities.

4.1 Physician

There is much variety in the way that the typical check out process can occur after a teledermatology visit. In some clinics, this may include a nurse or medical assistant joining the virtual call to set up the next visit and payment details, while other practices may have the physician themself schedule a follow-up visit or even have the patient call the clinic after the visit to establish next visit details. Regardless of what this process looks like however, it is essential that the physician develops and communicates with the patient the status of their follow-up plan. This communication can occur orally at the end of the virtual visit or can be included in the visit summary or correspondence sent to the patient following the appointment. Cases when this communication is most crucial includes when an in-person follow-up appointment is indicated, for example if a biopsy, excision, or in-person treatment method is needed or when there are signs of significant exacerbation of dermatologic condition. In this case, the physician should ensure that the patient understands that their follow-up appointment will not be virtual and that the patient is comfortable and able to come in-person.

In addition to scheduling follow-up appointments, prescriptions and medication management should also be confirmed at the end of the virtual visit and double checked by the physician afterwards. Even after logging off, the physician should review the patient chart to ensure that all prescriptions have been ordered and if there are any indications for lab work. If in-person laboratory work is needed for the patient, the physician should ensure that this is explicitly communicated during the visit and in the visit summary. The visit summary is an ideal place to include all patient education information including but not limited to, pending prescriptions and their respective pharmacy, laboratory work, treatment regimen, and follow-up visit information. A clearly written and personalized post-visit summary can increase patient education rates and improve treatment adherence [16].

A second key responsibility of the physician, and any individual on the health care team, is to ensure that all medical records and images are stored in a secure and private location following every teledermatology visit. This includes deleting patient images or screenshots from personal devices and ensuring that they are only stored in the patient chart. This also applies to patient images that were emailed to a provider via a personal email account. This responsibility is essential in ensuring that teledermatology meets the confidentiality and privacy requirements set out in the law on protection of personal data [17].

Overall, post-visit physician responsibilities are similar to those of an in person visit and should be carried out in the same timely manner and with the same level of quality. Ensuring follow-up visits, prescription medication, and treatment regimen are established and clearly communicated to the patient is essential to optimizing virtual patient care. Additionally, assurance of patient privacy should be carried out by every teledermatologist by ensuring all patient information and images are deleted from personal devices and email accounts.

4.2 Patient

Teledermatology care can look different for every patient. It is for this reason that patients should ensure any and all of their questions are answered either during the virtual visit or through communication with the physician afterwards. With regards to after a visit, the most important information for the patient includes follow-up and treatment regimen. The follow-up patient responsibilities can be on a spectrum from virtual follow-up visit in six months to urgent in-person assessment. Although the physician is ultimately responsible for ensuring a patient receives adequate follow-up and monitoring, in order to best optimize their care, patients should also ensure that they are educated on and understand the following steps they must take in treatment.

The visit summary is an informative tool that is typically uploaded to a patient's portal or chart that offers information regarding what was discussed during the virtual visit and patient information and treatment going forward. Should a patient have any questions regarding their visit summary or information given during the visit, it is recommended that they reach out to the physician via their patient portal or clinic contact information. It is also notable that many dermatology clinics and services may have different websites and virtual platforms by which they operate. Therefore, patients should familiarize themselves with the resources available to access their own patient information and the methods by which to contact their provider directly.

Lastly, in certain cases of ongoing treatment and monitoring, it may be helpful for patients to continue imaging concerning skin lesions (i.e. pigmented lesions, rashes, hair loss, etc.) and uploading images to their portal or saving these images for their follow-up visit.

5 Conclusion

Teledermatology has long served as a virtual option for the field of dermatology, making it a more accessible, economical, and faster means of dermatologic care for many patients. Since the COVID-19 pandemic, teledermatology rates have increased significantly. Most notably synchronous, or "live real-time virtual visits", appeared to be more commonly implemented than asynchronous visits, such as store-and forward teledermatology [18].

As an emerging field of dermatologic care, it is essential that quality improvement and optimization techniques are constantly being evaluated and implemented in order to best care for patients. This chapter includes the most updated information in optimization of dermatologic care by means of synchronous teledermatology. Aspects of teledermatology patient care begin before the virtual meeting and continue until after the virtual visit has ended.

Methods to optimize teledermatology before patient appointments include: ensuring virtual setup is adequate, private, and functioning properly, and that the patient's chart and most updated information has been reviewed. In terms of patient responsibilities prior to their visit, patients should: ensure their virtual setup is functioning properly and that they have uploaded any images or information to their patient portal that they would like the physician to access.

Methods to optimize teledermatology during patient appointments include: conveying physician expectations, reassuring the patient of the privacy and security measures being taken, and establishing physician–patient trust. The virtual physician–patient relationship is crucial for ensuring patient adherence to treatment and follow-up. Successful methods to build this relationship include maintaining eye contact through the web camera and utilizing small talk and pleasantries [14].

Methods to optimize teledermatology after patient appointments include: ensuring patient follow-up and treatment (including prescriptions) have all been documented and explained to the patient. The "visit summary" is a helpful correspondence that physicians may use to ensure all information is outlined clearly for patients. Additionally, it is essential that following every teledermatology visit, physicians ensure that no private patient information (including images without patient identifying information) remain on any personal devices or email accounts.

The methods outlined in this chapter are just broad guidelines in the optimization of virtual patient care. It is highly recommended that dermatologists continue to monitor and improve their own teledermatology techniques and patient care.

Conflicts of Interest The authors have no conflicts of interest to declare.

References

1. Pala P, Bergler-Czop BS, Gwiżdż JM. Teledermatology: idea, benefits and risks of modern age—a systematic review based on melanoma. Postepy Dermatol Alergol. 2020;37(2):159–67. https://doi.org/10.5114/ada.2020.94834.
2. Eber EL, Janda M, Arzberger E, et al. Survey on the status of teledermatology in Austria. J Dtsch Dermatol Ges. 2019;17(1):25–31. https://doi.org/10.1111/ddg.13729.
3. Ibrahim AE, Magdy M, Khalaf EM, et al. Teledermatology in the time of COVID-19. Int J Clin Pract. 2021;75(12):e15000. https://doi.org/10.1111/ijcp.15000.
4. Cohen JM, Bunick CG, Perkins SH. The new normal: an approach to optimizing and combining in-person and telemedicine visits to maximize patient care. J Am Acad Dermatol. 2020;83(5):e361–2. https://doi.org/10.1016/j.jaad.2020.06.075.
5. Naik PP. Rise of teledermatology in the COVID-19 era: a pan-world perspective. Digit Health 2022;8:20552076221076671. https://doi.org/10.1177/20552076221076671.
6. Thomas J, Kumar P. The scope of teledermatology in India. Indian Dermatol Online J. 2013;4(2):82–9. https://doi.org/10.4103/2229-5178.110579.
7. Prasad A, Brewster R, Newman JG, et al. Optimizing your telemedicine visit during the COVID-19 pandemic: practice guidelines for patients with head and neck cancer. Head Neck. 2020;42(6):1317–21. https://doi.org/10.1002/hed.26197.
8. Dhaduk K, Miller D, Schliftman A, et al. Implementing and optimizing inpatient access to dermatology consultations via telemedicine: an experiential study. Telemed J e-Health. 2021;27(1):68–73. https://doi.org/10.1089/tmj.2019.0267.
9. McKoy K, Antoniotti NM, Armstrong A, et al. Practice guidelines for teledermatology. Telemed J e-Health. 2016;22(12):981–90. https://doi.org/10.1089/tmj.2016.0137.
10. Agha Z, Roter DL, Schapira RM. An evaluation of patient-physician communication style during telemedicine consultations. J Med Internet Res. 2009;11(3):e36. https://doi.org/10.2196/jmir.1193.
11. Arimany-Manso J, Pujol RM, García-Patos V, et al. Medicolegal aspects of teledermatology. Actas Dermosifiliogr (Engl Ed). 2020;111(10):815–21. https://doi.org/10.1016/j.ad.2020.08.008.
12. Stevenson P, Finnane AR, Soyer HP. Teledermatology and clinical photography: safeguarding patient privacy and mitigating medico-legal risk. Med J Aust. 2016;204(5):198–200e1. https://doi.org/10.5694/mja15.00996.
13. Piccolo D, Smolle J, Wolf IH, et al. Face-to-face diagnosis vs telediagnosis of pigmented skin tumors: a teledermoscopic study. Arch Dermatol. 1999;135(12):1467–71. https://doi.org/10.1001/archderm.135.12.1467.

14. Claypool B. Telemedicine and COVID-19: 6 tips to ace your first visit. Wiley Periodicals, Inc., A Wiley Company; 2020.
15. Edison KE, Fleming DA, Nieman EL, et al. Content and style comparison of physician communication in teledermatology and in-person visits. Telemed J e-Health. 2013;19(7):509–14. https://doi.org/10.1089/tmj.2012.0227.
16. Zirwas MJ, Holder JL. Patient education strategies in dermatology: part 2: methods. J Clin Aesthet Dermatol. 2009;2(12):28–34.
17. Moreno-Ramírez D, Romero-Aguilera G, Pasquali P, et al. Position statement of the Spanish academy of dermatology and venereology on teledermatology. Actas Dermosifiliogr (Engl Ed). 2018;109(1):4–5. https://doi.org/10.1016/j.ad.2017.09.004.
18. Loh CH, Chong Tam SY, Oh CC. Teledermatology in the COVID-19 pandemic: a systematic review. JAAD Int. 2021;5:54–64. https://doi.org/10.1016/j.jdin.2021.07.007.

Tele-Education in Dermatology

Soraya Azzawi and Keyvan Nouri

Abstract The social-distancing mandates of the COVID-19 pandemic have radically transformed the medical education infrastructure. While online platforms have been gaining traction for some time, the sudden transition to virtual modalities highlights the benefits of these platforms as well as barriers to effective implementation (Hollander and Sites in NEJM Catal Innov Care Deliv, 2020 [1], Keesara et al. in N Engl J Med 382:e8, 2020 [2]). Given that SARS-CoV-2 is anticipated to enter long-term circulation in the population, telecommunications will likely become a permanent fixture within the landscape of medicine, both for education and care delivery (Kissler et al. in Science 368:860–868, 2020 [3], Ko et al. in Int J Dermatol. 59, 1539–1540, 2020 [4]).

Keywords Tele-education · Medical education · Health professions education · Whole slide imaging · Curriculum design · Flipped classroom

1 Introduction

Despite the global trend towards an increasing burden of skin and subcutaneous disease [5], many medical students received an unfortunately narrow exposure to dermatology even prior to the COVID19 pandemic [6]. Of 33 allopathic medical schools surveyed, 40% reported that dermatologic lectures should be required for medical students [7]. These curricula contained a median of 10 h of dermatology instruction. According to 85% of the respondents, the time devoted to teaching dermatology has either decreased or remained the same over the last 5 years. To evaluate the quality of medical student dermatologic education, Ulman and colleagues administered a 15-item quiz to 85 students in 2014 [8]. On average, students received scores of 49.9% and 43.2% on diagnostic and treatment items, respectively. Inadequate

S. Azzawi (✉) · K. Nouri
Dr. Phillip Frost Department of Dermatology and Cutaneous Surgery, Miller School of Medicine, University of Miami, Miami, FL, USA
e-mail: soraya.azzawi@jhsmiami.org

K. Nouri (ed.), *Telemedicine and Technological Advances in Dermatology*,
https://doi.org/10.1007/978-3-031-69091-4_10

preparation can lead to a lack of familiarity with the management of common dermatologic diseases [8, 9]. Compounding these present gaps in dermatologic education, the COVID19 pandemic has limited opportunities to learn through clinical rotations and conservatorships [6, 10]. From this nexus, tele-education has emerged as an ideal approach to not only preserving, but enhancing dermatologic instruction.

2 Electronic Didactic Modalities

Foundational knowledge in dermatology includes taking a targeted history and physical exam. Morphologic description is one of the hallmarks of dermatology education. Because this proficiency is rooted in visual recognition, it can feasibly be translated into electronic media. Many departments have adapted lectures designed in PowerPoint (Microsoft, Redmond, WA) and disseminated them through telecommunications like Zoom (Zoom Video Communications, San Jose, CA), while also being recorded for future use, creating a repository of knowledge. Online modules or quizzes administered after these lectures can quantitatively assess the educational value of the material and a given student's comprehension of it [11]. With respect to clinical education in dermatology, several online resources are readily available, including the American Academy of Dermatology basic curriculum, Visual Dx, NEJM Photo Challenge and Fig. 1.

Electronic educational media offer several unique benefits. While the breadth of diseases encountered through traditional clinical rotations is often limited by the patient population and geographic location, tele-education enables a broader range of instruction. Dermatoses like psoriasis and mucocutaneos lichen planus have demonstrated unequal geographic distributions [12, 13], restricting knowledge gained through clinical encounters within a given academic or community medical facility. Similarly, exposure to skin of color in clinical scenarios is often dictated by the area a trainee is receiving education in, meaning that medical students and residents are subject to inconsistent instruction in this regard. Pre-existing disparities in clinical training are exacerbated by the well-documented absence of skin of color from dermatology educational materials [14–18]. This conspicuous gap in training results in substandard expertise when treating dermatologic diseases in skin of color patients. In evaluating the prevalence of skin of color among 5026 clinical images from two standard dermatology textbooks, Lester and colleagues found that only 22–32% reflected disease as manifested in skin of color [16]. One study discovered that 47% of dermatologists and dermatology residents believed their training was insufficient to educate them on diagnosing conditions in skin of color [18].

Telecommunications enable the collaboration between experts across distant sites, and by extension, sharing clinical images of rare dermatoses or unique presentations in skin of color. By enabling collaboration between experts across distant sites, tele-education can help address a notable deficit in diagnostic training. Guest lectures via tele-conferencing from renowned experts would bestow residents and medical students with a diverse range of expertise beyond that of their home institution. This interfacing with communities from different academic institutions can facilitate research collaboration and promote the advancement of the field as a whole.

Key Points

- Electronic didactic modalities can create easily accessible repositories of knowledge and address existing challenges within medical school curricula.

3 Virtual Clinical Rotations

Although electronic didactic media afford several key benefits, one persistent criticism is the potential loss of bedside manner and subsequent dehumanization of patient care. The advent of teledermatology directly addresses this concern and greatly augments the field of tele-education. Both synchronous, in which the provider and patient interact in real-time, and asynchronous, in which the provider and patient exchange information in a deferred manner, modalities of teledermatology have demonstrable educational benefits [9, 19, 20]. In response to limitations set by the COVID19 pandemic, the Department of Dermatology at Brigham and Women's Hospital designed a clinical rotation interweaving both asynchronous and synchronous teledermatology to satisfy 12 of the 13 Association of American Medical Colleges Core Entrustable Professional Activities, key proficiencies for medical students to develop prior to beginning residency [21].

Epic, (Epic Systems Verona, WI), one of the most widely used electronic medical record software applications, incorporates real-time, virtual visits with patients. Both the desktop and the Epic Haiku mobile application contain a "multi-provider" feature that enables several remote providers to communicate with the patient concurrently, and have helped preserve trainee education in the wake of the COVID19 pandemic [20]. Under the auspices of the attending provider and with consent of the patient, both residents and medical students can be integrated into the clinical encounter, cultivating vital skills by leading the history taking and conducting a physical examination when possible. If the patient permits, the trainee may volunteer a differential diagnosis and provide an assessment and plan that the attending can modify as needed. Depending on the particular scenario, this also allows the trainee to learn from the attending's approach to clinical counseling and preferred treatment regimens. Following the patient leaving the encounter, additional discussion about the case may be continued in the virtual room.

Asynchronous teledermatologic modalities can also be adapted for medical student and resident education. eConsults describe a specialist providing recommendations about a particular clinical case to an inquiring physician, while eVisits implement store-and-forward technology such that physicians evaluates a case and then relay recommendations to the patient at a separate time. Both of these approaches allow medical students and residents to practice critical skillsets such as describing morphologies, structuring succinct oral presentations and producing differential diagnoses. Through eConsults, trainees may develop the capacity to both give and receive a patient handoff. The offline nature of asynchronous teledermatology offers a distinct pedagogic benefit, allowing the time for trainees to conduct literature reviews exploring novel therapeutic options for rare or refractory conditions. Furthermore, store-and-forward teledermatologic inpatient consultation has been found to have high diagnostic and therapeutic concordance with in-person inpatient dermatology consultation, highlighting the educational value of asynchronous teledermatology [22].

Although teledermatology is a useful educational adjunct, several limitations exist. Firstly, physical assessment is restricted to visual observation, which can impede a trainee's capacity to describe and evaluate a lesion's texture. Teledermatology precludes the performance of ancillary in-office testing, such as potassium hydroxide preparations, scabies mite preparations, Tzanck preparations and Wood's lamp exams. Similarly, opportunities to perform procedure like biopsies, cryotherapy, excisions, flap or graft repair and incision and drainage are hindered [21, 23].

Key Points

- Virtual clinical rotations can help overcome the physical constraints of the pandemic and connect students in remote locations to the expert educators. Although this modality holds promise, it is still limited by incomplete physical assessments and reduced procedural exposure.

4 Teledermoscopy

Given detailed exploration of the technologic advancements relevant to teledermoscopy a dedicated chapter, discussion here will be focused on the contributions of teledermoscopy to tele-education. The value of dermsoscopy as an economic approach to skin cancer screening is increasingly being appreciated. As part of the first consensus-based educational foundation in dermoscopy, a recent modified Delphi survey of pigmented lesion experts resulted in a list of 116 key diagnostic features for resident physicians to recognize [24].

Teledermoscopy describes the use of digital dermoscopic images to enhance remote evaluation of pigmented and nonpigment lesions [25, 26]. Analogous to the classification of teledermatology, teledermoscopy can be divided into synchronous and asynchronous modalities. Digital teledermoscopy refers to the acquisition and transmission of clinical images through non-mobile digital devices, whereas mobile dermoscopy relies on mobile devices to accomplish the same. The advent of mobile teledermoscopy in particular makes image acquisition intuitive and economically viable [27]. Given its ease of use, teledermoscopy has demonstrated moderate to excellent interobserver concordance [25]. Online lectures and case-based learning have resulted in notable increases in diagnostic accuracy when assessing a dermoscopic image [28].

It bears mention that although mobile teledermoscopy is highly sensitive for the detection of skin cancers, it missed a greater proportion of skin cancers when compared to traditional in-person evaluation [29].

Key Points

- Dermoscopy is well-suited to dissemination via Teleeducation and can enhance recognition of malignant lesions and improve confidence in diagnosing benign lesions.

5 Dermatopathology

Historically, the teaching of dermatopathology is a communal experience, whereby faculty leads the discussion of cases on a multi-headed scope shared by multiple trainees. This conventional approach has been precluded by the pandemic, leading to exploration of other forums to impart dermatopathological knowledge from a distance. Virtual dermatopathology presents another avenue through which tele-education can enrich dermatology training [30]. Utilizing digital whole slide imaging (WSI), virtual dermatopathology generates composite images from glass slides scanned at 40× magnification [31–33]. Selected sites of interest can be zoomed in for closer examination without jeopardizing image resolution. To illustrate the presence of microorganisms, scanning can also be performed in 100× magnification. One particularly appealing feature of virtual dermoscopy is the annotation of key findings, which can expedite dermatopathologic pattern recognition for the untrained eye [31–34]. Slides can be uploaded onto a cloud server, forming a space-efficient repository of digital slides. Several studies have attested to the diagnostic accuracy if virtual dermatopathology, which is equivalent when compared to traditional glass microscopy [35–37]. To date, there are two commercial WSI systems approved by the U.S. Food and Drug Administration: the Philips IntelliSite Pathology Solution (Philips, Amsterdam, Netherlands) and Leica Aperio AT2 DX System (Leica Biosystems, Buffalo Grove, Illinois, USA) [38, 39].

The educational value of virtual dermatopathology is reinforced by the findings of several studies [32, 33, 40–45]. Firstly, virtual dermatopathology also circumvents the need for routine replacement of glass slides as they deteriorate with age. Histologic findings of uncommon diseases that are scarcely observed in clinic can thus be preserved for posterity through digital libraries [32, 33]. Unfettered by the number of heads available at a traditional microscope, digital slide libraries can be accessed by an essentially unlimited number of trainees. Enabling remote access from mobile devices is of particular importance for trainees from geographic areas lacking experienced dermatopathologists, and therefore helps eliminate educational disparities [32]. Furthermore, remote access permits education tailored to the needs of the student. In evaluating the access patterns of students users of a digital slide library, Ordi and colleagues determined that 57.5% access requests occurred during the holiday season and 41.9% occurred after work hours [30, 41]. In addition to providing the opportunity for an individualized training regimen, the pedagogical approach of virtual microscopy was found to be modestly superior to that of optical microscopy and preferred by learners [45]. It bears mention that the American Board of Dermatology has "increased the ratio of virtual DP items to glass slides on the exam", highlighting the necessity of integrating virtual dermatopathology into curricula to cultivate familiarity with this technology [30, 31].

Despite its many benefits, virtual dermatopathology is hindered by the lofty cost of the requisite hardware and digital image storing software. Additional barriers to adoption include technical difficulty with scanning cytologic specimens and legal quandaries in certain regions [46, 47]. A plethora of digital slide repositories exist presently to enrich medical student and resident training [48].

Key Points

- Given that many areas are deprived of expertise in pathology, virtual dermatopathology is a tremendous educational asset, with numerous resources currently available for self-directed learning.

6 Procedural Skillsets

Remotely gaining proficiency in procedural skills poses a challenge, but may still be feasible through creative use of tele-education. Instructional videos on identifying surgical anatomy, prepping a patient and suture technique can be pre-recorded [11]; this serves as a valuable educational tool, allowing the student to rewind, slow or pause the video as necessary and individualizing surgical guidance. Moreover, visual learning can be supplemented by numerous commercially available skin substitutes. Further discussion of telesurgery is reserved for its designated chapter in this text.

Key Points

- Although procedural knowledge is unquestionably impacted by physical constraints, teleeducation a provides creative solution to overcome some of these hurdles through instructional videos and commercially available skin substitutes.

7 Residency and Professional Interviews

Dermatology is widely considered to have one of the most expensive application processes. Given the highly competitive nature of the specialty, prospective candidates are often forced to apply to a large number of programs to optimize their chances of matching [49]. In addition to the direct costs of submitting a residency application, candidates face the added costs of audition rotations and interviews. One assessment conducted in 2014 found that the total cost of application per applicant was higher for matched ($11,324) compared to non-matched ($9058) applicants, raising concerns of financial barriers excluding qualified candidates from the field [6, 50].

Transitioning the interview process to online platforms would greatly alleviate the financial burden and stress on applicants, enabling a more diverse applicant pool. Tours of the facility could also be conducted virtually.

Given that trainees spend a significant amount of time in residency training, it is important for them to enjoy the location in which they live. With a growing body of literature highlighting the staggering rates of burnout and a greater emphasis on wellness, it is critical for applicants to be able to experience potential residency locations. Virtual interviews may make it challenging to acquaint oneself with a city's character.

Key Points

- By negating the cost of travel, virtual interviews empower applicants to apply to institutions that may have otherwise been precluded by financial burden, thereby helping mitigate disparities in dermatology.

8 Virtual Society Meetings, Conferences, Journal Clubs and Webinars

Similarly to residency and professional interviews, virtual academic meetings obviate the cost and logistical challenges of travel for participants [51]. Capitalizing on tele-education modalities would reduce carbon emissions, thereby avoiding the substantial environmental impact that professional conferences can incur [52]. While traditional meetings can reach a saturation point, due to venue capacity for example, virtual conferencing enables broader participation [53]. Furthermore, virtual formats are able to accommodate translation into different languages more easily than traditional meetings, sometimes in real-time such as with the First Virtual Cardiology Conference.

A major limitation to consider is that online modalities may detract from organic networking opportunities. Meeting quality is often subject to the robustness of the telecommunications modality being used. Finally, virtual meetings can unintentionally promote groupthink or become dominated by a few opinionated individuals.

Key Points

- Virtual professional events reduce environmental impact and cost of travel while enabling broader participation, although organic networking opportunities may be more limited.

9 Conclusions

Given the visual and tactile nature of dermatologic diagnosis, there have been understandable concerns with implementing tele-education. Technologic advances, in addition to experience gleaned from the COVID19 pandemic, have enabled the adaptation of dermatologic pedagogy to online platforms. Didactics that emphasize visual media such as kodachromes and case-based clinicopathological correlation are particularly relevant. Broader adoption of tele-education can augment curricula by allowing experts to guest lecture and facilitate research collaboration among remote sites institutions. Both synchronous and asynchronous modalities can be adapted to incorporate medical student and resident education, for which teledermoscopy serves as an important adjunctive diagnostic tool. Finally, virtual interview and conferencing platforms reduce participant cost and environmental impact.

Key Concepts

- Teleeducation mitigates pre-existing disparities in educational opportunities, producing well-rounded clinicians in diverse areas to benefit of patients. While foundational knowledge can easily be adapted into this format using current technology, procedural and physical examination skillsets are more challenging to integrate.
- Virtual clinical rotations, interviews and meetings enable a larger and more diverse range of participants while diminishing the environmental impact and cost of travel. In spite of these benefits, accessing professional events remotely can detract from informal networking and collaboration opportunities.

References

1. Hollander JE, Sites FD. The Transition from reimagining to recreating health care is now. NEJM Catal Innov Care Deliv. 2020. https://doi.org/10.1056/CAT.20.0093. Published 8 Apr 2020. https://doi.org/10.1056/CAT.20.0093.
2. Keesara S, Jonas A, Schulman K. Covid-19 and health care's digital revolution. N Engl J Med. 2020;382(23):e82. https://doi.org/10.1056/NEJMp2005835. Epub 2 Apr 2020. PMID: 32240581.
3. Kissler SM, Tedijanto C, Goldstein E, Grad YH, Lipsitch M. Projecting the transmission dynamics of SARS-CoV-2 through the postpandemic period. Science. 2020;368(6493):860–8. https://doi.org/10.1126/science.abb5793. Epub 14 Apr 2020. PMID: 32291278; PMCID: PMC7164482.
4. Ko LN, Chen ST, Huang JT, McGee JS, Liu KJ. Rethinking dermatology resident education in the age of COVID-19. Int J Dermatol. 2020;59(12):1539–40. https://doi.org/10.1111/ijd.15235. Epub 7 Oct 2020. PMID: 33026650; PMCID: PMC7675434.
5. Laughter MR, Maymone MBC, Karimkhani C, et al. The burden of skin and subcutaneous diseases in the United States from 1990 to 2017. JAMA Dermatol. 2020;156(8):874–81. https://doi.org/10.1001/jamadermatol.2020.1573.

6. Oki O, Shah S, Scrivens L, Guckian J. COVID-19: challenges and solutions for the future of UK dermatology undergraduate curriculum delivery. Clin Exp Dermatol. 2021;46(1):171–3. https://doi.org/10.1111/ced.14386. Epub 26 Aug 2020. PMID: 32779782; PMCID: PMC7404844.
7. McCleskey PE, Gilson RT, DeVillez RL. Medical student core curriculum in dermatology survey. J Am Acad Dermatol. 2009;61(1):30-35.e4. https://doi.org/10.1016/j.jaad.2008.10.066. Epub 1 May 2009. PMID: 19410336.
8. Ulman CA, Binder SB, Borges NJ. Assessment of medical students' proficiency in dermatology: are medical students adequately prepared to diagnose and treat common dermatologic conditions in the United States? J Educ Eval Health Prof. 2015;17(12):18. https://doi.org/10.3352/jeehp.2015.12.18.PMID:25989840;PMCID:PMC4536337.
9. Loh TY, Hsiao JL, Shi VY. COVID-19 and its effect on medical student education in dermatology. J Am Acad Dermatol. 2020;83(2):e163–4. https://doi.org/10.1016/j.jaad.2020.05.026.
10. Goh P, Sandars J. A vision of the use of technology in medical education after the COVID-19 pandemic. MedEdPublish. 2020;9:49.
11. Patel PM, Tsui CL, Varma A, Levitt J. Remote learning for medical student-level dermatology during the COVID-19 pandemic. J Am Acad Dermatol. 2020;83(6):e469–70. https://doi.org/10.1016/j.jaad.2020.08.033. Epub 14 Aug 2020. PMID: 32798574; PMCID: PMC7426218.
12. Shavit E, Hagen K, Shear N. Oral lichen planus: a novel staging and algorithmic approach and all that is essential to know. F1000 Res. 2020;9:206. Published 24 Mar 2020. https://doi.org/10.12688/f1000research.18713.1.
13. Parisi R, Iskandar IYK, Kontopantelis E, et al. National, regional, and worldwide epidemiology of psoriasis: systematic analysis and modelling study. BMJ. 2020;369:m1590. Published 28 May 2020. https://doi.org/10.1136/bmj.m1590.
14. Ebede T, Papier A. Disparities in dermatology educational resources. J Am Acad Dermatol. 2006;55:687–90.
15. Nijhawan RI, Jacob SE, Woolery-Lloyd H. Skin of color education in dermatology residency programs: does residency training reflect the changing demographics of the United States? J Am Acad Dermatol. 2008;59:615–8.
16. Lester JC, Taylor SC, Chren MM. Under-representation of skin of colour in dermatology images: not just an educational issue. Br J Dermatol. 2019;180(6):1521–2. https://doi.org/10.1111/bjd.17608. PMID: 31157429.
17. Desai SR, McMichael AJ, Khanna R. Coronavirus disease 2019 and race in dermatology. Dermatol Clin. 2021;39(4):569–74. https://doi.org/10.1016/j.det.2021.05.003.
18. Buster KJ, Stevens EI, Elmets CA. Dermatologic health disparities. Dermatol Clin. 2012;30(1):53-viii. https://doi.org/10.1016/j.det.2011.08.002.
19. Su MY, Lilly E, Yu J, Das S. Asynchronous teledermatology in medical education: lessons from the COVID-19 pandemic. J Am Acad Dermatol. 2020;83(3):e267–68. https://doi.org/10.1016/j.jaad.2020.06.033. Epub 14 Jun 2020. PMID: 32553635; PMCID: PMC7293835.
20. Oldenburg R, Marsch A. Optimizing teledermatology visits for dermatology resident education during the COVID-19 pandemic. J Am Acad Dermatol. 2020;82(6): e229. https://doi.org/10.1016/j.jaad.2020.03.097.
21. Ashrafzadeh S, Imadojemu SE, Vleugels RA, Buzney EA. Strategies for effective medical student education in dermatology during the COVID-19 pandemic. J Am Acad Dermatol. 2021;84(1):e33–4. https://doi.org/10.1016/j.jaad.2020.08.068. Epub 20 Aug 2020. PMID: 32828857; PMCID: PMC7439964.
22. Keller JJ, Johnson JP, Latour E. Inpatient teledermatology: diagnostic and therapeutic concordance among a hospitalist, dermatologist and teledermatologist using store-and-forward teledermatology. J Am Acad Dermatol. 2020;82(5):1262–7.
23. Bari AU. Dermatology residency training in COVID-19 pandemic: transition from traditional to online teaching. J Coll Physicians Surg Pak. 2020;30(6):63–66. https://doi.org/10.29271/jcpsp.2020.Supp1.S63. PMID: 32723455.
24. Fried LJ, Tan A, Berry EG, Braun RP, Curiel-Lewandrowski C, Curtis J, Ferris LK, Hartman RI, Jaimes N, Kawaoka JC, Kim CC, Lallas A, Leachman SA, Levin A, Lucey P, Marchetti MA,

Marghoob AA, Miller D, Nelson KC, Prodanovic E, Seiverling EV, Swetter SM, Savory SA, Usatine RP, Wei ML, Polsky D, Stein JA, Liebman TN. Dermoscopy proficiency expectations for US dermatology resident physicians: results of a modified Delphi survey of pigmented lesion experts. JAMA Dermatol. 2021;157(2):189–97. https://doi.org/10.1001/jamadermatol.2020.5213.PMID:33404623;PMCID:PMC7788510.
25. Lee KJ, Finnane A, Soyer HP. Recent trends in teledermatology and teledermoscopy. Dermatol Pract Concept. 2018;8(3):214–223. Published 31 Jul 2018. https://doi.org/10.5826/dpc.0803a13.
26. Uppal SK, Beer J, Hadeler E, Gitlow H, Nouri K. The clinical utility of teledermoscopy in the era of telemedicine. Dermatol Ther. 2021;34(2):e14766. https://doi.org/10.1111/dth.14766. Epub 21 Jan 2021. PMID: 33421232.
27. Börve A, Dahlén Gyllencreutz J, Terstappen K, et al. Smartphone teledermoscopy referrals: a novel process for improved triage of skin cancer patients. Acta Derm Venereol. 2015;95(2):186–90. https://doi.org/10.2340/00015555-1906.
28. Seiverling E, Ahrns H, Stevens K, et al. Dermoscopic lotus of learning: implementation and dissemination of a multimodal dermoscopy curriculum for primary care. J Med Educ Curric Dev. 2021;8:2382120521989983. Published 1 Feb 2021. https://doi.org/10.1177/2382120521989983.
29. Janda M, Horsham C, Vagenas D, Loescher LJ, Gillespie N, Koh U, Curiel-Lewandrowski C, Hofmann-Wellenhof R, Halpern A, Whiteman DC, Whitty JA, Smithers BM, Soyer HP. Accuracy of mobile digital teledermoscopy for skin self-examinations in adults at high risk of skin cancer: an open-label, randomised controlled trial. Lancet Digit Health. 2020;2(3):e129–37. https://doi.org/10.1016/S2589-7500(20)30001-7. Epub 20 Feb 2020. PMID: 33334577.
30. Shahriari N, Grant-Kels J, Murphy MJ. Dermatopathology education in the era of modern technology. J Cutan Pathol. 2017;44:763–71.
31. Khullar G, Chandra M. Virtual dermatopathology: a potential educational tool during COVID-19 pandemic. Dermatol Ther. 2020;33(4):e13755. https://doi.org/10.1111/dth.13755. Epub 12 Jul 2020. PMID: 32495961; PMCID: PMC7300523.
32. Saco A, Bombi JA, Garcia A, Ramírez J, Ordi J. Current status of whole-slide imaging in education. Pathobiology. 2016;83(2–3):79–88. https://doi.org/10.1159/000442391. Epub 26 Apr 2016. PMID: 27101397.
33. Pantanowitz L, Valenstein PN, Evans AJ, Kaplan KJ, Pfeifer JD, Wilbur DC, Collins LC, Colgan TJ. Review of the current state of whole slide imaging in pathology. J Pathol Inform. 2011;2:36. https://doi.org/10.4103/2153-3539.83746. Epub 13 Aug 2011. PMID: 21886892; PMCID: PMC3162745.
34. Marsch AF, Espiritu B, Groth J, Hutchens KA. The effectiveness of annotated (vs. non-annotated) digital pathology slides as a teaching tool during dermatology and pathology residencies. J Cutan Pathol. 2014;41(6):513–8. https://doi.org/10.1111/cup.12328. Epub 7 Apr 2014. PMID: 24620842.
35. Koch LH, Lampros JN, Delong LK, et al. Randomized comparison of virtual microscopy and traditional glass microscopy in diagnostic accuracy among dermatology and pathology residents. Hum Pathol. 2009;40:662.
36. Mooney E, Hood AF, Lampros J, et al. Comparative diagnostic accuracy in virtual dermatopathology. Skin Res Technol. 2011;17:251.
37. Berger WA, Townsend Kraft M, Murphy MJ, Elaba Z. Randomized comparison of virtual microscopy and glass microscopy among dermatology and pathology residents during a simulated in-training examination. J Cutan Pathol. 2017;44:409.
38. Food and Drug Administration. Intellisite pathology solution (PIPS, Philips medical systems); 2017. https://www.fda.gov/drugs/resources-information-approved-drugs/intellisite-pathology-solution-pips-philips-medical-systems.
39. Food and Drug Administration. 510(k) summary aperio AT2 DX system. U.S. Department of Health and Human Services; 2019.
40. Boyce BF. Whole slide imaging: uses and limitations for surgical pathology and teaching. Biotech Histochem. 2015;90:321.

41. Ordi O, Bombí JA, Martínez A, et al. Virtual microscopy in the undergraduate teaching of pathology. J Pathol Inform. 2015;6:1.
42. Horn AJ, Czarnecki D, Lele SM. Interactive case vignettes utilizing simulated pathologist-clinician encounters with whole slide imaging and video tutorials of whole slide scans improve student understanding of disease processes. J Pathol Inform. 2012;3:34.
43. Dziegielewski M, Velan GM, Kumar RK. Teaching pathology using 'hotspotted' digital images. Med Educ. 2003;37:1047.
44. Kumar RK, Velan GM, Korell SO, Kandara M, Dee FR, Wakefield D. Virtual microscopy for learning and assessment in pathology. J Pathol. 2004;204:613.
45. Wilson AB, Taylor MA, Klein BA, Sugrue MK, Whipple EC, Brokaw JJ. Meta-analysis and review of learner performance and preference: virtual versus optical microscopy. Med Educ. 2016;50:428.
46. Morrison AO, Gardner JM. Microscopic image photography techniques of the past, present, and future. Arch Pathol Lab Med. 2015;139(12):1558–64. https://doi.org/10.5858/arpa.2014-0315-RA. Epub 19 May 2015. Erratum in: Arch Pathol Lab Med. 2016;140(7):618. PMID: 25989285.
47. Farahani N, Parwani A, Pantanowitz L. Whole slide imaging in pathology: advantages, limitations, and emerging perspectives. Pathol Lab Med Int. 2015;7:23–33.
48. Shahriari N, Grant-Kels J, Murphy MJ. Dermatopathology education in the era of modern technology. J Cutan Pathol. 2017;44(9):763–71. https://doi.org/10.1111/cup.12980. Epub 18 Jul 2017. PMID: 28612388.
49. Korman AM, Grant-Kels JM. Applying to dermatology residency: an ethical approach to an inherently unethical process. Int J Womens Dermatol. 2018;4(3):176–178. Published 26 May 2018. https://doi.org/10.1016/j.ijwd.2018.01.001.
50. Mansouri B, Walker GD, Mitchell J, Henderson RA. The cost of applying to dermatology residency: 2014 data estimates. J Am Acad Dermatol. 2016;74(4):754–6. https://doi.org/10.1016/j.jaad.2015.10.049. PMID: 26979356.
51. Pacher A, García Rojo M, Mola S, Torres G, Rioja Alcubilla C. Efficiency and cost—benefit ratio of biomedical virtual conferences. In: Presented at the fifth internet world congress for biomedical sciences (INABIS'98), 7–16 Dec 1998.
52. Raby CL, Madden JR. Moving academic conferences online: aids and barriers to delegate participation. Ecol Evol. 2021;11(8):3646–55. Published 16 Mar 2021. https://doi.org/10.1002/ece3.7376.
53. Lecueder S, Manyari DE. Virtual congresses. J Am Med Inform Assoc. 2000;7(1):21–7. https://doi.org/10.1136/jamia.2000.0070021.

Teledermatology in Skin of Color

Jacob Beer, Francelia J. Eckembrecher, Daphne G. Eckembrecher, Hemali Shah, and Heather Woolery-Lloyd

Abstract Although telemedicine has been used in dermatology since the 1970s, its utility has increased dramatically since the COVID-19 pandemic. While it is assumed that teledermatology increases access to healthcare, it may exacerbate health disparities in certain populations (Bakhtiar et al. in J Am Acad Dermatol 83(5):e345–e346, 2020 [1]). Some skin of color populations may face challenges when it comes to teledermatology (Sanchez et al. in J Drugs Dermatol 21(7):793–794, 2022 [2]). There is an increase in access to younger patients but there continues to be barriers in access in older patients, those with a lower education status, patients that lack computer internet access at home, or have limited smartphone proficiency which may greatly affect some SOC populations (Bakhtiar et al. in J Am Acad Dermatol 83(5):e345–e346, 2020 [1]).

Keywords Teledermatology · Skin of color · FST IV–VI · Access to care

1 Brief Introduction

Telemedicine has been used in dermatology since the 1970s. Its utility has increased dramatically since the COVID-19 pandemic and has allowed patients to continue seeing their providers in the setting of global shutdowns. Teledermatology has improved access to individuals that were may have not previously had easy access to healthcare. Although teledermatology is often regarded as increasing access to healthcare in theory, in practice it can exacerbate health disparities in certain populations [1]. Some authors suggest that the skin of color (SOC) populations may be more vulnerable to health disparities in teledermatology [2]. This is critical to address, as it is projected that by 2050, 50% of the population will be comprised of individuals

J. Beer (✉) · F. J. Eckembrecher · D. G. Eckembrecher · H. Woolery-Lloyd
Dr. Phillip Frost Department of Dermatology and Cutaneous Surgery, University of Miami Miller School of Medicine, Miami, FL, USA
e-mail: jbeermd@beerdermatology.com

H. Shah
Albany Medical College, Albany, NY, USA

K. Nouri (ed.), *Telemedicine and Technological Advances in Dermatology*,
https://doi.org/10.1007/978-3-031-69091-4_11

with SOC [3]. This chapter will provide insights into teledermatology care for SOC patients. We will discuss the challenges, advantages, diagnostic concordance, and future directions. This chapter will review the conflicting research on telemedicine in SOC populations as some studies show improved utilization in SOC populations while others show disparities. Understanding this conflicting data will help us understand how to improve telemedicine utilization in many SOC populations.

1.1 Teledermatology in SOC: Challenges

One well-known barrier to dermatological care is difficulty obtaining appointments due to long wait times; teledermatology has the potential to address this [4]. Teledermatology may offer the opportunity for faster and more efficient scheduling especially for patients who need to be seen quickly [5]. Studies have shown that teledermatology decreases morbidity and mortality and enhances the quality of dermatologic care [4]. However, some barriers to teledermatology access include older age, education status, and lack of home internet access. In contrast, certain younger skin of color populations are more likely to use telemedicine for their medical care than Asians, non-English language speakers, and Medicaid users [6].

1.1.1 Desktop/Laptop Portals for Telehealth

Teledermatology has the potential to exacerbate disparities for certain populations, especially for SOC patients [1, 5]. Having reliable home internet access has been reported in certain populations in the US. One study reported African American and Hispanic patients owned computers but were less likely to have broadband internet compared to the national average [7]. In 2019, 26% of Americans earning less than $30,000 per year lacked high quality internet access and relied on their smartphones [1]. Furthermore, 37% of adults living in rural areas and 25% of adults in urban areas lack broadband internet [5]. In New York City alone, 50% of low-income households lack home internet access [1]. Brownsville, a city in Miami-Dade County with predominantly African American residents, reported only 51% of households as having home internet subscriptions between 2015 and 2019 compared to 80% in the overall population [2]. SOC populations may be at risk since areas with lower rates of home internet access often have higher proportion of SOC residents.

1.1.2 Smartphones Use in SOC

Although SOC patients are less likely to have desktop internet access, 94% of Hispanic and 94% of Black individuals use their smartphones for internet access [8]. According to the Pew Research Center around 73% of both Hispanic and Black smartphone users use their phones to research health conditions. Even though 79%

of Latinx and 80% of Black users own smartphones, lower-income smartphone users are more likely to cancel or discontinue service due to cost [9].

1.1.3 Telemedicine in SOC

A primary care study with a cohort of 148,402 patients looked at telemedicine completed visits. Asian race, non-English language as the patient's preferred language, and Medicaid were independently associated with fewer completed telemedicine visits [6]. Older age, female sex, Black race, Latinx ethnicity, and lower household income were associated with lower use of video for telemedicine care [6]. Studies have explored reasons for telemedicine utilization disparities. Some reasons offered were decreased access, cultural and community norms, decreased preferences for digital resources, and mistrust [9].

1.2 Teledermatology in SOC: Advantages

Although some studies have shown underutilization of telemedicine in SOC populations, other studies have shown greater utilization in this population. A retrospective chart review was conducted at the University of Massachusetts during the months of May and June of 2019 and 2020 [10]. The study showed that telehealth visits had lower no-show rates compared to in-person visits and that the greatest reduction was seen in African American, Latinx, and primary non-English speaking patients. These findings suggest that in University of Massachusetts hospital system, offering telemedicine may increase access to healthcare for African American, Latinx, and primary non-English speaking patients. Additionally, the study also noted that there was an increase in Medicaid enrollees seeking dermatologic care via telemedicine visits [10].

Another review examining the impact of teledermatology on healthcare disparities described how a California Medicaid-managed care plan found a 64% increase in patients visiting dermatologists [4]. The same study also confirmed that Medicaid-insured patients had increased access to dermatologic care [4]. Another retrospective cohort study in Connecticut demonstrated that teledermatology decreased the no-show rates among Medicaid-insured patients from 84 to 24% [4].

1.2.1 Dermatology Specific Limitations of Telehealth

Equity in teledermatology is also impacted by patients' camera quality. When a patient submits an image, it is crucial that they have a clear picture, as the dermatologist is relying on this visual to examine the lesion and provide a diagnosis. In a systematic review conducted in Australia, it was reported that teledermatological accuracy was 66% for poor quality images compared to 87% with adequate quality images [11]. The authors noted that image quality increased significantly with newer phone cameras [11].

1.2.2 Telemedicine Exposure/Education in Residency Training

Telemedicine is not a milestone in dermatology per the Accreditation Council of Graduate Medical Education (ACGME) as of the 2020 Milestones National Report, which is the most recently available for dermatology [12]. Seven specialties mention utilizing telehealth or telemedicine in their supplemental milestone guides, including Surgery, Transitional Year, Regional Anesthesiology and Acute Pain Management, Pathology, Hospice and Palliative Medicine, and Addiction Medicine. A full analysis of the ACGME milestones revealed that only Child and Adolescent Psychiatry included "telehealth" in the document [13].

With the lack of requirement or recommendation from the residency training governing body, exposure to telemedicine during dermatology residency may be limited which could hamper residents' comfort level and diagnostic accuracy. The resident may feel less prepared for these types of encounters and the resident may be less prepared. Residents that are not exposed or have limited exposure to SOC patients during residency, both in-person and through telemedicine may not feel comfortable seeing these patients. It is important to have these encounters for their future as dermatologists.

Studies have shown there is value to the implementation of teledermatology into dermatology residency programs through providing care and dermatologic training for residents [14]. This value stems from enhanced learning opportunities via increased case volume with the ability to review with attendings with less time constraints, particularly during the COVID-19 pandemic [14]. Many residency programs have modified telehealth clinics so that residents have the opportunity to participate in enriching clinical experiences [15]. Moreover, the University of California reported that having virtual consults with residents, attendings, and patients was an effective way to educate dermatology residents [14]. Overall, education with teledermatology is complex but undergoing major improvements secondary to the pandemic. Further research is warranted to examine the scope of telemedicine education within dermatology residency.

1.3 Diagnostic Concordance

Diagnostic concordance, or agreement in diagnoses between teledermatology and in-person visits, is important in teledermatology; numerous studies have analyzed this concept in various patient populations. A meta-analysis from 2021 identified that diagnostic concordance in teledermatology is significantly lower than in-person diagnoses, suggesting that there is room for improvement in teledermatology [16]. The study also highlighted that during teledermatology visits, dermatologists are more likely to order biopsies that may be unnecessary due to concerns of missing a malignancy or due to inadequate visualization of a rash [16].

In contrast, another systematic review suggested that diagnostic concordance is comparable between teledermatology and in-person consultations. This study looked specifically at skin cancer diagnosis and wound management. Despite concordance demonstrated in this study, subjective clinician confidence remained lower in teledermatology [17]. This may be due to concerns about misdiagnosis, legal repercussions, or due to the lack of information about long-term outcomes with teledermatological management [17].

While concordance has shown varying results overall, a limited number of these studies look at different. One prospective study including different racial/ethnic groups looked at the accuracy of store- and forward teledermatology. Photographs were taken by patients and sent to clinicians along with a written history of present illness and no live interaction [18]. This study reported excellent diagnostic concordance between in-person and teledermatology. In this study, 13.1% of subjects were Black (1.9%), Latino (7.8%), Asian (1.5%), or Other (1.9%). In another prospective study also evaluating store- and forward teledermatology, the reliability, diagnosis, and management recommendations were assessed [19]. Of 232 patients, 47% of the patients were FST I–III and 53% were FST IV–VI. The study revealed that the concordance among diagnosis, diagnostic testing, and clinic-based therapy were similar for both groups which is a promising finding [19].

1.4 Future Directions

The demand for dermatologic care is growing; however, there is an inadequate supply of dermatologists, contributing to the widening gap in health care access. Teledermatology may be able to minimize this gap by increasing access to care [4]. Teledermatology can increase access to dermatology care therefore, it should be of increased priority in dermatology residency training. Dermatologic training with SOC continues to improve [1]. Adding teledermatology to dermatology training may increase access for dermatologic care for some SOC patients.

2 Conclusion

Teledermatology has changed how dermatology is practiced and it has the potential to positively impact patients. Patients that are Fitzpatrick IV–VI may benefit from teledermatological visits but there are many barriers that need to be addressed. Some studies suggest that for some younger SOC populations telehealth increases access as younger patients have better understanding of how to navigate the internet [20]. In other studies some racial/ethnic groups may underutilize telehealth visit. It is important to note that the impact of telehealth on healthcare access is nuanced and cannot be generalized across all SOC populations.

Conflicts of Interest The authors have no conflicts of interest to declare.

References

1. Bakhtiar M, Elbuluk N, Lipoff JB. The digital divide: how COVID-19's telemedicine expansion could exacerbate disparities. J Am Acad Dermatol. 2020;83(5):e345–6.
2. Sanchez C, et al. Teledermatology and skin of color patients. J Drugs Dermatol. 2022;21(7):793–4.
3. Nijhawan RI, Jacob SE, Woolery-Lloyd H. Skin of color education in dermatology residency programs: does residency training reflect the changing demographics of the United States? J Am Acad Dermatol. 2008;59(4):615–8.
4. Maddukuri S, Patel J, Lipoff JB. Teledermatology addressing disparities in health care access: a review. Curr Dermatol Rep. 2021;10(2):40–7.
5. Yeboah CB, et al. The impact of COVID-19 on teledermatology: a review. Dermatol Clin. 2021;39(4):599–608.
6. Eberly LA, et al. Patient characteristics associated with telemedicine access for primary and specialty ambulatory care during the COVID-19 pandemic. JAMA Netw Open. 2020;3(12): e2031640.
7. Hadeler EK, Beer J, Nouri K. Teledermatology: improving access or widening healthcare disparities? J Drugs Dermatol. 2020;19(12):1248.
8. Atske S, Perrin A. Home broadband adoption, computer ownership vary by race, ethnicity in the U.S. Pew Research Center; 2021.
9. Haynes N, et al. "Can you see my screen?" Addressing racial and ethnic disparities in telehealth. Curr Cardiovasc Risk Rep. 2021;15(12):23.
10. Franciosi EB, et al. Understanding the impact of teledermatology on no-show rates and health care accessibility: a retrospective chart review. J Am Acad Dermatol. 2021;84(3):769–71.
11. Coustasse A, et al. Use of teledermatology to improve dermatological access in rural areas. Telemed J E Health. 2019;25(11):1022–32.
12. Education ACGME. Dermatology milestones. Chicago, IL; 2020.
13. Pourmand A, et al. Lack of telemedicine training in academic medicine: are we preparing the next generation? Telemed J E Health. 2021;27(1):62–7.
14. Mahmood F, et al. Teledermatology utilization and integration in residency training over the COVID-19 pandemic. J Cutan Med Surg. 2022;26(2):135–42.
15. Svoboda SA, et al. Inspired by COVID-19 isolation: evolving educational techniques in dermatology residency programs. Clin Dermatol. 2021;39(1):41–4.
16. Bastola M, Locatis C, Fontelo P. Diagnostic reliability of in-person versus remote dermatology: a meta-analysis. Telemed J E Health. 2021;27(3):247–50.
17. Trettel A, Eissing L, Augustin M. Telemedicine in dermatology: findings and experiences worldwide—a systematic literature review. J Eur Acad Dermatol Venereol. 2018;32(2):215–24.
18. Clarke EL, et al. The utility of teledermatology in the evaluation of skin lesions. J Telemed Telecare. 2023;29(5):382–9.
19. Altieri L, et al. Interobserver reliability of teledermatology across all Fitzpatrick skin types. J Telemed Telecare. 2017;23(1):68–73.
20. Evans YN, et al. Using telemedicine to reach adolescents during the COVID-19 pandemic. J Adolesc Health. 2020;67(4):469–71.

The Effect of Teledermatology on Access to Care

Edward Hadeler and Keyvan Nouri

Abstract The use of teledermatology has rapidly increased during the COVID-19 pandemic. While teledermatology presents promise, concerns over its impact on health care disparities for underserved populations have arisen. In this chapter, we discuss the early usage of telemedicine, including the populations that have historically utilized the service least. We then discuss data describing the impact of teledermatology on healthcare access across practices that have recently adopted teledermatology during the pandemic. We expand upon the various barriers patients may face in accessing a teledermatology appointment. We then discuss limitations to provider implementation of telemedicine that may exacerbate disparities in care for patients. Finally, we describe the necessary steps that must be taken to ensure equitable digital care moving forward.

Keywords Access to care · Health equity · Teledermatology · Telemedicine · Technology · Digital divide · Underserved · Barriers to care · Disparities · Healthcare access

1 Access to Care and Teledermatology: A Historical Perspective

Underserved patients struggle to obtain access to dermatologic care. Lower socioeconomic status, place of residence, and race/ethnicity have all been linked with reduced access to in-person care [1].

Despite a recent surge in its use, teledermatology is one of the earlier technological advancements of dermatology, with its use dating back to the mid-1990s [2]. Teledermatology was developed with the goal of extending care to underserved populations, showing promise in reducing patient travel and waiting times, triaging dermatology visits, and improving access to care for underserved populations [2].

E. Hadeler (✉) · K. Nouri
Miller School of Medicine, University of Miami, Miami, USA
e-mail: ehadeler@gmail.com

K. Nouri (ed.), *Telemedicine and Technological Advances in Dermatology*,
https://doi.org/10.1007/978-3-031-69091-4_12

In one instance, teledermatology was effectively used in a community setting to triage care for a patient with Reed Syndrome [3]. Despite its potential promise and goals, national data from the Census Bureau's 2011 Computer and Use Supplement Survey, which includes data from over 53,000 households in the United States, demonstrated that historically underserved populations were some of the least likely to use telemedicine [4]. Survey participants with an income of less than $25,000, no high school diploma, inhabitants of rural areas, and those over the age of 65, were least likely to use telemedicine [4]. A study conducted by George Washington University later confirmed these results [5]. While they found a dramatic increase in the use of telemedicine between 2013 and 2016 across multiple population groups, including patients with limited mobility (including people with self-reported physical or mental health concerns that limit their activities and Medicare beneficiaries younger than 65), underserved patients including Medicaid, low-income, and rural populations still utilized telemedicine the least [5]. One potential barrier to the early adoption of telemedicine may be attributed to the simple lack of offering of telemedicine services. In 2016, the American Telemedicine Association found that only 38% of community health centers, a significant care provider for underserved populations, offered telemedicine services [5, 6]. Further, Park et al. highlights that policies may be necessary to incentivize providers and health systems to increase telemedicine use, including financial incentives, organizational culture shifts to accept telemedicine, and removing consumer barriers such as telemedicine copayments for low-income populations [5].

2 Access to Care and Teledermatology: Revisiting the Topic During COVID-19

With the onset of the COVID-19 pandemic in March 2020, emergency legislative changes expanded the implementation and use of teledermatology across practices. The increased utilization of telemedicine provided researchers a unique opportunity to compare access to virtual care with in-person care, evaluating its impact on underserved populations.

Studies have provided varying results on the influence of technology on healthcare access. At UMass Memorial Hahnemann, Franciosi et al. compared no-show rates for in-person visits in 2018 to telemedicine visits in 2020. They documented increased access to appointments for Black, Latinx, and non-English speaking patients [7]. Furthermore, a higher percentage of Medicaid patients also accessed telemedicine appointments compared to in-person care. Given that lack of access to private transportation, childcare, and busy work schedules can decrease in-person attendance for underserved communities [7, 8], Franciosi et al. postulate that telemedicine may provide a suitable option that is readily accepted by patients if offered [7].

On the other hand, studies showed that telemedicine worsened access to care for certain populations. Blundell et al. retrospectively compared pediatric teledermatology visits in 2020 with in-person appointments in 2019 and found that Spanish-speaking patients had scheduled significantly fewer telemedicine appointments in 2020 (9% vs. 5% [$p < 0.001$]). Concerningly, Spanish-speaking patients lacked many of the necessary key items to successfully coordinating a virtual care visit. These include having an email address documented in their health record and access to an activated online patient portal (45% vs. 62% [$p = 0.017$], and 23% vs. 66% [$p < 0.001$], respectively) [9]. Additionally, Chunara et al. highlighted that Black patients had a significantly lower odds of accessing telemedicine appointments compared to White patients (OR 0.6, 95% CI: 0.58–0.63]) [10]. However, since the researchers did not compare these results to the odds of accessing in-person care, it is unclear if the odds of accessing telemedicine was better or worse than accessing in-person care for Black patients.

3 Barriers to Digital Care

Overall, the use of telemedicine across practices surfaced concerns regarding its impact on healthcare access for underserved populations. Specifically, researchers termed this disparate access to technology the "digital divide", which ultimately describes the varying use of technology among patients of diverse socioeconomic, racial, ethnic, financial, and language groups [10]. Furthermore, patient's digital literacy, the ability to which they can effectively utilize and access information through technology, also varies across demographic groups [10] and studies have reported that patients from underserved communities have lower digital literacy [11].

Multiple factors must be considered in understanding differences in healthcare access across populations. While access to technology has increased in 2021, with 85% of the population reported to own a smartphone by the Pew Research Center [12], an estimated 21 million people in the United States lack access to high-quality internet [13, 14].

Furthermore, as the Blundell et al. study suggests, lacking access to patient portals may result in barriers to coordinating virtual care across populations. Health portals are online platforms where patients can access personal health information, including visit summaries, lab results, medication information, appointments, and messages with healthcare staff. Studies have highlighted that underserved patients are less likely to have access to healthcare portals, including patients with Medicaid insurance and those without a high school diploma [15]. Portal designs that fail to account for patients' language and cultural needs may contribute to their variable usage, as one study highlighted frustration with designs as a barrier to portal usage in a diverse study population [16].

Lack of parity in reimbursement for phone and video visits may also serve as a barrier to providers adopting telemedicine, subsequently decreasing access to care for patients [17]. Eberly et al. discussed in their study that patients who utilized video visits over telephone only visits were less likely to be Black and more likely to have a higher median household income [17]. As Park et al. previously highlighted, lack of financial incentives for providers continues to prohibit equal access to virtual care [5]. Without equal reimbursement for these visits, providers are less likely to accept telephone only visits, even if it is the only form of virtual visit a patient has access to.

4 Steps for Equitable Digital Care Moving Forward

Given its promise and the continued expansion of technology development in the healthcare space, we anticipate the use of teledermatology to continue to expand beyond the pandemic. However, it is essential that the continued implementation of technology into the healthcare space does not create new or exacerbate previously existing barriers to care for underserved populations. Ensuring equal access to virtual care will be an ongoing task for the years to come, and will require changes on a technology design, staffing, financial, and policy level to ensure its success.

Patient health portals should be designed for ease of use across multiple populations, accounting for digital literacy, cultural and language needs of patients. Accounting for patient preference for online communication modality is also a necessity in improving access to remote dermatologic care. For example, studies have reported that certain patient populations, including Spanish-speaking patients are less likely to engage in patient portal communications and may prefer text messaging [18]. Therefore, utilizing text messaging may serve as a more accessible line of communication for connecting with underserved patients.

Staffing clinics with information technology (IT) staff may prove beneficial in assisting patients with low digital literacy access virtual appointments. A study in San Diego demonstrated that IT members on their staff were beneficial in providing virtual care to underserved communities, assisting patients in accessing virtual visits and providing technical assistance as needed [19].

Policy changes can improve digital care for providers and patients. With the expanding use of technology in healthcare, it is important that policymakers continue to identify ways to expand access to the internet for all populations. Furthermore, providing improved financial incentives and parity across virtual visit types may encourage providers to utilize teledermatology and provide it as an option to underserved patients who request it. Extending lifted regulations on state-level licensure requirements that emerged from the pandemic will ensure patients from rural areas can access virtual care across state borders beyond the pandemic.

As the digital world continues to evolve, it is essential that we continue to explore ways to leverage technology to improve delivery of care for underserved populations.

References

1. Cortez JL, Vasquez J, Wei ML. The impact of demographics, socioeconomics, and health care access on melanoma outcomes. J Am Acad Dermatol. 2021;84(6):1677–83.
2. Tensen E, van der Heijden JP, Jaspers MWM, Witkamp L. Two decades of teledermatology: current status and integration in national healthcare systems. Curr Dermatol Rep. 2016;5:96–104.
3. Da Silva DM, Roth RR, Simpson CL. Teledermatology leading to an important diagnosis in an underserved clinic. Dermatol Online J. 2018;24(4).
4. Exploring the Digital Nation: America's Online Experience.
5. Park J, Erikson C, Han X, Iyer P. Are state telehealth policies associated with the use of telehealth services among underserved populations? Health Aff (Millwood). 2018;37(12):2060–8.
6. Washington J. Survey reveals strong demand for telehealth despite access and cost confusion [Internet]. 2016. Available from: http://www.americantelemed.org/blogs/jessica-washington/2016/10/04/wego-ata-survey-results.
7. Franciosi EB, Tan AJ, Kassamali B, O'Connor DM, Rashighi M, LaChance AH. Understanding the impact of teledermatology on no-show rates and health care accessibility: a retrospective chart review. J Am Acad Dermatol. 2021;84(3):769–71.
8. Sharp DJ, Hamilton W. Non-attendance at general practices and outpatient clinics. BMJ. 2001;323(7321):1081–2.
9. Blundell AR, Kroshinsky D, Hawryluk EB, Das S. Disparities in telemedicine access for Spanish-speaking patients during the COVID-19 crisis. Pediatr Dermatol. 2021;38(4):947–9.
10. Chunara R, Zhao Y, Chen J, Lawrence K, Testa PA, Nov O, et al. Telemedicine and healthcare disparities: a cohort study in a large healthcare system in New York City during COVID-19. J Am Med Inform Assoc. 2021;28(1):33–41.
11. Chang BL, Bakken S, Brown SS, Houston TK, Kreps GL, Kukafka R, et al. Bridging the digital divide: reaching vulnerable populations. J Am Med Inform Assoc. 2004;11(6):448–57.
12. Pew Research Center. Mobile fact sheet [Internet]. Available from: https://www.pewresearch.org/internet/fact-sheet/mobile/.
13. Monica A. Mobile technology and home broadband 2019. [Internet]. Pew Research Center. Available from: https://www.pewresearch.org/internet/2019/06/13/mobile-technology-andhome-broadband-2019/.
14. Rodriguez JA, Clark CR, Bates DW. Digital health equity as a necessity in the 21st century cures act era. JAMA. 2020;323(23):2381–2.
15. Anthony DL, Campos-Castillo C, Lim PS. Who isn't using patient portals and why? Evidence and implications from a national sample of US adults. Health Aff. 2018;37(12):1948–54.
16. Sarkar U, Gourley GI, Lyles CR, Tieu L, Clarity C, Newmark L, et al. Usability of commercially available mobile applications for diverse patients. J Gen Intern Med. 2016;31(12):1417–26.
17. Eberly LA, Khatana SAM, Nathan AS, Snider C, Julien HM, Deleener ME, et al. Telemedicine outpatient cardiovascular care during the COVID-19 pandemic: bridging or opening the digital divide? Circulation. 2020;142(5):510–2.
18. Amin MD, Bundogji NK, Zamora SM, Magit AE. A survey of adult preferences regarding recruitment for pediatric research. Int J Pediatr Otorhinolaryngol. 2020;135: 110108.
19. Falicov C, Niño A, D'Urso S. Expanding possibilities: flexibility and solidarity with under-resourced immigrant families during the COVID-19 pandemic. Fam Process. 2020;59(3):865–82.

Global Dermatology and Telehealth

Bianca Sanabria and Carrie Kovarik

Abstract The global burden of skin disease is often compounded by the lack of access to dermatology expertise, particularly in low-resource settings. The most significant gap in access to dermatologic care exists in low and middle income countries. With recent advancements in telecommunications, teledermatology is a potential tool that may assist in narrowing these gaps. Although several methods of teledermatology exist, understanding the technological requirements and limitations of the participating site will allow for selection of the best suited modality. Recognizing the benefits and risks of implementing these modalities, as well as the challenges experienced when scaling teledermatology to a sustainable practice, is imperative in ensuring high quality, equitable and efficient care. In this chapter, we explore the advancements of telemedicine globally, focusing on low-resource settings, in the field of dermatology.

Keywords Teledermatology · Global dermatology · Telehealth

Learning Objectives

- Understand how teledermatology services are used in low-resource settings to address challenges in dermatological care
- Explain the different modalities of teledermatology
- Recognize the barriers of implementing teledermatology and understand ways to scale sustainable teledermatology programs.

B. Sanabria
Rutgers-Robert Wood Johnson Medical School, Piscataway, NJ, USA
e-mail: bianca.sanabria@rutgers.edu

C. Kovarik (✉)
Perelman School of Medicine at the University of Pennsylvania, Philadelphia, PA, USA
e-mail: Carrie.Kovarik@pennmedicine.upenn.edu

K. Nouri (ed.), *Telemedicine and Technological Advances in Dermatology*,
https://doi.org/10.1007/978-3-031-69091-4_13

1 Introduction

Skin and subcutaneous disorders have the potential to create a significant burden on a patient's well-being, lead to disability, and cause socioeconomic issues in low-resource settings. In 2010, skin diseases were the 4th leading cause of nonfatal disease worldwide [1]. As a result of infectious diseases, genetics, culture, and environmental factors, there are significant regional variations in the presentation and distribution of skin diseases, affirming the role for dermatology expertise in global health [2]. Despite this clear need for skilled dermatology providers, billions of people lack access to basic care for skin diseases. In many countries, there may be a rural–urban imbalance in availability of dermatologists or no dermatologists at all [3]. Telemedicine has the potential to bridge this gap in providing care to populations that do not have access to care [3]. When delivered properly, telemedicine can be an effective modality of providing quality care at a distance through the use of digital and communication technologies. Improvements in internet connectivity and digital infrastructure have led to opportunities for telemedicine use around the world. Telemedicine can also create collaborative efforts, which transcend borders, between specialists, facilitating complex care in underserved regions [4].

2 Types of Teledermatology

Telemedicine is the utilization of modern communication technology to deliver health care services at a distance and exchange information for diagnostic and management of care [5]. Teledermatology can be classified by its purpose such as consultation, triage, follow-up, and education. However, teledermatology is typically classified by its delivery modality, which includes store-and-forward (SAF), real-time (RT), and hybrid.

Store-and-forward teledermatology consists of clinicians utilizing technology to capture digital samples (text files, images, video audio) and other relevant data from a patient to compile a case in one location [6]. That same digital device is used to upload the data into a secure system to allow transmission to a remote site for consultation by dermatologist. In this method, the electronic transmission of patient data via email, SMS, phone application, or web-based interfaces requires no direct interaction between the providers and patients, separated by time and location [7].

Traditionally, SAF (asynchronous) modalities relied on the use of computer desktops and web-based programs, which posed challenges in areas with limited internet access and computer resources [8]. With the expansion of mobile telecommunications globally, many web-based platforms developed mobile applications, allowing providers to use mobile smartphones to transmit photos and patient information for remote consultations [8]. Mobile applications (apps), solely for the use of telemedicine, have also been developed, and established communication platforms, such as Whatsapp, have been used for teleconsultation. The ability to utilize the users' own phone as well as wireless connectivity has allowed dermatology to reach remote areas globally [9]. This modality is commonly referred to as mobile Health (mHealth).

Real-time teledermatology (synchronous) uses live videoconferencing modalities so a patient and dermatologist meet virtually in different locations [3]. This method is location independent but not time independent [10]. Hybrid, is a modality blending the advantages of SAF and real-time dermatology [11, 12]. The use of real-time teledermatology can be difficult in low-resource settings, given issues surrounding internet connectivity and bandwidth.

2.1 *Teledermatopathology*

Histologic analysis of the skin plays an important role for the diagnostic confirmation of certain dermatological conditions, thus different methods of delivering dermatopathology services in low-resource settings globally have been created [8]. The simplest method, with low budget requirements, is static imaging. In this method, photographs of histological slides are obtained at different magnifications, using either a smartphone or digital camera with an adapter, and transmitted to a remote dermatopathologist using secure file-sharing platforms [8]. For dynamic imaging systems, histological slides are viewed in real time using a live microscopy viewing platform and robotic microscope, so a remote dermatopathologist can control the live streaming of histological images. Although these systems have been used in low-resource settings with success, the function of the system is limited by the speed and reliability of the internet connection [13]. Virtual slide microscopy creates the best quality images for telepathology, and slides are scanned and stored for review by the consulting pathologist. These systems are difficult to implement in low-resource settings due to the high cost of the equipment and high bandwidth requirements. In addition, all methods of teledermatopathology require local partners who desire histology consultation and have the ability to deliver quality processed glass slides for evaluation.

3 Example Uses of Teledermatology Globally

3.1 *Médecins Sans Frontières*

Médecins Sans Frontières (MSF) is an international, independent, and medical humanitarian organization that responds to emergency situations and provides medical assistance to people affected by armed conflict, epidemics, natural disasters, and exclusion from healthcare. In 2009, MSF launched a telemedicine service connecting field staff with experts around the world. The use of the telemedicine service, which often includes teledermatology, enables MSF to provide specialty care in low-resource settings. Specialists are able remotely assist medical teams through SAF methods via the receipt of patient's history, details of treatment, photos, and videos. Consultations for complex cases are also conducted using videoconference platforms, which enable discussion between physicians. [14].

3.2 Swinfen Charitable Trust

The Swinfen Charitable Trust (SCT), is a telemedicine system based in the UK, created in 1999, to connect specialists to low-resource settings, mostly in Africa, Asia, and Australasia. This system has enabled health professionals in low-resource countries and areas of conflict, like Iraq, to obtain specialty medical advice. In a study conducted by Patterson et al. teleconsultation referrers found the advice useful and claimed it provided cost saving which benefited patients, hospitals, and clinics. Cost-savings resulted from few doctors' visits, fewer drugs needed, saved in-country travel, saved internal travel, avoided investigations and surgeries. [15]

3.3 Asia

3.3.1 China

Where a large number of populations live in rural areas, like China, telemedicine is implemented to reduce geographic barriers by providing specialized medical services at a distance [16]. For example, the People's Liberation Army, established telemedicine networks to connect military hospitals, civil hospitals, and specialists, permitting access to specialty care for civilians and military personnel in urban and rural areas [17]. The rapid expansion of smartphone use in China also paved the way for the development of mHealth solutions to provide care to underserved populations; however, a recent review showed that 90% of mHealth initiatives are in urban areas [18]. Mobile health resources may need to be redirected to serve the more vulnerable populations.

3.3.2 Vietnam

Globally, mHealth solutions may provide an opportunity for increased access to specialty care like dermatology. In remote areas of Vietnam, numerous mHealth solutions have been implemented to improve access to care for vulnerable and hard-to-reach populations [19]. One example includes an initiative to increase general health education, including safe sexual practices, for ethnic minority populations through SMS. Challenges for sustainability and progression to more advanced care include language barriers, sociocultural issues, and sustainable funding.

3.3.3 Mongolia

Mobile phone platforms, especially for SAF teledermatology modalities, have been used to increase access to specialty care in remote and medically underserved areas in rural Mongolia. Open source technology, including OpenMRS and Sana Android Client, were used to develop the technology for this system. This program was shown to reduce referrals to tertiary care centers, total costs for the patients and healthcare center, and time to receive dermatologic care. [20]

3.3.4 Afghanistan

Teledermatology services expanded in Afghanistan using a free SAF email service beginning in 2013 [21]. Primary care providers sent cases to a dermatologist in Kabul, and 326 cases were answered over 4 years [21]. This service fostered partnerships between remote primary care providers and a dermatology consultant, and enhanced both patient care as well as provider education.

3.3.5 Nepal

Specialists, such as dermatologists, are primarily in Nepal's urban areas, limiting access to rural populations [22]. With the help from the government of Nepal, Nepal Research and Education Network (NREN) and the South Asian Association for Regional Cooperation (SAARC) telemedicine project, telemedicine services have been provided to rural areas of Nepal [22]. Teledermatology has also been coordinated by individual institutions, including Communication Health Education Services by Telehealth (CHEST) and Patan Academy of Health Sciences [22]. These services include SAF techniques, live videoconferencing, and hybrid [22]. Although the focus of teledermatology has been on the rural community, the increased use of mobile devices has led to a rise in teledermatology in rural and urban settings [22, 23].

3.4 The Americas

3.4.1 Mexico

A program called Community Dermatology, in the state of Guerrero, was established in Mexico to bring specialized medical services to marginalized groups that lacked access. The program was initially founded in 1991 with the goal of improving the dermatological health of remote, marginalized inhabitants of the state of Guerrero through on-site basic dermatology training for local providers, and free medical consultation and treatment for local patients. With the improvement in local telecommunication technology, telemedicine was a natural extension to the program, and allowed for continued training and care. The program initiated a telemedicine network through the telemedicine office of the Ministry of Health, and this allowed for greater reach while minimizing costs of transportation and improving the safety of the participants. [24]

3.4.2 Argentina

The COVID-19 pandemic created challenges for dermatological outpatient visits in the public sector of Argentina. This led to the development of a teledermatology program in the area of connective tissue diseases in the Dermatology Division of the José María Ramos Mejía Acute Hospital, in Buenos Aires. Through email or WhatsApp, patients were able to send information for consultation. After information was sent, direct telephone contact was established or videoconference was generated. When the consultation was complete, medical indications and corresponding orders were sent via email. In a study of 120 cases received, 57.5% were from patients of the outskirts of Buenos Aires and 47.5% of consultations were from patients with no medical insurance. Of the total, only 17 (14.2%) required referral to a health center. [25]

3.4.3 French Guiana

French Guiana, a tropical region covered by rainforest in the north coast of South America, has a significant burden of infectious and tropical skin diseases. Diagnosing these infectious skin diseases can be challenging in remote areas with limited access to dermatologists. With most settlements located on the coast, where access to interior land is accessible only by boat or plane, dermatological care is inaccessible. Thus, teledermatology was introduced to alleviate this inequity by facilitating care between the main hospital in Cayenne and remote health centers in French Guiana. A study of this system analyzed 254 cases over an 18 month period. Infectious diseases represented the most common reason for requests (46%), and the majority of users felt the system was fast and educational. However, the consultation has to be done on a clinic computer, and exchanges are limited to those that have the consultation software and training. [26]

3.4.4 Brazil

In the city of Sao Paulo, Brazil, basic skin conditions, which could be manageable within a primary care setting, are unnecessarily referred to a dermatologist due to the lack of general dermatology training of primary care professional. An increase demand of dermatological consultations created a waiting list, with up to a one year wait time in 2017. This led the municipal health department of Sao Paulo to implement a teledermatology project at the Hospital Israelita Alberta Einstein, which is a large private hospital. The goal of the program was to provide dermatological support via teledermatology to free up dermatological appointments and create shorter wait times for patients who require face-to-face dermatological care. The Hospital Israelita Albert Einstein developed a platform and app for mobile devices which allowed health technicians to use a digital camera to take photographs and upload them with patient data and a short clinical history, which is accessible to certified dermatologist recruited for the project. The use of the teledermatology project in a pediatric primary care setting reduced the mean wait time from 6.5 to 1.5 months (78%) for an in-person dermatology appointment. The project was also able to optimize in-person consultations for more serious, surgical, or complex skin illnesses. [27]

3.5 Africa

3.5.1 Africa Teledermatology Project

Dermatologists and dermatopathologists are scarce in sub-Saharan Africa. Thus, the Africa Teledermatology Project was initiated to create a global collaborative effort between many countries, including but not limited to, Botswana, Kenya, Uganda, Swaziland, Lesotho, Tanzania, Austria, and the United Sates. This project created a SAF method, where clinical photographs and patient history can be uploaded onto a web-based, and more recently mobile-based, application and reviewed securely by teledermatologists for diagnosis and management of care. For cases in which clinical diagnosis is challenging and stakeholders are in agreement, skin biopsy specimens can be collected and sent to the United States for processing and diagnosis. [28]

3.5.2 Botswana

In Botswana, there are very little dermatologists in the public sector and many dermatology patients live 5–8 h away from clinics. Due to the difficulty of in-person visits, WhatsApp was integrated into clinical practice for dermatological care. WhatsApp is a free instant messaging mobile application that allows people to exchange text, photos, videos, audio, and documents. WhatsApp has become a reliable modality of communication because users can send or view messages when the device receives WIFI connectivity, and without using cellular connectivity. The use of WhatsApp in clinical practice has enabled patients to reach clinicians directly, share photos of their skin, and adjust management plans. It has also become a tool for streamlining clinic flow and optimizing clinic visits. WhatsApp has also become a method of remote teaching of the referring physicians, by feedback on performing skin exams, triaging skin conditions, and explaining diagnoses and treatment plans in their own patients. It has also facilitated cross-specialty communication via the creation of "group chats", connecting clinicians and creating multidisciplinary care teams. [29]

3.5.3 South Africa

South Africa suffers from a wide burden of skin diseases, including cutaneous manifestations of HIV/AIDS, skin cancer, and burn wounds [30–32]. However, there's an acute shortage of dermatologists, with most of South Africa's registered dermatologists in private practice or in urban hospitals [30, 33]. Therefore, since 1999, South Africa has implemented teledermatology services in three of its provinces: Eastern Cape, Western Cape, and KwaZulu-Natal (KZN). In Eastern Cape two teledermatology modalities were initiated, however, they are no longer active. A SAF email based teledermatology service was initiated in KZN in 2001. However, this teledermatology service became labor intensive since doctors had to use at home dialup modems after hours, due to lack of connectivity in hospitals. This service ended in 2002 but another service begun in 2003, which used synchronous teledermatology, which enhanced outreach, supplemented continuing medical education programs, and reduced referral rates. In 2013, another teledermatology service, started, utilizing smartphones. This service allowed rural physicians and residents/registrars undergoing dermatology training to connect with dermatologist at the University of KwaZulu-Natal via the transmission of images and data. In Western Cape, a collaborative asynchronous service started between University of Cape Town's Department of Dermatology and University of Washington. A mobile device teledermatology program, similar to the one created in KZN, was also initiated in the Overberg District of Western Cape. Status of these programs are based on a study conducted by Walters et al., which are based on publication date, not current state. [30]

4 Benefits and Limitations of Teledermatology

4.1 Benefits

Collaboration between primary care providers, specialties, and subspecialties can be facilitated by teledermatology globally [4]. Teledermatology has the potential to decrease barriers to multispecialty care, especially in hard-to reach areas experiencing a high burden of chronic dermatologic conditions [4]. Facilitating access to dermatology experts can mitigate the maldistribution of specialties, allowing for more equitable access to dermatological care [34].

Inequalities also exist between rural and urban settings, as people in rural areas may experience significant geographic, physical, and logistical barriers to accessing dermatological care [35]. Teledermatology through its various modalities may increase care in rural settings by connecting patients and their specialists virtually, eliminating the need for transportation. Connecting patients from rural geographical regions to major urban medical centers has the potential for high quality care through the consultation of professional dermatology expertise [35]. Remote access to dermatologists may also reduce wait times and unavoidable visits to urgent care and emergency departments through teletriage and telecare. In addition, teledermatology can be utilized in follow-up visits for medical dermatology, postoperative care for surgical procedures, or management of wounds [35].

Teledermatology services have the potential to be cost-effective modalities for care in low-resource settings, with both patients and health professionals experiencing savings. With advances in the internet, mobile phone technology, and the rising number of mobile broadband phone subscriptions globally, pre-existing infrastructure can now be used to deliver telemedicine without the purchase of expensive equipment. This allows for more cost-effective solutions, minimizes necessary training, and may even engage patients in the teledermatology workflow. WhatsApp is an example of a secure communication platform that is popular globally, can be downloaded on personal smartphones for free, and is a potential cost-effective method of teledermatology consultation in low-resource setting [36]. The AccessDerm application, supported by the American Academy of Dermatology, can also be downloaded and used on personal smartphones in low-resource settings in the United States. A retrospective study of 700 teledermatology cases submitted by the Philadelphia city health clinics using AccessDerm was conducted. Within these Philadelphia community health centers, 48% of the patients are covered by Medicaid, and approximately 35% are uninsured patients. The study showed that a percentage of both in person and emergency room visits could have been avoided, providing cost savings for the health care systems and likely the patients [37].

4.2 *Limitations*

Face to face encounters with a specialist are the "gold-standard" for many patients. Shifting face-to-face interactions via the use of teledermatology does not allow for complete history taking (when using SAF), full-body examinations, and procedures [38]. The proliferation of these telecommunications, especially the use of telemedicine, can threaten traditional physician–patient relationships, as some patients believe the use of electronic evaluation to be insufficient, ultimately decreasing patient satisfaction [35].

Sufficient dermatology evaluations via telemedicine depends on the ability of the dermatology provider to evaluate the skin through a video visit and/or submitted photos. Poor quality images threaten diagnostic confidence [38]. Unclear or misleading photos can thus lead to medical errors, the inability to make a diagnosis, and delays in care [39]. The capturing, transmission, and storage of images can also risk patient privacy [40]. The risk associated with failure to ensure patient privacy through Health Insurance Portability and Accountability Act (HIPAA) and other legal frameworks gets complicated when telemedicine is implemented across borders [40]. With no uniform standard globally, patient privacy is addressed differently by individual countries.

Legal and ethical frameworks should be considered when evaluating potential risk of teledermatology. No matter where teledermatology is practiced, it is important that the patient is informed of the process and consented properly. Eliminating face-to-face interactions without patient knowledge or bypassing informed consent for the transmission of medical information for store-and-forward modalities, poses a risk to autonomy [39]. Patients are disempowered when they are not able to exercise their right to choose the type of care they receive.

Providers who have limited experience with practicing care in unfamiliar geographical regions can find the practice of global dermatology challenging. Although these issues can occur with face-to-face interactions, telemedicine may exacerbate these issues. Providers may not be familiar with local cultures and religious beliefs which can impact patient physicians' relationships [41]. In addition, providers may not be familiar with local disease prevalence, treatment options, health care coverage, and referral patterns, making customized recommendations difficult. It is often recommended that those practicing global teledermatology work on site first before providing teledermatology services.

5 Implementation Challenges

The global application of teledermatology has significant potential to create a virtual highway between providers; however, it is not a system without challenges [42]. To develop sustainable telemedicine networks that transcend borders it's imperative to understand the factors that influence the scalability of telemedicine.

5.1 Standards and Regulation

Globally, there are no standard guidelines or regulations for implementing telecommunications for specialty care. A lack of standards and regulations to the practice of teledermatology creates inconsistent documentation and imaging, leading to variable outcomes [40, 43, 44]. Due to the visual nature of dermatology, high picture quality, especially for SAF modalities is critical.

The lack of laws addressing medical licensures for telemedicine networks transcending borders is also a barrier to global implementation. Legal frameworks that don't address patient privacy and data security can also prevent effective implementation of telemedicine, when stakeholders across borders support different platforms with competing data-sharing policies [45]. Funding for teledermatology programs for low-resource settings is variable, with many running through the use of grant programs, volunteer physicians, and donations. However, contention between stakeholders can also arise due to the variety of options for reimbursement, including fee for service, per-case service, direct-to-consumer, and capitated service contracts [46]. Standardizing licensure, patient-privacy, and payments for telemedicine globally, is necessary in order to expand sustainable telemedicine services across borders.

5.2 *Infrastructure*

Internet connection accessibility is a technical factor that influences successful adoption and sustainability of global telemedicine networks. Underdevelopment of technological infrastructure and internet connectivity in low-resource regions hinder the establishment of telemedicine, especially for specialty care [9]. Lack of availability of hardware, such as computers, phones, and tablets, and necessary software or applications can also prevent the widespread use of teledermatology; however, utilizing technology that is already in place and is familiar to local providers will allow for the best success of the program [8]. Sustainability of the teledermatology program may be dictated by the enthusiasm of local providers to participate, as well as the ability to train them on the system. Rapid turnover of participating providers can threaten the program, and plans for continual training should be in place [8]. The economic status of patients impacts the utilization of telemedicine, especially in countries where patients cannot utilize the service if it is not cost-effective or free [41].

5.3 *Acceptance/Attitudes*

Successful teledermatology programs must be integrated into local healthcare systems and providers practicing care at a distance must be familiar with local disease, work flow, and cultures [8]. Dermatologists who lack local understanding, can negatively impact patient acceptance and attitudes to teledermatology care. Many unique, local socioeconomic factors influence the development of skin diseases, which must be considered for diagnosis and management. When these factors are neglected, the quality of care is impaired, affecting patient attitudes on the efficiency of teledermatology. The perceptions of teledermatology, as a suitable method of care, can also pose a challenge to use, especially in areas where patients expect face-to-face interactions or do not accept the practice of photographing skin [8]. Thus a consulting physician's understanding of their patient's culture, religion, and socioeconomic background influences the success of telemedicine [47].

6 Recommendations for Implementing/Scaling Effective Teledermatology

Acknowledging and understanding barriers to effective and scalable teledermatology is important when creating developmental models [47]. It is imperative to ensure that the implementation of teledermatology involves local partners who understand local infrastructure, cultures, technological literacy [8]. Conducting a local needs assessment is necessary to ensure that the modality used for teledermatology can effectively be implemented and is practical in addressing the dermatological needs for the population [8]. For telemedicine networks that will transcend borders, understanding differences in workflow and infrastructure across health systems is essential. This will require local partnerships that support the implementation of teledermatology [8].

When local community partnerships are identified, they must be involved every step of the implementation process. Clear roles and responsibilities should be established between all stakeholders. Benefits expected from both sides need to be transparent and dialogue must include how resources, manpower, and information exchange should be shared to achieve these benefits [48]. Engagement with community members enables an understanding of the socioeconomic influences on the utilization of teledermatology and unique barriers to receiving dermatology care. Understanding community perspectives and their challenges will allow for the development of telecommunication infrastructure and a framework that is useful and culturally sensitive.

Due to the lack of global legal or ethical frameworks for implementing teledermatology programming, stakeholders must establish policies and standards that support the practice of teledermatology in all the health systems involved. To scale a sustainable teledermatology network, the technological model involved must abide by standards of patient privacy and information in exchange in the involved health care environments [8]. This is challenging especially when telemedicine networks transcend borders. However, through collaborative efforts between local, national, and private stakeholders, regulatory frameworks can be developed which support the needs of all parties.

A developmental model facilitating local, national, and private collaboration is essential to address barriers in implementing scalable telemedicine networks. In global networks, public and private partnerships have been successful in serving as a framework for implementing telemedicine programs that can improve access to care in hard-to-reach regions around the world. Public–private partnerships are established partnerships between the public and private sector to accomplish a common interest [48]. These partnerships can be rooted from the goal of gaining access to products or services that may not be otherwise be accessible as well as improve infrastructure [48]. On the global level, public private partnerships typically involve collaborative efforts between multinational companies with public entities such as governmental systems on the national, state, or local level, as well as public organizations like colleges, associations, and community based organizations [48]. This is why many areas of public health have utilized this developmental model when developing efforts to expand access to health services. Using this model also allows geographical regions with limited funding to harness private funds and access to infrastructure needed for the implementation of teledermatology [49]. Using a public–private partnership may not only enable the introduction of new technologies but facilitate the development of relationships, expectations, and responsibilities amongst global stakeholders in teledermatology [47]. Thus, it can serve as a development model to scale teledermatology initiatives into sustainable efforts.

Case Example: Botswana

Botswana is a middle-income country in sub-Saharan Africa with a shortage of medical specialists, including dermatologists. This has made specialty care almost inaccessible to rural populations, given the few dermatologists are located predominantly in the urban areas. Historically, patients have been required to travel long distances before receiving care for complex dermatological issues. To improve access to specialized healthcare services throughout Botswana, in 2012, the Botswana-University of Pennsylvania Partnership (BUP) began scale-up of four telemedicine referral programs in Botswana, in conjunction with the Ministry of Health (MoH). [50]

Due to improvements in mobile telecommunications in Botswana, healthcare workers were able to use smart phones equipped with a built-in-camera and SIM card, donated by the Orange Foundation in Botswana, to submit telemedicine consults. After obtaining patient consent, health practitioners utilized smartphones to collect clinical history and images. Patient data collected were sent for consultation to a medical specialist in country. Using the data obtained, specialists were able to provide a diagnosis and recommendations on the course of treatment. Local physicians in Botswana also had access to physicians at the University of Pennsylvania for consultation. This form of asynchronous, SAF telemedicine was managed by an organizational team that included in-country medical specialists, international specialists (only positions not held by a Ministry of Health employee), referring health care workers, and a referral site coordinator. [50]

BUP's collaboration with local partners in the four specialty programs, including dermatology, radiology, cervical cancer screening, and oral medicine, allowed patients to avoid long waiting times for hospital treatment and reduce travel time and distance, which permitted quicker medical attention with improved medical outcomes. These benefits resulted in the Ministry of Health to "scale-up" the project by adopting the "Kgonfalo" mobile telemedicine system. To scale a sustainable solution, financial factors were addressed through a collaborative effort between the public and private sector. The Ministry of Health in Botswana committed to a recurrent budget and collaborated with 5AM Solutions, a private software development and integration company, to ensure necessary technology is provided. [50]

A Memorandum of Understanding (MOU) was signed between Botswana's Ministry of Health and the Orange Foundation of Botswana, a non-profit organization. The MOU established roles and other legal units for each partner, including the Orange Foundation's commitment to all mobile devices with customized SIM cards. Additionally, based on community engagement from the pilot project, BUP provided recommendations to the Orange Foundation on the specifications needed for mobile devices in each specialty to ensure the Foundation designed a device that respects the cultures, religions, and health needs in Botswana. In general, the long term roles, responsibilities, and benefits of all stakeholders, which were established in the formal agreements, were a crucial step in ensuring the scale-up and sustainability of the BUP pilot project to a national service. [50]

7 COVID-19 and Teledermatology

To minimize transmission of COVID-19, maintain social distancing, and limit unnecessary contact, the COVID-19 pandemic shifted traditional face-to-face care to virtual teleconsultations. Although telemedicine has existed in the field of dermatology for years, the pandemic accelerated the development of virtual clinics globally, especially as travel restrictions and the emergency of variants impose a barrier to global dermatological care. Additionally, COVID-19's disruption on healthcare systems and its exacerbation on healthcare disparities led to widespread collaborative efforts in scaling telemedicine networks.

In response to the public health emergency, the increased emphasis on teledermatology resulted in many changes. Prior to the pandemic, the most used teledermatology modalities were SAF models [51]. However, regulatory changes led to an increase in the use of live-interactive visits [51]. In the United States, reimbursement restrictions were eased to decrease barriers to utilization. Additionally, licensure requirements for out-of-state telehealth clinicians were waived at the height of the pandemic, and patients were permitted to initiate electronic visits. [52]

Prior to the COVID-19 pandemic, many countries lacked standard guidelines for using teleconsultations, which has significantly changed since. During the pandemic, the Medical Council in India, instituted guidelines for practice by adding Regulation 3.8, "Consultation of Telemedicine" and telemedicine practice guidelines in appendix 5 of the 2002 Medical Council in India regulations [53]. The American Academy of Dermatology and British Association of Dermatologists also released guidelines for the management of teledermatology [53–55]. In Brazil, where the use of teledermatology was often viewed with reservations, the rapid transmission of COVID-19 led to the Federal Council of Medicine to recognize the potential of telemedicine and the establishment of temporary guidelines for remote consultations via the Ordinance No. 467 of Ministry of Health and Law 13,989 [56].

The COVID-19 pandemic did not mitigate all implementation barriers to teledermatology. However, it highlighted its potential for triaging urgent cases, maintaining follow-up care, and providing care for people of different socioeconomic backgrounds [57]. Thus, the pandemic created opportunities for health systems around the world to explore the use of teledermatology by adopting its practice [57]. As the COVID-19 pandemic changed the practice of medicine and healthcare technologies continue to advance, a pathway was paved for the use of telemedicine and other technologies in the practice of dermatology [53].

Although COVID-19 increased the use of teledermatology globally, its wide scale adoption also highlighted issues with health disparities. Vulnerable patients, including those of lower socioeconomic standing, older individuals, and non-English-speaking patients, may experience increased barriers to accessing teledermatology. There may be lower rates of reliable internet connection, decreased digital device availability, and issues with digital literacy. When a patient consents for a teledermatology visit, steps should be taken to ensure a successful visit and optimal outcome.

8 Conclusion

The proliferation of telemedicine is reconfiguring health practices as a method to address the most pressing issues in healthcare delivery and organization, including the global healthcare worker shortage and long distances to health facilities [47]. In doing so, telemedicine is not only introducing new technologies but is building new relationships, expectations, and responsibilities amongst global stakeholders [47]. It is also connecting providers both within and across borders, as well as enhancing the way we exchange knowledge by facilitating faster communication. Using effective developmental models for scaling information technologies for telemedicine can reshape healthcare and improve access to specialty care such as dermatology globally. In many countries where access to a dermatologist is limited, telemedicine may be able to bridge this gap when implemented appropriately.

References

1. Hay RJ, Johns NE, Williams HC, Bolliger IW, Dellavalle RP, Margolis DJ, et al. The global burden of skin disease in 2010: an analysis of the prevalence and impact of skin conditions. J Invest Dermatol. 2014;134(6):1527–34.
2. Williams VL, Kovarik CL. The Growing Importance of Dermatology on the Global Stage. Dermatol Clin. 2021;39(1):xiii–xiv.
3. Desai B, McKoy K, Kovarik C. Overview of international teledermatology. Pan Afr Med J. 2010;6:3.
4. Madu PN, Chang AY, Kayembe MK, Kovarik CL. Teledermatology as a means to provide multispecialty care: a case of global specialty collaboration. Pediatr Dermatol. 2017;34(2):E89–92.
5. Sood S, Mbarika V, Jugoo S, Dookhy R, Doarn CR, Prakash N, et al. What is telemedicine? A collection of 104 peer-reviewed perspectives and theoretical underpinnings. Telemed J E Health. 2007;13(5):573–90.
6. Store and Forward Center for Connected Health Policy, the National Telehealth Policy Resource Center. Available from: www.cchpca.org/.
7. Trettel A, Eissing L, Augustin M. Telemedicine in dermatology: findings and experiences worldwide—a systematic literature review. J Eur Acad Dermatol Venereol. 2018;32(2):215–24.

8. Williams V, Kovarik C. Long-range diagnosis of and support for skin conditions in field settings. Trop Med Infect Dis. 2018;3(3):84.
9. Tran K, Ayad M, Weinberg J, Cherng A, Chowdhury M, Monir S, et al. Mobile teledermatology in the developing world: implications of a feasibility study on 30 Egyptian patients with common skin diseases. J Am Acad Dermatol. 2011;64(2):302–9.
10. Tensen E, van der Heijden JP, Jaspers MW, Witkamp L. Two decades of teledermatology: current status and integration in national healthcare systems. Curr Dermatol Rep. 2016;5:96–104.
11. Pearlman RL, Le PB, Brodell RT, Nahar VK. Evaluation of patient attitudes towards the technical experience of synchronous teledermatology in the era of COVID-19. Arch Dermatol Res. 2021;313(9):769–72.
12. Kanthraj GR. Classification and design of teledermatology practice: what dermatoses? Which technology to apply? J Eur Acad Dermatol. 2009;23(8):865–75.
13. Micheletti RG, Steele KT, Kovarik CL. Robotic teledermatopathology from an African dermatology clinic. J Am Acad Dermatol. 2014;70(5):952–4.
14. Bonnardot L, Liu J, Wootton E, Amoros I, Olson D, Wong S, et al. The development of a multilingual tool for facilitating the primary-specialty care interface in low resource settings: the MSF tele-expertise system. Front Public Health. 2014;2:126.
15. Patterson V, Wootton R. A web-based telemedicine system for low-resource settings 13 years on: insights from referrers and specialists. Glob Health Action. 2013;6:21465.
16. Jha AK, Sawka E, Tiwari B, Dong H, Oh CC, Ghaemi S, et al. Telemedicine and community health projects in Asia. Dermatol Clin. 2021;39(1):23–32.
17. Lian P, Fu Z, Ning Y, Zhai X. The telemedicine network of the people's liberation army. J Telemed Telecare. 2001;7(4):187–92.
18. Yang X, Kovarik CL. A systematic review of mobile health interventions in China: identifying gaps in care. J Telemed Telecare. 2021;27(1):3–22.
19. Lam JA, Dang LT, Phan NT, Trinh HT, Vu NC, Nguyen CK. Mobile health initiatives in Vietnam: scoping study. JMIR Mhealth Uhealth. 2018;6(4):e106.
20. Byamba K, Syed-Abdul S, Garcia-Romero M, Huang CW, Nergyi S, Nyamdorj A, et al. Mobile teledermatology for a prompter and more efficient dermatological care in rural Mongolia. Br J Dermatol. 2015;173(1):265–7.
21. Ismail A, Stoff BK, McMichael JR. Store-and-forward teledermatology service for primary care providers in Afghanistan. Int J Dermatol. 2018;57(11):e145–7.
22. Paudel V. The increasing scope of teledermatology in Nepal. JNMA J Nepal Med Assoc. 2020;58(232):1100–2.
23. Telemedicine Services in Nepal: South Asia Subregional Economic Cooperation (SASEC) Information Highway Project. Available from: http://www.sasecrtn.edu.np/index.php/en/resources/usefulinfo/information-on-e-health-and-telemedicine/telemedicine-services-in-nepal
24. Chavez-Lopez MG, Estrada-Chavez GE, Orozco-Figueroa M, Solis-Rivera A, Solchaga-Rosas J, Armendariz-Valle F, et al. Avances recientes en dermatologia comunitaria 2016–2017. Teledermatologia, un modelo de ensenanza y asistencia en atencion primaria a la salud. Gac Med Mex. 2018;154(Supp 2):S36–40.
25. Debernardi ME, Bordon MP, Campastri A, Chequim A, Cilio AM, Fava MV, et al. Teledermatology during de COVID-19 pandemic in a public hospital. Medicina (B Aires). 2020;80(Suppl 6):18–24.
26. Messagier AL, Blaizot R, Couppie P, Delaigue S. Teledermatology use in remote areas of French Guiana: experience from a long-running system. Front Public Health. 2019;7:387.
27. Bianchi MG, Santos AP, Cordioli E. The majority of skin lesions in pediatric primary care attention could be managed by teledermatology. PLoS ONE. 2019;14(12):e0225479.
28. Tsang MW, Kovarik CL. The role of dermatopathology in conjunction with teledermatology in resource-limited settings: lessons from the african teledermatology project. Int J Dermatol. 2011;50(2):150–6.
29. Williams V, Kovarik C. WhatsApp: an innovative tool for dermatology care in limited resource settings. Telemed E-Health. 2018;24(6):464–8.

30. Walters LE, Mars M, Scott RE. A review and critique of teledermatology in the South African public health sector. Stud Health Technol Inform. 2016;231:143–51.
31. WHO. South Africa: WHO statistics profile, Country statistics and global health estimates: WHO and UN Partners; 2015. Available from: http://www.who.int/gho/countries/zaf.pdf?ua=1
32. Mars M, Scott RE. Spontaneous telemedicine services—what can we learn? 2015;8:229–32.
33. Carruthers J. Dermatology in South Africa. Dermatology World. 2013;14–6.
34. Walters LEM, Scott RE, Mars M. Teledermatology scale-up frameworks: a structured review and critique. BMC Health Serv Res. 2018;18(1):613.
35. Vyas KS, Hambrick HR, Shakir A, Morrison SD, Tran DC, Pearson K, et al. A systematic review of the use of telemedicine in plastic and reconstructive surgery and dermatology. Ann Plas Surg. 2017;78(6):736–68.
36. Hogan SC, van Hees C, Asiedu KB, Fuller LC. WhatsApp platforms in tropical public health resource-poor settings. Int J Dermatol. 2019;58(2):228–30.
37. Yang X, Barbieri JS, Kovarik CL. Cost analysis of a store-and-forward teledermatology consult system in Philadelphia. J Am Acad Dermatol. 2019;81(3):758–64.
38. Landow SM, Mateus A, Korgavkar K, Nightingale D, Weinstock MA. Teledermatology: key factors associated with reducing face-to-face dermatology visits. J Am Acad Dermatol. 2014;71(3):570–6.
39. Rismiller K, Cartron AM, Trinidad JCL. Inpatient teledermatology during the COVID-19 pandemic. J Dermatolog Treat. 2020;31(5):441–3.
40. Wang RH, Barbieri JS, Nguyen HP, Stavert R, Forman HP, Bolognia JL, et al. Clinical effectiveness and cost-effectiveness of teledermatology: where are we now, and what are the barriers to adoption? J Am Acad Dermatol. 2020;83(1):299–307.
41. Ly BA, Labonte R, Bourgeault IL, Niang MN. The individual and contextual determinants of the use of telemedicine: a descriptive study of the perceptions of Senegal's physicians and telemedicine projects managers. PLoS ONE. 2017;12(7):e0181070.
42. Telemedicine opportunities and developments in member states. World Health Organ; 2010.
43. Position statement on teledermatology [press release]. Am Acad Dermat; 2021.
44. Peart JM, Kovarik C. Direct-to-patient teledermatology practices. J Am Acad Dermatol. 2015;72(5):907–9.
45. Coates SJ, Kvedar J, Granstein RD. Teledermatology: from historical perspective to emerging techniques of the modern era: part II: emerging technologies in teledermatology, limitations and future directions. J Am Acad Dermatol. 2015;72(4):577–86 quiz 87-8.
46. Weig EA, Tull R, Chung J, Wanat KA. Inpatient teledermatology: current state and practice gaps. J Am Acad Dermatol. 2020;83(3):797–802.
47. Sanabria B. Public–private partnerships: a development model for creating sustainable telemedicine networks in low-income and low-middle income countries. (Unpublished masters essay): Columbia University Graduate School of Arts and Sciences 2018.
48. Mitchell M. An overview of public private partnerships in health.
49. Sekhri N, Feachem R, Ni A. Public–private integrated partnerships demonstrate the potential to improve health care access, quality, and efficiency. Health Aff (Millwood). 2011;30(8):1498–507.
50. Ndlovu K, Littman-Quinn R, Park E, Dikai Z, Kovarik CL. Scaling up a mobile telemedicine solution in Botswana: keys to sustainability. Front Public Health. 2014;2:275.
51. Kennedy J, Arey S, Hopkins Z, Tejasvi T, Farah R, Secrest AM, et al. Dermatologist perceptions of teledermatology implementation and future use after COVID-19: demographics, barriers, and insights. JAMA Dermatol. 2021;157(5):595–7.
52. Armstrong AW, Singh I. Economics of teledermatology-does the math add up? JAMA Dermatol. 2021;157(1):27–8.
53. Ashique KT, Kaliyadan F. Teledermatology in the wake of COVID-19 scenario: an Indian perspective. Indian Dermatol Online J. 2020;11(3):301–6.
54. Teledermatology toolkit American academy of dermatology association. Available from: https://www.aad.org/member/practice/telederm/toolkit

55. COVID-19: clinical guidelines for the management of dermatology patients remotely: British association of dermatologists. Available from: https://www.bad.org.uk/healthcare-professionals/covid-19/remote-dermatology-guidance
56. Silva DLF, Gameiro L, Massuda JY, Magalhaes RF, da Costa Franca AFE. Teledermatology before and after coronavirus. An Bras Dermatol. 2021;96(2):248–50.
57. Gupta R, Ibraheim MK, Doan HQ. Teledermatology in the wake of COVID-19: advantages and challenges to continued care in a time of disarray. J Am Acad Dermatol. 2020;83(1):168–9.

Conducting Clinical Research Remotely Through Technology

Edward Hadeler and Keyvan Nouri

Abstract Conducting research remotely is an area of ongoing interest in dermatology. Significant interruptions in research amid physical distancing requirements during the COVID-19 pandemic drove the development of technologies aimed at conducting remote clinical research. Remote clinical research has several potential benefits. Moving clinical research to patient homes may expand the number of patients willing to participate in research by improving its convenience and reducing travel burdens. The incorporation of technologies such as artificial intelligence may also improve the objectivity of clinical research. However, challenges exist, and research technologies should be designed with these challenges in mind. In this chapter, we provide some background on the importance of implementing remote research modalities. We discuss the pros and cons of moving clinical research to patient homes, and the necessary technological components needed to effectively conduct research remotely.

Keywords Research · Technology · Smartphone · Mobile · Teledermatology · Store-and-forward · Live-interactive

1 Remote Dermatology Clinical Research: Navigating the COVID-19 Pandemic and Beyond

The COVID-19 pandemic resulted in dramatic declines in clinical research participation and progress [1]. From April 2019 through May 2020, researchers reported 92 of 1010 (9.1%) of dermatology-related clinical trials were suspended, withdrawn, or terminated [2]. Fifty-seven (62%) of the suspensions, withdrawals, and terminations occurred between March and May of 2020, affecting an estimated 7141 patients [2]. The resulting deficits in clinical research, which affected primarily phase 2 or 3 clinical trials, was twofold. Thousands of enrolled research patients were directly

E. Hadeler (✉) · K. Nouri
Miller School of Medicine, University of Miami, Miami, USA
e-mail: ehadeler@gmail.com

K. Nouri (ed.), *Telemedicine and Technological Advances in Dermatology*,
https://doi.org/10.1007/978-3-031-69091-4_14

affected, and potentially even more patients were affected by the delays in drug development. Without technology readily available to conduct research remotely, many clinical trials were unable to navigate physical distancing requirements implemented during the pandemic.

2 Remote Research: Modalities

Teledermatology can occur through two primary modalities. Live-interactive teledermatology occurs through synchronous platforms, such as a live video conference, while store-and-forward teledermatology occurs asynchronously, through phone or web-based applications. Remote research could be performed through either modality, or a combination of the two.

Previous studies have evaluated the efficacy of teledermatology in clinical care [3, 4], showing that adequate assessments, including efficacy and safety measurements, could be performed remotely. Furthermore, Gelfand and Hefele discuss the successful enrollment of new patients in the LITE study utilizing teledermatology during the COVID-19 pandemic [1]. In their model, the patient signed consent at home while the study coordinator completed baseline activities at a separate location [1].

The widespread use of smartphone technology may also accelerate the use of remote research modalities. With smartphone ownership now listed at 85% in 2020 [5], these devices may be some of those most amenable to facilitate clinical research. Recent reviews have assessed the use of mobile applications in the clinical care space [6, 7], however, limited information exists on the use of mobile applications specifically designed for clinical research, warranting further research on the topic.

3 Conducting Research Remotely: The Pros

In addition to protecting research from future pandemics, conducting research remotely provides several other benefits that promote its implementation beyond the COVID-19 pandemic. Diversity in research participation is a longstanding issue in dermatology. Previous studies have highlighted that a low number of nonwhite patients have been cited in psoriasis trials [8]. Additionally, the challenges of balancing transportation, busy work schedules, and childcare has led to higher no-show rates for minority and Medicaid patients in the clinic space [9, 10]. Improving the convenience of clinical research and moving it to patient homes may help patients who would otherwise struggle to attend monthly, and sometimes weekly, research appointments.

Furthermore, clinical research often imposes significant travel burdens on patients. In 2018, Borno et al. reported that among 1600 research patients, the median unidirectional distance traveled to a study site was 25.8 miles, and this distance increased to as high as 39.4 miles for trials sponsored by the National Institutes of Health (NIH)

[11]. Additionally, patients from lower-income areas traveled longer distances than patients from higher-income areas (58.3 vs. 17.8 miles, respectively; $p < 0.001$) [11]. Allowing patients to participate in research remotely may encourage patients who face significant travel barriers to participate in research, especially patients from low-income areas. Remote research could also help mitigate the potential costs associated with traveling long distances.

In addition to improving the generalizability of clinical research through expanded patient participation, new technologies may also enhance the objectivity of clinical research. Artificial intelligence (AI) has emerged as a technology capable of evaluating clinical image characteristics [12, 13]. Designing algorithms that can objectively rate clinical characteristics such as skin erythema or induration, clinical factors that are key measures of treatment effectiveness in dermatology clinical research, may improve the objectivity of skin evaluations. Recognizing changes in clinical measures can also be challenging across different skin color tones, and artificial intelligence algorithms may provide more objective skin evaluations in patients with skin of color.

4 Conducting Research Remotely: The Cons

While remote clinical research may expand the pool of participants and improve the generalizability of clinical research, the cost of obtaining technology to participate in research remotely may be prohibitive. These technologies include laptops, desktop computers, smartphone devices, cameras, and high-quality internet connections. The Pew Research Center, a nonpartisan American think tank based in Washington D.C., reports that of U.S. adults who earn less than $30,000 annually in 2019, only 56% had access to home broadband internet [14].

Similarly, if technology is not designed with care and consideration for the cultural and language needs of research participants, research participation may be limited. A previous study of clinical care applications showed that only 43% of participants from a racially and ethnically diverse population were able to complete tasks across 11 applications [15]. Additionally, navigating technology can be difficult for participants with low digital literacy. Digital literacy refers to an individual's ability to effectively utilize digital platforms to find, evaluate, and communicate information [16]. Ultimately, it is essential that the cultural, digital literacy, and language needs of a diverse group of patients influence the design of remote research applications. Additional staffing or increased availability of information technology personnel may also be necessary to assist patients with low digital literacy in remote research.

5 The Necessary Technological Components of Remote Clinical Research

Considering every aspect of clinical research, from recruitment to study close out, is important in designing technology for research.

Through their computer or smartphone device, participants should be able to easily survey research studies of interest to them, with ample information available to educate them about the studies. Once a participant has demonstrated interest in a research study, they should be able to provide informed consent and be screened for eligibility through the technology.

The technology should be capable of acquiring a variety of information, including personal medical information (medications, past medical history, etc.), demographics, and other survey data.

Facilitating high quality photograph acquisition is one of the greatest challenges of conducting research remotely. The technology should guide participants in taking high-quality photographs. Patients should be thoroughly instructed on proper positioning, the need for good lighting, and any other specific maneuvers that may assist them in taking photographs independently if necessary. Once completed, these photographs should then be uploaded and organized on a digital platform that is easily accessible by the study team for evaluation.

Communication between study personal and participants is key, especially for reporting of adverse events during the study. Therefore, the technology should provide a communication portal, for general inquiries and risk assessments.

In all, the patient should have access to a digital platform and central dashboard where they can track their study progress, provide data (medications, medical history, etc.), complete study tasks (photograph taking, questionnaire completion, etc.), and communicate with the study team. The study team should have access to a platform where they can easily track the study participant's progress, evaluate images, review data, and communicate with patients.

Finally, study teams will need to account for data storage and appropriate software capable of encrypting and safely storing patient related health information.

6 The Future of Remote Research

The expansion of remotely driven research has become an area of vested interest in the medical industry. Two corporations, Medable and Science 37, received substantial investments to design phone and web-based applications to enhance clinical research [17, 18]. Furthermore, some researchers have also reported the successful implementation of remote research methods utilizing technology [1].

Conducting research remotely with technology has promise. If challenges in its adoption are appropriately addressed and digital platforms are designed with careful consideration of a diverse study population, they have the potential to expand the participant pool in clinical research and improve the research experience for providers and patients.

References

1. Gelfand JM, Hefele BE. Clinical research after COVID-19: embracing a new normal. J Investig Dermatol. 2021;141(3):481–3.
2. Desai S, Manjaly P, Lee KJ, Li SJ, Manjaly C, Mostaghimi A. The Impact of COVID-19 on dermatology clinical trials. J Investig Dermatol. 2021;141(3):676–8.
3. Armstrong AW, Chambers CJ, Maverakis E, Cheng MY, Dunnick CA, Chren M-M, et al. Effectiveness of online vs in-person care for adults with psoriasis: a randomized clinical trial. JAMA Netw Open. 2018;1(6):e183062.
4. Armstrong AW, Johnson MA, Lin S, Maverakis E, Fazel N, Liu F-T. Patient-centered, direct-access online care for management of atopic dermatitis: a randomized clinical trial. JAMA Dermatol. 2015;151(2):154–60.
5. Pew Research Center. Mobile Fact Sheet [Internet]. Available from: https://www.pewresearch.org/internet/fact-sheet/mobile/.
6. Glines KR, Haidari W, Ramani L, Akkurt ZM, Feldman SR. Digital future of dermatology. Dermatol Online J. 2020;26(10).
7. Clark AK, Bosanac S, Ho B, Sivamani RK. Systematic review of mobile phone-based teledermatology. Arch Dermatol Res. 2018;310(9):675–89.
8. Reddy VD, Myers BA, Chan SY, Thibodeaux QG, Brownstone ND, Bhutani T, et al. A review of current phase III clinical trials of plaque psoriasis: under-representation of nonwhite participants and need for reform. Br J Dermatol. 2021;184(2):348–50.
9. Syed ST, Gerber BS, Sharp LK. Traveling towards disease: transportation barriers to health care access. J Community Health. 2013;38(5):976–93.
10. Dantas LF, Fleck JL, Cyrino Oliveira FL, Hamacher S. No-shows in appointment scheduling—a systematic literature review. Health Policy. 2018;122(4):412–21.
11. Borno HT, Zhang L, Siegel A, Chang E, Ryan CJ. At what cost to clinical trial enrollment? A retrospective study of patient travel burden in cancer clinical trials. Oncologist. 2018;23(10):1242–9.
12. Chan S, Reddy V, Myers B, Thibodeaux Q, Brownstone N, Liao W. Machine learning in dermatology: current applications, opportunities, and limitations. Dermatol Ther (Heidelb). 2020;10(3):365–86.
13. Partl R, Jonko B, Schnidar S, Schöllhammer M, Bauer M, Singh S, et al. 128 shades of RED: objective remote assessment of radiation dermatitis by augmented digital skin imaging. Stud Health Technol Inform. 2017;236:363–74.
14. Monica A. Mobile technology and home broadband 2019. [Internet]. Pew Research Center. Available from: https://www.pewresearch.org/internet/2019/06/13/mobile-technology-andhome-broadband-2019/.
15. Sarkar U, Gourley GI, Lyles CR, Tieu L, Clarity C, Newmark L, et al. Usability of commercially available mobile applications for diverse patients. J Gen Intern Med. 2016;31(12):1417–26.
16. American Library Association. Digital literacy [Internet]. 2021. Available from: https://literacy.ala.org/digital-literacy/.

17. Hall C. Medable secures $78M series c extension to scale digital clinical trials program [Internet]. 2021. Available from: https://news.crunchbase.com/news/medable-secures-78m-series-c-extension/.
18. Ben A. Virtual trial specialist and big pharma-backed science 37 nabs $40M funding round [Internet]. 2020. Available from: https://www.fiercebiotech.com/cro/virtual-trial-specialist-and-big-pharma-backed-science-37-nabs-40m-funding-round.

Geriatric Teledermatology

Jaya Manjunath and Carrie Kovarik

Abstract Teledermatology can be a highly effective health-care tool, and it has increased in demand since the onset of the COVID-19 pandemic. Older adults are an important subset of patients who have the potential to benefit from teledermatology services. We discuss the current state of teledermatology in older adults in general, as well as unique populations including nursing home residents and aging veterans. Few studies have systematically evaluated teledermatology in older patients, and a limited number of published teledermatology reports include a significant proportion of older adults (65 + years old). Store-and-forward was the preferred modality in these studies, and the majority of dermatology visits could be completed via teledermatology alone, with no in-person consultation needed. These teledermatology studies demonstrated good diagnostic accuracy (88%) and treatment accuracy (70–90%). Teledermatology was found to offer many potential additional benefits for older patients, including reduced transportation costs, time savings, reduced wait times, as well as increased accessibility to dermatology care for underserved patients. Some limitations include low technological capabilities in a subset of older adults, poor image quality, difficulty in taking photos, and issues with digital literacy. For older adults facing technological barriers, teledermatology visits should be assisted by the patient's personal support network. For those with more severe physical or cognitive conditions, assistance from nurses at long-term care facilities or home health aides is recommended.

Keywords Geriatric teledermatology · Teledermatology · Older adults · Store-and-forward · Digital divide

---

J. Manjunath
The George Washington University School of Medicine and Health Sciences, Washington, DC, USA
e-mail: jayamanjunath@gwmail.gwu.edu

C. Kovarik (✉)
Department of Dermatology, University of Pennsylvania Perelman School of Medicine, 3600 Spruce St. 2 Maloney Building, Philadelphia, PA 19104, USA
e-mail: carrie.kovarik@pennmedicine.upenn.edu

K. Nouri (ed.), *Telemedicine and Technological Advances in Dermatology*,
https://doi.org/10.1007/978-3-031-69091-4_15

Key Questions

- What is Geriatric Teledermatology?
- What types of teledermatology services are utilized by older adults? What are unique older adult sub-populations to consider?
- What are the distinct challenges of teledermatology in nursing homes?
- What are some solutions for the digital divide that occurs among a subset of older adults?
- How can we increase access to teledermatology services for older adults?

1 Brief Introduction to Geriatric Teledermatology

Telemedicine has emerged as a critical health care tool and continues to transform delivery of services to millions of people globally. Teledermatology is a sub-specialty of telemedicine that utilizes technology to remotely provide dermatologic diagnoses, treatment, and education. The visual nature of dermatology has allowed it to be particularly suited to the use of telemedicine, as several diagnoses can be made based on skin images and clinical history. The use of teledermatology skyrocketed during the COVID-19 pandemic to facilitate access to care and reduce strain on the healthcare system. In fact, an online survey of 184 dermatologists in 2020 revealed the use of teledermatology by 163/184 (88.5%) dermatologists in their practice [1].

Chronological aging of the skin can lead to structural and functional changes, leaving older adults susceptible certain issues, such as contact dermatitis, pruritus, drug eruptions, and autoimmune blistering diseases. The overwhelming majority of non-melanoma skin cancers occur in the older adult population, particularly in those with other risk factors [2]. While many older adults opt for and succeed with teledermatology, others may require it by necessity. This could be due to travel difficulties (due to health restrictions, disability, lack of transportation), hospitalization, or other issues. Some of these patients may struggle with technological, financial, or health literacy issues, which can make a successful virtual visit challenging [3]. This chapter introduces the types of teledermatology services used by older adults and discusses possibilities for the expansion of teledermatology in this population.

2 Teledermatology and the Various Delivery Methods

Teledermatology is typically delivered in either synchronous live visits, through asynchronous store-and-forward virtual visits, or a hybrid of both [4]. In synchronous sessions, the dermatologist conducts a live virtual visit with the patient where they may examine the patient's skin, clarify clinical history, and provide recommendations [4]. However, high-resolution images are typically superior to video visit examinations for making accurate diagnoses [5]. Hence, a hybrid visit, where an asynchronous store-and-forward system permits patient images and clinical history to be forwarded to the dermatologist before a live virtual visit (video chat or telephone), allows better visualization of the skin [5]. When used alone, asynchronous store-and-forward virtual visits may provide a cost-effective and flexible solution, with diagnostic accuracy that can exceed that of low-resolution live visits without photos [5].

Teledermatology (primary) consists of direct communication between the patient and dermatologist [6]. This was the most common type of teledermatology during the COVID pandemic. In secondary teledermatology, a patient communicates with a primary care provider or nurse who then consults a dermatologist, seeking advice on behalf of the patient [6]. In tertiary teledermatology, dermatologists may consult another specialist, for example a dermatologic surgeon, to aid in the clinical diagnosis or management [6].

Geriatric patients may use multiple modalities in their teledermatology care, including store-and-forward teledermatology, live virtual visits, and hybrid. Here is an example of a primary teledermatology workflow, which utilizes a patient uploading photos and a triage system: (1) Patient or patient assistant photographs the skin (2) Skin images and clinical history are sent/uploaded (3) Dermatologist reviews the case (4) Dermatologist decides whether a diagnosis can be made virtually or requests an in-person evaluation. In patient-assisted teledermatology, patients photograph their own skin and upload skin images before a virtual visit with a dermatologist. Alternatively, older adults may receive assistance from family members, friends, technicians, nurses, or home health aides in photographing skin images and navigating teledermatology portals.

3 Effectiveness and Barriers of Teledermatology in Older Adults

Teledermatology in the general population has been widely deemed effective, with concordance reports for the diagnosis and treatment of skin conditions ranging between 60 and 100% [7]. Multiple studies have found teledermatology to be a successful way to triage patients [7, 8]. After receiving images and patient history, a dermatologist may either provide recommendations virtually or request an in-person clinic visit for further evaluation. This triage process identifies high-priority patients in a more efficient manner and reduces the number of unnecessary clinic visits [7].

Older adults (age 65 +) in general have the potential to benefit from teledermatology services. In addition, approximately 1.3 million older adults live in nursing homes [9] and by 2030, older adults are expected to account for 20% of our population [10]. Many have physical limitations, restricting travel to in-person dermatology visits, or may live in rural areas with limited access to dermatological care. Thus, teledermatology has the potential to improve access to care. Additionally, teledermatological monitoring of post-surgical wounds or long-term wound care, with the assistance of home care nurses, has been found to be effective. According to one study, 71% of leg ulcers decreased in size after teledermatology visits [11]. Teledermatology is particularly well suited for follow-up appointments of chronic conditions such as psoriasis, leg ulcers and vitiligo and those with physical travel restrictions in the older adult population [12].

Important to note, there are barriers to teledermatology adoption in a subset of the older adult population, as some older adults have historically adapted late to technology and geriatric patients may face additional challenges navigating a teledermatology visit. For example, while 92% of older adults have a cellphone, only 61% have a smartphone, which could create difficulties in navigating teledermatology [13]. In addition, in 2018, 41.4% of Medicare beneficiaries did not have access to a computer with internet [14]. Addressing this "digital divide" may provide several benefits to older adults, as telehealth is effective in improving self-monitoring behaviors, self-care skills and independence in older adults [15].

Studies on teledermatology in the older adult population have yielded promising results. For instance, in one study in Sao Paolo, an in-person consultation was not required in 67% of dermatological diagnoses [16]. Interestingly, several previous studies explored teledermatology usage in certain subgroups of older adult populations such as nursing home residents and veterans. The diversity of teledermatology options among the older adult population is crucial to convey, and it is important to recognize the barriers to care within each subgroup of older adults. For example, in nursing homes, understaffing, inadequate nurse training, poor organizational leadership and unclear workflows are unique factors that can significantly reduce effectiveness of teledermatology programs [17].

In the upcoming sections, we describe in more detail the current state of teledermatology in the general older adult population, nursing home residents and veterans, emphasizing the barriers to care within each population. At the end of the chapter, we provide areas for potential growth of teledermatology in the older adult population.

4 Teledermatology in the General Older Adult Population

In response to the coronavirus disease 2019 (COVID-19) pandemic, the Centers for Medicare and Medicaid Services expanded telemedicine access for Americans aged older than 65. This shifted many patient encounters to virtual visits, and teledermatology transitioned to a patient-to-provider workflow. Despite a shift back to in-person care, teledermatology continues to be of great benefit to many patients, particularly in the older population.

Teledermatology in the general older adult population is typically carried out through patient-assisted teledermatology services or with the assistance of a patient's personal support network or health technicians. In a study of teledermatology in 130 geriatric patients with skin diseases in Italy in 2009, clinical history and images were taken at the department of dermatology [18]. Both face-to-face examination and store-and forward teledermatology were completed and diagnostic agreement, confidence and therapeutic agreement were evaluated [18]. Overall, 87.7% of patients were diagnosed with the same ICD-9 code and agreement between therapies was seen in 69.6% of patients who underwent both an in-person consultation and teledermatology visits [18]. Important to note, diagnostic confidence was significantly higher in the face-to-face examination compared with the teledermatology examination [18]. In another study completed in 2017–2018, 6633 patients over the age of 60 were enrolled in a medical center in Sao Paulo to determine the proportion of dermatology diagnoses that could be managed through teledermatology [16]. Health technicians assisted in the uploading of photographs and clinical history [16]. Dermatologists triaged the patients, first deciding if the image quality was satisfactory for diagnostic purposes [16]. If the photo quality was satisfactory, patients were either referred for a biopsy, dermatology consultation or back to the primary care provider with management recommendations [16]. This triage method was highly effective and decreased mean waiting times from 6.7 months prior to the study to 1.5 months during the study [16]. Additionally, it was found that 66.66% (8408/12,614) of dermatological diagnoses did not require an in-person consultation [16]. Teledermatology with technician assistance for skin image photography and history upload was highly effective, accurate and well received in this general older adult population (Table 1).

In a teledermatology study monitoring leg ulcers in 2007, home-care nurses assisted patients in completing teledermatology follow-ups from home [11]. Patients were between 47 and 86 years old and the median age was 73. [11] Overall, 644/724 (89%) of dermatological images were of sufficient quality and 71% of ulcers decreased in size [11]. Training for home-care nurses in image capture and navigating the teledermatology platform was essential to the success of the program [11]. Most patients (12/16) believed that teledermatology could replace the in-person consultation. Also, the acceptance of teledermatology was high in the home-care nurse population [11]. The results from this study suggest a tremendous potential for teledermatology for follow-ups of previously diagnosed skin-conditions, particularly chronic wounds.

Patient-assisted teledermatology services are an excellent method for patients to send and receive data without provider support. This remains a feasible option for older adults who meet technological requirements and are technologically proficient. For those who may need additional assistance, more patient-friendly resources should be presented. For example, one study described methods to optimize virtual care for geriatric patients including using user-friendly telemedicine platforms, more descriptive, clear language with videos and screenshots, encouraging the use of larger user-friendly devices, and allowing trusted family members/advocates during the visit [19]. Most importantly, instructions for image capture must be clear and well described [19]. Also, an opt-in text message system where patients can text skin images rather than upload images into a more complex portal system would increase access for patients without a computer. Family and friends are an optimal first line of support to assist patients in photography and maneuvering teledermatology portals. It is important to encourage older adults to maintain as much independence as possible to improve self-efficacy [20]. Assistance from nurses and home health aides may

Table 1 Review of teledermatology in general older adult population, nursing homes and veterans

Author	Year	Population	Modality	Method	Outcome
General older adult population					
Binder et al. [11]	2007	• Graz, Austria • 16 patients with 45 leg ulcers	SFT*	• Home care nurses captured images and uploaded them • Experts provided assessments within 24 h	• 32 (71%) of ulcers decreased in size • 14 (31%) of ulcers healed completely • 10 (22%) of ulcers increased in size • Transportation costs reduced by 46%
Rubegni et al. [18]	2011	• Italy • 130 patients	SFT	• Dermatologists completed both face-to-face and telederm assessments • Diagnosis, diagnostic confidence & therapy logged	• 114/130 (87.7%) patients were diagnosed with same ICD-9 code • Treatment agreement in 69.6% • Diagnostic confidence significantly higher in face-to-face examination
Bianchi et al. [16]	2020	• São Paulo, Brazil • 6633 patients	SFT	• Health technicians uploaded skin images, clinical history and patient data • Dermatologists triaged patients	• 66.7% (8408/ 12,614) of dermatoses did not require in-person evaluation • Mean waiting time decreased from 6.7 to 1.5 months
Nursing homes					

(continued)

Table 1 (continued)

Author	Year	Population	Modality	Method	Outcome
Zelickson et al. [22]	1997	• Minneapolis, USA • 29 residents	SFT	• Nurses collected and uploaded images • Teledermatology diagnosis plans were compared to in-person plans	• > 85% of cases could be diagnosed and treated via teledermatology • Correct diagnosis made in 88% • Correct treatment given in 90% • Cost savings of $34-$224
Janardhanan et al. [17]	2008	• Singapore • 50 residents	SFT	• Nurses captured/uploaded skin images & clinical history • Dermatologist submitted diagnosis report • Resident prescribed meds	• 54% of patients were recommended for in-person consultation but could not attend • All patients were diagnosed and treated via teledermatology alone
Veteran population					
Bezalel et al. [26]	2015	• Florida, USA • 2012: 28 SFT consults • 2013: 608 SFT consults	SFT	• Retrospective study • Compare 2012 and 2013 (when SFT was heavily used)	• Significant decrease in no-shows and wait-times for new patients • Correlation between the number of SFTs and the % of new patients

(continued)

Table 1 (continued)

Author	Year	Population	Modality	Method	Outcome
Bertrand et al. [28]	2019	• Providence VHA, USA • 460 tele-consultations	SFT	• Retrospective chart review • 5 locations for skin imaging • Patients referred to primary care with recommendations or received in-person derm eval	• Face-to-face consultations were not required in 51% of cases • 99% of teledermatology consultations were performed within 1 week of completed imaging
Peracca et al. [29]	2021	• 16 hub facilities in USA	SFT	• Funding was provided to 16 VA hub facilities • First 2 years of program was compared to the year before funding began	• Teledermatology encounters and # of unique patients increased in each of the first 2 years • The number of unique rural patients served increased • Faster treatment

* Store and forward teledermatology

be a more appropriate option for patients facing cognitive impairment or health limitations.

Overall, teledermatology is an excellent option for many older adults to receive timely access to high quality dermatological care. However, we must continually assess the needs of older adult patients and provide assistance as required. Issues related to technology, digital literacy, device ergonomics, ability to photograph, and internet connectivity should be addressed before expanding teledermatology in this population. Previous teledermatology studies completed in the older adult population demonstrated that most dermatology consultations could be conducted via teledermatology alone; however, many were done using trained staff to collect photographs. Finally, while teledermatology may serve as a useful diagnostic tool, it is important to keep in mind that many dermatological diagnoses, such as skin cancer, may require in-person visits for definitive diagnosis and treatment.

5 Teledermatology in Nursing Homes

Teledermatology has tremendous potential in nursing homes and long-term care facilities, where many residents face travel restrictions. Skin cancer, actinic keratosis, pressure ulcers and skin infection are extremely common dermatological diagnoses among nursing home residents [21]. In fact, a study of 10 long-term care facilities in Germany found that almost every resident (n = 223) had at least one dermatological condition, and almost 1 in 5 residents had actinic keratosis [21]. Residents with physical limitations may face scheduling difficulties and increased wait-times. Teledermatology with nurse assistance is a practical method to triage nursing home residents to limit unnecessary travel and improve access to high quality dermatological care.

Previously, two studies evaluated store-and-forward teledermatology in nursing homes. In one study, a teledermatology system was implemented in a nursing home in Singapore between 2005 and 2007[17]. In this system, nurses entered patients' medical records, uploaded skin images and requested diagnoses and treatment plans for patients[17]. Dermatologists then uploaded a diagnosis/treatment report into the teledermatology system (DPHIMS). Resident doctors used this report to prescribe medications [17]. Then, nurses and nurse aides administered medications and monitored residents. Patient cases were reuploaded into the DPHIMS system for follow-up as needed. Although 54% of nursing home residents were recommended for an in-person consultation, these residents could not attend due to financial reasons so they continued to receive care through the DPHIMS platform [17]. In both phases of the study, most nurses (80–100%) were satisfied with the performance of the teledermatology system and would recommend it to other nurses [17]. In a second study, 29 nursing home residents in Minneapolis were enrolled in nurse assisted teledermatology [22]. 85% of cases could be diagnosed and treated using teledermatology alone. The correct diagnosis was made for 88% of patients and the correct treatment was selected for 90% of patients. The cost of each consult was $34–$224 cheaper than the in-person consultation [22]. Overall, teledermatology was found to be accurate, cost-effective, and efficient in these nursing homes (Table 1).

However, the implementation of teledermatology in nursing homes poses several challenges. Foremost, the success of the teledermatology programs was dependent on the ability of nurses to photograph patients, enter clinical histories and request appointments in a timely manner. In the study conducted in Singapore, nurses faced several barriers including administrative problems such as the lack of overtime pay and technological challenges when using computers and teledermatology software [17]. It became evident that the entire nursing home administration needed to embrace teledermatology to promote efficient workflow and to ensure formal training of nurses [17].

Importantly, nurses were responsible for photographing the patient's skin and obtaining high-resolution, quality images, one of the most important tasks in the workflow. The uploading of poor-quality images can impede the workflow and increase wait times. A study of teledermatology in Dutch Nursing Homes suggested the following tips for photographing a patient's skin: use a minimum resolution of

1.2 MP, provide a solid contrasting background different than the patient's skin color, do not use flash, avoid shadowing, and potentially include a tape measure in photos. [23]

Given the extensive training required for nurses and the high dermatology case load in nursing homes, we recommend designating a small number of nurses for teledermatology tasks. These nurses should be trained in high-resolution image photography, navigating the telehealth software, and training new staff. For the teledermatology workflow, we recommend the initial use of nurse-assisted store-and-forward teledermatology; however, we encourage setting up a virtual visit between the dermatologist and patient when possible, once the photos have been reviewed. In the study completed in Singapore, the dermatologist submitted a report without consulting the patient on next steps, and this workflow did not provide patients an opportunity to ask questions or directly communicate with the dermatologist [17].

When setting up a teledermatology framework in a nursing home, several considerations should be made including:

- Insurance coverage
- Reimbursement for different types of teledermatology visits
- Training nurses in image capture
- Teledermatology software and medical record navigation/integration.
- Clear designation of tasks to nurses and provision of schedules.
- Clear communication between nurses, dermatologists, and primary care.
- Confirming a mode of transport for patients with physical limitations to dermatology office if in-person visit is recommended.

Overall, teledermatology should be generally available in nursing homes. It is an excellent tool to triage and select high-priority patients requiring an in-person visit. For residents with skin conditions that could be diagnosed via image and history alone and for residents attending follow-up visits, teledermatology, if implemented appropriately, is an efficient, cost-effective, and appealing choice of care. Teledermatology offers a practical solution for nursing home residents, as it may not always be feasible to transfer a patient to a dermatology office or for a dermatologist to visit a nursing home.

6 Teledermatology in the Veteran Population

The veteran population is an important population to consider in this chapter as 47% of veterans are older adults [24] and the median age of veterans is 65 [25]. Dermatology is considered one of the highest in demand specialties in the Veterans Health Administration (VHA) system and teledermatology has been well established in the VHA system for many years [26]. In a study examining teledermatology in the VHA system between 2002 and 2014, initially most veterans using teledermatology services lived in rural locations; however, by 2012, more veterans living in urban locations were using teledermatology services [27].

There are several important points to consider from the implementation of teledermatology systems in the VHA population. In a study evaluating the Providence Veterans Affairs Medical Center (PVAMC) in 2016, it was found that 51% of patients did not require an in-person dermatology consultation [28]. Additionally, teledermatology was found to reduce wait times as 99% of teledermatology consultations were performed within 1 week of image upload [28]. In a study of the implementation of store-and-forward teledermatology in a VA Medical Center in Tampa in 2013, the percentage of no shows and new patient wait-times decreased [26]. Most importantly, teledermatology was found to improve patient access as a correlation was established between the number of store-and-forward teledermatology visits and the percentage of new patients seen [26]. In a study implementing teledermatology for rural veterans in 16 hub facilities in 2017, teledermatology was found to be effective in serving remote patients as the number of teledermatology encounters and unique patients increased in the first 2 years of the program (Table 1) [29].

The VHA has established an excellent teledermatology service "VA Telederm App", that has integrated referring clinicians, teledermatology imagers and readers into the application system [30]. Additionally, the VHA system has created a rigorous training curriculum to train teledermatology imagers and a standardized operation manual for store-and-forward teledermatology, thus improving image quality and efficiency [27]. While teledermatology increased access to care and decreased waiting times in the VA population, there were mixed reviews regarding the implementation of patient-assisted teledermatology models. Many VA patients did not meet the technological requirements (having a computer/tablet/phone with internet connection) for teledermatology and many were unable to navigate the teledermatology software [28]. One study suggested that it remains unclear whether the older veteran population would benefit from patient-assisted teledermatology [31]. The provision of financial assistance for those without technological device/internet access could mitigate the digital divide. Programs such as "Tech for Troops" donate refurbished computers to veterans in need [32]. Also, formal education programs could be offered at VA centers to teach patients the technological skills required to navigate the teledermatology platform. This may be particularly useful for those without a strong social support network to help navigate the virtual encounters. The program may improve the patient-assisted teledermatology model, allowing veterans to maintain their independence.

7 Discussion

In summary, teledermatology, when implemented appropriately, is an accurate, efficient, and effective health-care service option for many older adults. Studies described in this chapter found that most dermatology visits (51–100%) could be conducted via teledermatology alone, with no in-person consultation necessary. In these studies, dermatologists triaged patients and either diagnosed and treated the patient virtually, sent the patient for biopsy or recommended an in-person visit. Teledermatology visits tend to be shorter than in-person consultations, as dermatologists can review images and history prior to the meeting. However, technological issues, problems navigating the devices/software, and other issues can increase the visit length. Overall, with the proper preparedness, teledermatology may improve access to care and decrease clinic wait times [33] (Table 2).

This chapter describes teledermatology services in the general older adult population and two unique groups containing a significant proportion of older adults: nursing home residents and veterans (Fig. 1). In all eight studies identified in this population, only store-and-forward teledermatology was utilized. Many older adults struggled with navigating technology systems and image upload. For older adults with technological limitations, we recommend the use of teledermatology assisted by family members or friends. If the patient is willing to improve technological skills, they could transition to patient-assisted teledermatology once they achieve technological proficiency. In addition, using easily accessible telehealth platforms and providing clear written instructions with screenshots and videos may assist older adults in navigating telehealth software [19]. In the future, systems may be able to assist patients with photography, using artificial intelligence (AI) to improve image quality through feedback [34]. For those that require them, the ability to add interpreters to a virtual visit could also improve accessibility and patient comfort [35]. For those facing significant physical or cognitive issues, assistance from health aides at home and nurses in the nursing home environment would be more appropriate.

To ensure the success of teledermatology, high resolution image quality must be ensured. The VA system has an excellent model to provide teledermatology services, as skin photographs or dermoscopic images are captured by trained imagers at imaging centers. Creating a standardized method for image photography and employing well-trained image photographers increases the image quality and efficiency of teledermatology workflow. Although in-person photo imaging centers with trained imagers in primary care offices and hospitals could help with image quality, this may not be feasible due to cost and difficulty of patients to travel to these sites. If patients opt for taking photos themselves, they should receive adequate simple

Table 2 Potential benefits and limitations of teledermatology for older adults

Benefits	Limitations
Transportation cost savings	Technological barriers (issues with patient portal, digital devices, internet)
Healthcare option for older adults with physical limitations	Difficulty taking photos, poor image quality
Decreases in wait times	Issues with digital literacy
Effective method of triaging patients	Physical/cognitive conditions makes navigating visit difficult
Improves access to care, especially in remote locations	Lack of personal support network

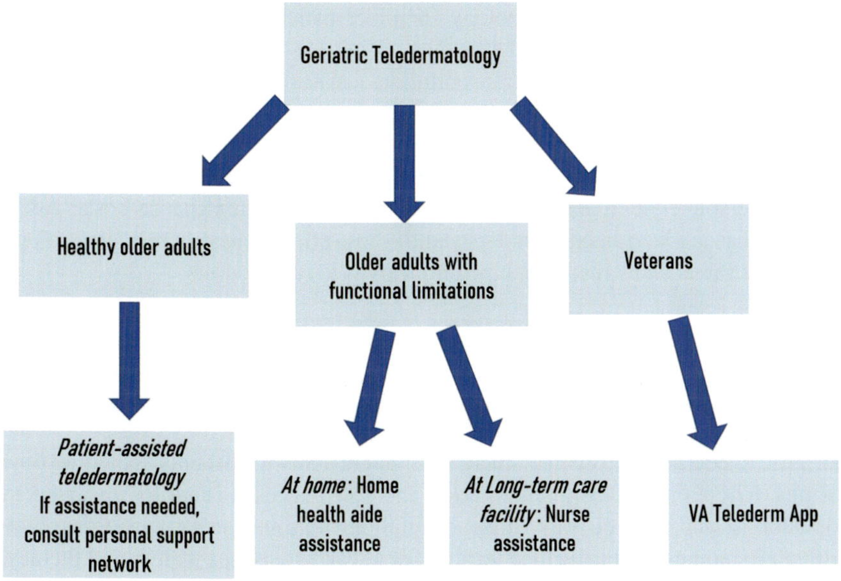

Fig. 1 Teledermatology in the older adult population

instructions that will lead to success. If they are unable, a proxy should be chosen to assist them with the photography.

An effort should be made to increase awareness regarding teledermatology access for patients in remote locations or for those with travel restrictions. One strategy is bridging partnerships between dermatologists and primary care physicians [29]. For example, in one study, 49.8% of teledermatology patients were referred to primary care with guidance on the management of the most likely diagnosis, without a face-to-face dermatology consultation [16]. These relationships are essential in providing a holistic approach to caring for geriatric patients. When caring for geriatric patients through virtual visits, additional factors such as polypharmacy, cognition, mobility, caregivers, and social support must be taken into consideration [36]. Primary care physicians can refer patients who need access to teledermatology services, particularly elderly patients with physical restrictions.

There are additional limitations to providing teledermatology in this population (Table 2). One of the major concerns of teledermatology is the inability to complete a full-body skin examination, thus increasing the chance that concerning lesions may not be identified [33]. Also, making virtual diagnoses can be challenging, especially if sufficient information is not provided or a proper examination cannot be performed. It is important for patients to be aware that an in-person visit may be required for further evaluation or treatment. A current general limitation to consider includes the fluid changes in regulations during the COVID pandemic. These include issues related to malpractice insurance coverage, licensure, reimbursement for teledermatology services, and use of non-HIPAA secure platforms [33, 35].

Implementation of teledermatology for older patients may be cost saving for some individual patients but could have larger initial start-up costs for larger facilities. There could be significant transportation cost savings, with one geriatric teledermatology study reporting a 46% reduction in transportation costs for patients [11]. However, in nursing homes and assisted living facilities, there are significant costs associated with the implementation of large teledermatology services, training personnel such as technicians and nurses, and maintenance costs. Additional studies are warranted to understand the cost-effectiveness of teledermatology in these facilities and to determine potential areas to reduce costs.

8 Conclusion

Geriatric teledermatology offers many potential benefits for patients, including time savings, reduction in transportation costs, increased access to care for underserved populations, and reduced wait times. Limitations that may make teledermatology difficult for some patients include technological barriers, issues with digital literacy, issues taking skin photographs, physical or cognitive conditions, and lack of a support network (Table 2).

Key Points

1. Teledermatology is a healthcare tool that can be used to improve access to dermatology among older adults.
2. Store-and-forward teledermatology was used in all teledermatology studies with a significant older adult population. It has been found to reduce waiting-times, number of no-shows, and travel costs.
3. Teledermatology may be particularly well suited to older adults with physical restrictions and those with follow-up visits for previously diagnosed dermatological conditions.
4. Limitations of teledermatology in a subset of the older adult population include limited ability to navigate teledermatology services, difficulty taking high quality images resulting in less-effective workflows, and the extensive training requirements of nurses and staff in nursing home settings.

Suggested Reading

- Rubegni P, Nami N, Cevenini G, et al. Geriatric teledermatology: store-and-forward vs. face-to-face examination. *J Eur Acad Dermatol Venereol.* 2011;25(11):1334–1339.
- Simpson CL, Kovarik CL. Effectively engaging geriatric patients via teledermatology. *J Am Acad Dermatol.* 2020;83(6):e417–e418.

- Bianchi M, Santos A, Cordioli E. Benefits of Teledermatology for Geriatric Patients: Population-Based Cross-Sectional Study. *J Med Internet Res.* 2020;22(4):e16700.
- Zelickson BD. Teledermatology in the nursing home. *Curr Probl Dermatol.* 2003;32:167–171. https://doi.org/10.1159/000067357
- Janardhanan L, Leow YH, Chio MT, Kim Y, Soh CB. Experience with the implementation of a web-based teledermatology system in a nursing home in Singapore. *J Telemed Telecare.* 2008;14(8):404–409.
- Binder B, Hofmann-Wellenhof R, Salmhofer W, Okcu A, Kerl H, Soyer HP. Teledermatological Monitoring of Leg Ulcers in Cooperation With Home Care Nurses. *Archives of Dermatology.* 2007;143(12):1511–1514.
- Fortugno AP, Dellavalle RP. Implementation of a patient-assisted teledermatology model in the Veteran Health Administration. *Dermatol Online J.* 2019;25(11).
- Bertrand SE, Weinstock MA, Landow SM. Teledermatology Outcomes in the Providence Veterans Health Administration. *Telemed J E Health.* 2019;25(12):1183–118
- Yeboah CB, Harvey N, Krishnan R, Lipoff JB. The Impact of COVID-19 on Teledermatology: A Review. Dermatol Clin. 2021.
- Farr MA, Duvic M, Joshi TP. Teledermatology during COVID-19: an updated review. *American Journal of Clinical Dermatology.* 2021:1–9.

References

1. Sharma A, Jindal V, Singla P, Goldust M, Mhatre M. Will teledermatology be the silver lining during and after COVID-19? Dermatol Ther. 2020;33(4):e13643. https://doi.org/10.1111/dth.13643.
2. Garcovich S, Colloca G, Sollena P, Andrea B, Balducci L, Cho WC, et al. Skin cancer epidemics in the elderly as an emerging issue in geriatric oncology. Aging Dis. 2017;8(5):643–61. https://doi.org/10.14336/AD.2017.0503.
3. Maddukuri S, Patel J, Lipoff JB. Teledermatology addressing disparities in health care access: a review. Curr Dermatol Rep. 2021;10:40–7. https://doi.org/10.1007/s13671-021-00329-2.
4. Lee JJ, English JC 3rd. Teledermatology: a review and update. Am J Clin Dermatol. 2018;19(2):253–60. https://doi.org/10.1007/s40257-017-0317-6.
5. Brinker TJ, Hekler A, von Kalle C, Schadendorf D, Esser S, Berking C, et al. Teledermatology: comparison of store-and-forward versus live interactive video conferencing. J Med Internet Res. 2018;20(10):e11871. https://doi.org/10.2196/11871.
6. Pasquali P, Sonthalia S, Moreno-Ramirez D, Agrawal M, Gupta S, Kumar D, et al. Teledermatology and its current perspective. Indian Dermatol Online J. 2020;11:12. https://doi.org/10.4103/idoj.IDOJ_241_19.
7. Wang RH, Barbieri JS, Nguyen HP, Stavert R, Forman HP, Bolognia JL, et al. Clinical effectiveness and cost-effectiveness of teledermatology: where are we now, and what are the barriers to adoption? J Am Acad Dermatol. 2020;83(1):299–307. https://doi.org/10.1016/j.jaad.2020.01.065.
8. Barbieri JS, Nelson CA, James WD, Margolis DJ, Littman-Quinn R, Kovarik CL, et al. The reliability of teledermatology to triage inpatient dermatology consultations. JAMA Dermatol. 2014;150(4):419–24. https://doi.org/10.1001/jamadermatol.2013.9517.

9. Nursing Home Care. https://www.cdc.gov/nchs/fastats/nursing-home-care.htm (2021). Accessed 5 July 2021.
10. Fueled by aging baby boomers, nation's older population to nearly double in the next 20 years, Census Bureau Reports. https://www.census.gov/newsroom/press-releases/2014/cb14-84.html (2014). Accessed 5 July 2021.
11. Binder B, Hofmann-Wellenhof R, Salmhofer W, Okcu A, Kerl H, Soyer HP. Teledermatological monitoring of leg ulcers in cooperation with home care nurses. Arch Dermatol. 2007;143(12):1511–4. https://doi.org/10.1001/archderm.143.12.1511.
12. Garehatty K. Patient-assisted teledermatology practice: what is it? When, where, and how it is applied? Indian J Dermatol Venereol Leprol. 2015;81:136–43. https://doi.org/10.4103/0378-6323.152172.
13. Mobile Fact Sheet. https://www.pewresearch.org/internet/fact-sheet/mobile/ (2021). Accessed 11 July 2021.
14. Roberts ET, Mehrotra A. Assessment of disparities in digital access among medicare beneficiaries and implications for telemedicine. JAMA Intern Med. 2020;180(10):1386–9. https://doi.org/10.1001/jamainternmed.2020.2666.
15. Guo Y, Albright D. The effectiveness of telehealth on self-management for older adults with a chronic condition: a comprehensive narrative review of the literature. J Telemed Telecare. 2018;24(6):392–403. https://doi.org/10.1177/1357633x17706285.
16. Bianchi M, Santos A, Cordioli E. Benefits of teledermatology for geriatric patients: population-based cross-sectional study. J Med Internet Res. 2020;22(4):e16700. https://doi.org/10.2196/16700.
17. Janardhanan L, Leow YH, Chio MT, Kim Y, Soh CB. Experience with the implementation of a web-based teledermatology system in a nursing home in Singapore. J Telemed Telecare. 2008;14(8):404–9. https://doi.org/10.1258/jtt.2008.080105.
18. Rubegni P, Nami N, Cevenini G, Poggiali S, Hofmann-Wellenhof R, Massone C, et al. Geriatric teledermatology: store-and-forward vs. face-to-face examination. J Eur Acad Dermatol Venereol. 2011;25(11):1334–9. https://doi.org/10.1111/j.1468-3083.2011.03986.x.
19. Simpson CL, Kovarik CL. Effectively engaging geriatric patients via teledermatology. J Am Acad Dermatol. 2020;83(6):e417–8. https://doi.org/10.1016/j.jaad.2020.05.118.
20. Walters K, Kharicha K, Goodman C, Handley M, Manthorpe J, Cattan M, et al. Promoting independence, health and well-being for older people: a feasibility study of computer-aided health and social risk appraisal system in primary care. BMC Fam Pract. 2017;18(1):47. https://doi.org/10.1186/s12875-017-0620-6.
21. Akdeniz M, Hahnel E, Ulrich C, Blume-Peytavi U, Kottner J. Prevalence and associated factors of skin cancer in aged nursing home residents: a multicenter prevalence study. PLoS ONE. 2019;14(4):e0215379. https://doi.org/10.1371/journal.pone.0215379.
22. Zelickson BD, Homan L. Teledermatology in the nursing home. Arch Dermatol. 1997;133(2):171–4.
23. Lubeek SF, Mommers RJ, van der Geer ER, van de Kerkhof PC, Gerritsen MJ. Teledermatology within Dutch nursing homes. Tijdschr Gerontol Geriatr. 2016;47(3):117–23. https://doi.org/10.1007/s12439-016-0177-1.
24. Shay K. Aging veterans and the department of veterans affairs. https://www.aginglifecarejournal.org/aging-veterans-and-the-department-of-veterans-affairs/ (2015). Accessed 6 July 2021.
25. Census Bureau Releases New Report on Veterans. https://www.census.gov/newsroom/press-releases/2020/veterans-report.html (2020). Accessed 5 July 2021.
26. Bezalel S, Fabri P, Park HS. Implementation of store-and-forward teledermatology and its associated effect on patient access in a veterans affairs dermatology clinic. JAMA Dermatol. 2015;151(5):556–7. https://doi.org/10.1001/jamadermatol.2014.5272.
27. Landow SM, Oh DH, Weinstock MA. Teledermatology within the veterans health administration, 2002–2014. Telemed J E Health. 2015;21(10):769–73. https://doi.org/10.1089/tmj.2014.0225.

28. Bertrand SE, Weinstock MA, Landow SM. Teledermatology outcomes in the providence veterans health administration. Telemed J E Health. 2019;25(12):1183–8. https://doi.org/10.1089/tmj.2018.0242.
29. Peracca SB, Jackson GL, Lamkin RP, Mohr DC, Zhao M, Lachica O, et al. Implementing teledermatology for rural veterans: an evaluation using the RE-AIM framework. Telemed J E Health. 2021;27(2):218–26. https://doi.org/10.1089/tmj.2020.0013.
30. VA TeleDerm App User Manual. https://mobile.va.gov/sites/default/files/VA-TeleDerm-App-UM-508.pdf (2018). Accessed 23 July 2021.
31. Fortugno AP, Dellavalle RP. Implementation of a patient-assisted teledermatology model in the veteran health administration. Dermatol Online J. 2019;25(11):1.
32. Tech for Troops. https://techfortroops.org/ Accessed 24 July 2021.
33. Farr MA, Duvic M, Joshi TP. Teledermatology during COVID-19: an updated review. Am J Clin Dermatol. 2021;22:467–75.
34. Puri P, Comfere N, Pittelkow MR, Bezalel SA, Murphree DH. COVID-19: an opportunity to build dermatology's digital future. Dermatol Ther. 2020;33(6):e14149. https://doi.org/10.1111/dth.14149.
35. Yeboah CB, Harvey N, Krishnan R, Lipoff JB. The impact of COVID-19 on teledermatology: a review. Dermatol Clin. 2021. https://doi.org/10.1016/j.det.2021.05.007.
36. Linos E, Chren M-M, Covinsky K. Geriatric dermatology-a framework for caring for older patients with skin disease. JAMA Dermatol. 2018;154(7):757–8. https://doi.org/10.1001/jamadermatol.2018.0286.

Imaging Technology

Digital Photography

Loren Elizabeth de la Caridad Hernandez, Kayla Mashoudy, Daphne G. Eckembrecher, Francelia J. Eckembrecher, Noreen Mohsin, and Keyvan Nouri

Abstract Digital photography undoubtedly plays an important role in the field of dermatology, a visual specialty that relies on pattern detection to make a diagnosis. The use and interpretation of digital images enhances the visual literacy that is integral to dermatology. In this chapter, various technical aspects of digital photography and the many uses of digital images in dermatology are examined. After describing how digital cameras function, explaining relevant photography terms, and discussing important image storage formats, the chapter explores the many roles digital photography plays in patient care, medical academia, patient education, and research. Moreover, the importance of safeguarding patient privacy is highlighted in the sections discussing informed consent and HIPAA compliant regulations and practices. Finally, the topic of underrepresentation of skin of color in dermatology textbooks and medical literature is highlighted with focus on the lack of diversity that persists and needs to be addressed. In conjunction with these important considerations, the proper use of digital photography in the dermatology specialty is a powerful tool for enhancing the visual proficiency and scope of the field.

Keywords Digital photography · Skin of color · Photodocumentation · Camera

1 Introduction

Dermatology is a unique specialty in that diagnoses can be made via visual inspection. Dermatologists diagnose and treat diseases of the integumentary system, consisting of the skin and its derivatives such as nails, hair, and oil glands. The mnemonic ABCDE in the triaging of potential malignant nevi is one such example of dermatology's visual dependence. A refers to asymmetry, B to irregular borders, C to

L. E. de la Caridad Hernandez (✉) · K. Mashoudy · D. G. Eckembrecher · F. J. Eckembrecher · N. Mohsin · K. Nouri
Dr. Phillip Frost Department of Dermatology and Cutaneous Surgery, University of Miami Miller School of Medicine, 1600 NW 10Th Ave #1140, Miami, FL 33136, USA
e-mail: loren.hernandez@med.miami.edu

K. Nouri (ed.), *Telemedicine and Technological Advances in Dermatology*,
https://doi.org/10.1007/978-3-031-69091-4_16

variances in color, D to diameter greater than 6 mm, and E to evolution or progression of the suspicious lesion over time. Given that the skin is the largest organ in the human body, and the most visible, clinical photography plays a key role in the evaluation, diagnosis, and treatment of dermatological disorders. It is also important in documenting the progression of disease and efficacy of treatment, as well as the documentation of pre- and post-treatment results. This chapter will discuss digital photography and its applications in dermatology, recent advances in digital technology, important considerations such as informed consent, HIPAA security and compliance, and photodocumentation in persons of colored skin.

2 How Digital Cameras Work and Devices Used

In digital cameras, light enters the camera and strikes a sensor. The two types of sensors available include the charge-coupled device (CCD) and complementary metal-oxide semiconductor (CMOS). There are photodiodes present on both sensors which absorb photons and release electrons. The electrons produced are stored as an electric charge—the amount of charge that is produced is proportional to the amount of photons that initially hit the sensor. This charge is then converted to an analog voltage, which is subsequently sent to an analog to digital converter, which results in a number value. Each number represents the color, brightness, and location of a pixel, which produces an image. There are many types of camera devices available. They include digital single lens reflex (DSLR), mirrorless, compact (point and shoot), bridge, and smartphone cameras.

To understand DSLR cameras, one must understand the mechanism behind single-lens reflex (SLR) cameras. In SLR cameras, there is an internal reflex mirror present. Light reflects off the mirror to the optical viewfinder. This allows the user to visualize what the lens can see and thus, what will be captured by the camera. This same mechanism is the basis for DSLR cameras, one difference being that DSLR cameras capture images digitally whereas SLR cameras use film to record images. In contrast to DSLR cameras, mirrorless cameras do not have a reflex mirror nor an optical viewfinder. Compact (point and shoot) cameras also do not have a mirror system—light simply enters and creates an image on the camera's sensor. When using a mirrorless camera, one has the option to switch the camera's lens. This is not possible when using a compact digital camera. Bridge cameras fall in-between SLR cameras and compact cameras. They have an LCD (liquid crystal display) screen that allows the user to have a continuous live view. Bridge cameras also have an electronic viewfinder and a long-range zoom lens.

There are some differences between the cameras of smartphones and digital cameras. The main difference is the size of the camera sensor. In smartphones, the physical size of the sensor is much smaller than that of any other digital camera. A smartphone's lens is also much smaller than that of a digital camera and are typically made of molded plastic. These differences ultimately alter image quality and although smartphone cameras are becoming more prominent secondary to their convenience and ease of use, digital cameras remain superior in regards to image quality.

3 Important Terms and Definitions

Aperture: opening of the camera where light enters. The aperture ranges from f/1 and f/32, a wide and narrow aperture, respectively. F refers the f-number, discussed below. A narrow aperture results in a deep/large depth of field and a dim image. A wide aperture results in a shallow/small depth of field.

Depth of Field: difference in distance between closest and farthest objects in a photo that appear sharp and in focus. A shallow depth of field may blur the background thereby emphasizing the subject [1]. A deep depth of field may have multiple objects in focus [1].

Exposure: amount of light that reaches the camera sensors, helps to determine how bright or dark a photograph will be. If there is too much light, the photograph appears "burnt" or overexposed. If there is too little light, the photograph will appear too dark or underexposed. In the case of overexposure, details are lost and appear white, whereas in underexposure, details are lost and appear black.

Focal Length: optical distance from point of convergence of the lens and sensor recording the image. A parameter that is measured in millimeters. It can be divided into wide (28–35 mm), standard (38–70 mm), and long (80–200 mm) focal lengths. Standard focal lengths are the most used as they are similar to the human eye's angle of vision.

Focus: parameter that describes when a clear and defined image is present on a focal plane, results from the convergence of a lens' rays of light. Focus is typically automatic in most digital cameras, as pressing the push button triggers the camera to autofocus.

F-Number: ratio of focal length to aperture diameter. A small F-number implies a larger aperture, a brighter image, and a shallower depth of field.

ISO Sensitivity: ISO (International Standards Organization) is a measure of sensitivity of a digital camera's sensor to different lighting conditions. The quality of an image is inversely proportional to the sensitivity of the camera's sensor. An ISO speed of 100 is standard for normal daylight conditions. A higher ISO speed translates to greater sensitivity to light, but more of an image's texture.

Pixels: a pixel is the smallest unit of information that constitutes an image.

Resolution: the amount of detail an image holds.

Shutter Speed/Exposure Time: amount of time that the camera sensor is exposed to light when a picture is being taken. When a user decides to take a photograph, the shutter opens which allows light to enter the aperture of the camera's diaphragm. The shutter speed ranges from second to fractions of second. When taking photographs of moving subjects, a high shutter speed is preferred (above 1/250 s). When taking photographs of static subjects, a low shutter speed is preferred, typically 1/60.

There are four primary uses of digital photography in the medical field: medical consultation and documentation, medical education, patient and family education, and research. These four subdivisions of medical digital photography will be discussed in the following sections. Regardless of which subdivision of medical digital photography is being discussed, it is important to consider the following when photographs are taken for physician review. Appropriate image quality is pivotal to any form of medical photography. Without it, a physician's assessment becomes unclear and less reliable. It also becomes difficult to accurately assess progression of treatment and/or pathology. Here, we will touch upon how medical photography can be optimized.

When taking photographs, the patient should be positioned appropriately to eliminate distractions and properly focus on the area(s) of concern. One way this can be done is by placing the patient in front of a solid background, such as a solid-colored wall or cloth sheet. It has been shown that a light blue color background can provide contrast to an image and may be optimal as it prevents the intermixing of other colors [2, 3]. However, one must take into consideration that discoloration of the skin may be possible when using a light to medium blue-colored background [4]. In patients with Fitzpatrick skin types IV–VI, the optimal background colors for images are white and gray. These colors provide the most contrast, and the most ideal background color for an image is one that provides the greatest contrast [5].

It is also important to remove any extraneous distractions from the area itself such as chairs, tables, and lamps. As for the patient him/herself, depending on the site of the photograph, jewelry such as rings, necklaces, watches, and earrings should be removed. Busy patterns and/or bright-colored clothing may be distracting, and neutral, solid-colored clothing may be preferred. The patient should also be de-identified and the photograph(s) taken should not include any cosmetic markings, tattoos, birthmarks, identification tags, or any otherwise identifying features. However, this may not always be possible [6]. Currently, the standard practice when de-identifying a patient in medical photography is to crop the image to remove such features while maintaining the clinical components of the picture [6]. Patients should be advised to not wear face makeup, tinted skincare products, or body makeup prior to taking a photograph. If they are, they should be advised to remove it to optimize the photograph(s). The subject should show no facial expressions if the image's center of focus is the face. Expressions can emphasize facial wrinkles and lines, potentially distorting the image.

As for the camera settings and environment lighting, the following should be considered. The appropriate amount of exposure should be used when a photograph is being taken so that it is neither too dark nor too bright. If one is using a smartphone camera to take the photograph, tapping the touchscreen adjusts the exposure in an iPhone. Android smartphones have exposure sliders that may be adjusted when taking a photo. When photographing persons with skin of color, it is important to appropriately adjust the exposure so that the patient does not appear too dark or too light, thus obscuring the image. Given that dark skin absorbs more light and light skin reflects more light, one can slightly overexpose the image, which allows for appropriate image exposure. Focus can be adjusted by simply tapping on the touchscreen. Flash is another important component in medical photography. Flash refers to an artificial light that is in sync with the shutter of a camera. When a user presses the camera to take a photograph, the flash produces a rapid but powerful light. If the environment is dark, flash can improve an image's exposure and focus. In a standard examination room with adequate lighting, flash is not a necessity but may prevent a blurry image [4].

The orientation of the image in respect to the area of concern, the distance between the camera and the area being photographed, and the perspective of the camera are also pivotal in medical photography. The camera should be properly oriented. I.E. If a leg is being photographed, the image should be vertical. If a chin is being photographed, the image should be horizontal [4].

4 Storage and Image Formats

JPEG (Joint Photographic Experts Group), TIFF (Tagged Image File Format), and RAW are three file formats available in digital cameras. After a digital camera takes a picture, the image's data is recorded as a file in the camera's memory card. If all the data of the image is stored, this is considered a "lossless file." If only the portion of the data is stored in the camera's memory card, usually only the portion visible to the human eye, this file is referred to as a "lossy file." Given that in lossless files, all of the data is stored, the file tends to be much larger than lossy files. In contrast, conversion of an image into a "lossy" format results in some irreversible loss of image quality that accumulates with successive conversions.

JPEG or Joint Photographic Experts group is a "lossy" format meaning that the image is compressed to optimize storage on a memory card and create a smaller file. At lower compression ratios, image degradation is not evident to the human eye, but at higher ratios, image distortion and subsequent loss of detail becomes perceivable, especially along the edges of structures [7]. The main strength of this image format lies in its ability to reduce the size of larger image files which outweighs any minimal loss of perceivable detail at low compression levels [8]. Therefore, to minimize loss of detail, avoiding digital camera settings that apply a high level of compression is the best option. In addition to their excellent compatibility with most computer imaging software, JPEG files are very widespread on the Internet and a common format for digital cameras [7]. This makes them ideal for web use, non-professional printing, storage and transmission of photographic images, and PowerPoint presentations and provides an advantage for use in the electronic teaching environment.

TIFF, which stands for Tagged Image File Format, are "lossless" image files that support the full range of image sizes, color depths, and resolutions. They can also be saved in a "lossy" compression format and can contain multiple images in a single file [9]. TIFF allows for the preservation of all original image details and maintains high-quality images at the expense of producing very large files [7]. An advantage to using the TIFF capture format is that the images do not require conversion by special software after being downloaded on a computer. However, because file sizes are so large, memory cards will store fewer TIFF images and subsequent processing time is prolonged [10]. Therefore, it is not ideal for the digital educational environment but is an excellent format option for professional print publishing, high quality prints, and storing important images or archival copies.

RAW files are images generated by digital cameras that contain uncompressed, raw image data using a "lossless" format. Because they contain unaltered image data, RAW files produce high quality images that can be very large in size. After they are downloaded from a camera to a computer, RAW images need to be processed by image editing software such as Adobe Photoshop, Lightroom, or Phase One and converted to a standard image format like TIFF [10]. The unaltered images can then be adjusted for factors such as white balance, color depth, and exposure. These corrections are more effective when applied to unprocessed RAW data as compared with adjustments to images captured in JPEG or TIFF format [10]. Therefore, RAW capture mode is superior for producing larger prints with excellent image quality.

5 Digital Photography for Medical Consultation and Documentation

Photography has altered the way medical professionals document patient care and track progression of pathology and treatment. It has become nearly essential in the practice of dermatology and in other specialties that are highly dependent on visual inspection. This section will discuss digital photography's role in the diagnosis, treatment, and progression of disease status as well as its use in triaging patients for more immediate care.

5.1 *Diagnosing, Monitoring Progression and Treatment of Disease*

Areas of concern, given a patient's consent, should be photographed upon initial presentation as a baseline. If a physician is unsure of a patient's diagnosis, photographic documentation in conjunction with historical information can be used to communicate with peers and facilitate discussion. Serial images are helpful in monitoring the progression of a disease and to assess the effects of treatment. When taking serial photographs for these purposes, it is important to standardize how photographs are taken to maintain consistency, quality, and reproducibility of images [11]. This includes ensuring that the parameters mentioned in the previous section are maintained from photograph to photograph with as little fluctuation as possible. This allows for appropriate comparison of the images taken and assessment of pathology and/or efficacy of treatment. Digital photographs may also be used in the documentation of wound management and to assess the progression of wound healing. These consecutive photographs can be compared to one another and metrics such as size of the treated area, erythema, epithelialization, and wound contracture can be noted from digital images. Photographs also play a key role in the evaluation of efficacy of treatment. Patients can have a baseline photo taken as well as photos taken after treatment. By comparing these images, a clinician can determine if the treatment is improving the concern at hand. Patients can also note their progress and depending on results, conversations on treatment changes can be had.

5.2 *Triaging Patients*

Triaging is the process whereby patients are sorted according to their need for immediate medical treatment. Utilizing the store-and-forward method, also known as asynchronous telemedicine, patients can send their providers photographs and other data to be reviewed prior to their consultation. This is especially important in patients with suspicious nevi, lesions, and/or other skin concerns. Patients can take pictures of their skin concern(s) and send them to their dermatologist for review. Based on their assessment of the digital photograph sent, the clinician may schedule in-person or telehealth follow-up, prescribe medication, or recommend that the patient seek health care immediately.

An advancement in the field of medical photography in dermatology is "MedX," an innovative teledermatology screening tool. The SIAscope, a Class II A medical device, was created by MedX to provide more accurate imaging of suspicious lesions. It takes 5 images, including 4 spectrophotometric images, of 2 mm depth below the surface of the skin. This allows clinicians to better assess suspicious cutaneous pathologies, as more details are elucidated with the SIAscope. They also founded DermSecure™, a cloud-based telemedicine platform that can integrate with patient electronic medical records. Images are uploaded to patient profiles and can be stored for up to 10 years. According to MedX, lesions can be scanned via their medical device at low barrier-to-entry partners such as physician offices, pharmacies, medical clinics, and medical spas. Detailed assessment reports are created based on this imaging and within two business days is sent to patients and their physician.

6 Digital Photography for Medical Academia

Photographs play an important role in the training of medical students and physicians. In traditional medical education, studies are divided into pre-clinical and clinical divisions. Pre-clinical studies include the teaching of subjects such as anatomy and physiology, pathology, pharmacology, and microbiology. Clinical studies involve teaching students in the specialties of internal medicine, psychiatry, surgery pediatrics, and obstetrics and gynecology. Photographs are commonly used in didactic lectures and seminars to teach medical students and para-medical staff. Certain pathologies are rarely seen clinically but can still be taught to students via medical images. Photographs can help students with pattern recognition—an image shown in lecture and/or textbook materials may help a student recognize that same pathology clinically. Medical images may also help students to better remember the material being taught. It has been shown that colored photos are better remembered than those that are black and white [12].

7 Digital Photography for Patient and Family Education

Photographs may be used to help patients and their families better understand their disease process and the results of procedures and/or treatments. Educational information, such as pamphlets and brochures, many times include photographs of disease pathology. These materials can be found in physician offices and are oftentimes available online. Photographs may also be used to show patients the effects of procedures and/or treatments. By showing pre- and post-treatment images, patients can better understand the possibilities of treatment. This also provides physicians with an opportunity to manage expectations and provide patients with more information on treatment options.

8 Digital Photography for Research Purposes

Medical photography is important for research purposes. Photographs are vital in substantiating the claims of researchers as well as for the documentation of results in clinical research.

9 Important Considerations

9.1 Informed Consent

It is vital to obtain informed consent prior to taking a patient's photograph. A patient's consent should be obtained prior to taking the photo and the purpose of each photograph should be fully disclosed, as well. It must be divulged that their participation is completely voluntary and that they may withdraw consent at any time. Patients should also be informed that if they decline to have their photo taken and/or withdraw consent, that their care will not be impacted in any way. Of note, informed consent is typically discussed in reference to the discussion and treatment of disease—it is a legal standard. However, informed consent for medical photography has not been delineated in the courts. Regardless, it is only ethical for a physician to apply these standards when consenting a patient in respect to medical photography.

9.2 HIPAA Security, Compliance, and Protected Health Information (PHI)

HIPAA stands for the Health Insurance Portability and Accountability Act. It is a federal law created in 1996 to prevent the disclosure of patient health information without their consent or knowledge. There are three rules included in this law, they are the Privacy Rule, the Security Rule, and the Breach Notification Rule. The HIPAA Privacy Rule focuses on protecting an individual's protected health information (PHI). PHI includes any identifiable health information, some examples being a patient's name, phone number, social security number, and email address. It also includes full face photographs and other identifiable information such as tattoos, nevi, or birthmarks. The Privacy Rule must be upheld by certain individuals and organizations, these groups referred to as covered entities. They include healthcare providers, health plans, healthcare clearinghouses, and business associates. This rule allows for disclosure of PHI without a patient's permission for twelve national priority purposes.

The Security Rule allows for the establishment of standards to ensure the protection of any electronic PHI by a covered entity. Covered entities must be able to detect and protect against any potential security threats, maintain confidentiality of electronic PHI, prevent possible impermissible uses or disclosure of PHI, and ensure that employees are compliant. The Breach Notification Rule stipulates that upon the breach of unsecured PHI, covered entities must provide notification of the breach. Electronic protected health information (ePHI) may be accessed by health care providers, covered entities, and business associates on mobile devices, such as smartphones, if there are appropriate physical, technical, and administrative safeguards in place.

To mitigate the risks of data theft and HIPAA violations, methods of communicating, storing, and sharing patient photographs must be done in a HIPAA-compliant and safe manner. Although text messaging is a primary form of communication and common in the clinical workflow, most standard text messaging services are not HIPAA compliant because they are not encrypted and don't offer HIPAA-related Business Associate Agreements. In contrast to text messaging, the e-mail systems used by most healthcare organizations are secure and HIPAA compliant but have storage limitations and are difficult to organize. Conversely, electronic medical records are an ideal, HIPAA compliant storage method that is organized around patient identifiers but is impractical as a sharing medium due to its specialized software and login security. Electronic medical records are also valuable and common targets for remote data theft. Likewise, local drives including computer hard drives, flash drives, and external hard drives are prone to loss and theft. Unless they are encrypted and password protected, they are not HIPAA compliant and can be targeted because of their weak security. Considering these factors of capturing, sharing, storing, and minimizing the risk of data theft, an ideal solution can be accomplished through combining smartphone and cloud storage services [13]. Smartphones can be HIPAA compliant if they are encrypted and password protected and can be reset remotely by appropriate administrators. They can instantly upload photographs into a linked permanent cloud storage and remove local copies to minimize the risk of data theft. Lastly, if the storage of data and unnecessary third-party applications on the smartphone is avoided, this risk can be further minimized [13].

Any patient identifying photo including full-face photographs and photographs of distinctive features like tattoos or birthmarks all constitute PHI and are subject to HIPAA restrictions. Therefore, they must be used for permitted purposes and require the patient's written consent detailing the manner in which they will be used, especially for marketing and fundraising reasons [14]. Distribution of patient photographs to anyone outside of the healthcare facility for a permissible use also requires written consent from the patient. Although photographs used for payment, treatment, or healthcare operations don't require patients' written authorization, it is still advisable to obtain it [14]. Moreover, to limit the disclosure of patient images outside of a healthcare organization, providers should try to use facility-operated equipment instead of personal devices to take photographs and train staff on the organization's policy and HIPAA compliant procedures.

9.3 Photographic Representation of Skin Tones in Dermatology Journals and Textbooks

The United States of America is becoming more ethnically and racially diverse, with many ethnic and racial populations growing in number from the 2010 to 2020 census. It has been shown that there are some differences in how common skin diseases present in persons of skin of color[15, 16] and in the basic structure of skin itself [17, 18].

However, it has been shown that dermatology textbooks and online sources lack diversity in their representation of ethnic and darker skin tones. One study sought to assess representation of skin of color in Google image searches. A total of 3700 photographs were evaluated encompassing 71 skin conditions. After visually assessing and categorizing the images according to the Fitzpatrick scale, they found that less than 12% of photographs displayed dark skin [19]. Another study evaluated the representation of varying skin tones in three dermatology journals. They found that only 5.6, 4.1, and 8.3% of images in the Journal of the American Academy of Dermatology, JAMA Dermatology, and Pediatric Dermatology, respectively, were of patients with Fitzpatrick skin types V–VI [20]. It is evident that medical textbooks, dermatological journals, and resources need to include more patients of color.

The underrepresentation of skin of color in medical textbooks has larger implications for patient care. Because teaching images disproportionately depict lighter skin patients, medical students have been found to have a harder time identifying dermatologic conditions in skin of color than in light skin [21]. Moreover, the overrepresentation of lighter skin tones in dermatology texts does not accurately reflect skin color demographics seen in the United States and thus the patient population that American physicians serve [21]. Failing to expose medical students and physicians to a diverse range of clinical appearances creates the potential for inaccurate or delayed diagnoses of skin conditions in skin of color patients.

In addition to lost educational opportunities, the suboptimal confidence in diagnosing and providing medical care for patients of color can negatively impact the physician–patient relationship. Uncertainty in clinical diagnosis can contribute to the health disparities faced by communities of color in subtle but profound ways and strengthen their legacy of mistrust in the medical system [22]. Furthermore, the unequal visual representation of all skin color types can create feelings of job dissatisfaction and burnout in medical trainees during a time when calls for increased diversity in the field are being made [22]. This imbalance in image representation can also affect the integrity of the field such that the specialty has a diminished scope of practice and reduced impact. Therefore, it is important that the visual educational images from which physicians teach and learn reflect the diversity of their patient population. More efforts need to be made to actively take and include images of skin of color across common teaching platforms.

10 Key Points

- There are many types of camera devices and various image storage formats like JPEG, TIFF, and RAW that can be utilized for medical photography.
- The four primary uses of digital photography in clinical settings are medical consultation and documentation, medical education, patient and family education, and research.

- Prior to taking a patient's photograph, it is imperative to fully disclose the purpose of the photograph and to obtain informed consent.
- Employing the use of HIPAA compliant procedures with clinical photography will mitigate the risks of data theft and protect patient information.
- The historical trend of underrepresentation of darker skin tones in medical literature has negative impacts for both patient care and the field of dermatology.
- Greater attempts to equalize visual representation of all skin color types should be made to expand the field's scope of practice and reflect the diversity of patient populations.

11 Conclusions

This chapter discussed the many applications of digital photography to the field of dermatology. Due to the visual nature of the specialty, clinical photography is vital for the recognition, diagnosis, and treatment of dermatological conditions. When photographs are taken for clinical review, it is important to optimize image quality through important consideration of various factors such as patient orientation, background color, the site of the photograph, and camera settings like exposure, flash, and focus. Moreover, the patient should be advised to remove any face or body makeup and jewelry, asked to remain expressionless if the image's center of focus is the face, and de-identified whenever possible while preserving the clinical relevance of the picture. When using digital cameras, it is also necessary to be aware of the different storage formats such as JPEG, TIFF, and RAW which provide various options for image quality and transmission. Being knowledgeable about these image factors will assist clinicians in reliably utilizing digital photography for medical consultation, documentation, and treatment progression. Clinicians should also be aware of current HIPAA regulations and implement HIPAA-compliant methods to store and share patient photographs in conjunction with informed consent. Importantly, more efforts should be made to document images of skin of color to help address the underrepresentation of darker skin tones in medical literature and increase familiarity with disease presentation in those skin tones.

References

1. Taheri A, Yentzer BA, Feldman SR. Focusing and depth of field in photography: application in dermatology practice. Skin Res Technol. 2013;19(4):394–7.
2. DiBernardo BE. Standardized photographs in aesthetic surgery. Plast Reconstr Surg. 1991;88(2):373–4.
3. DiBernardo BE, Adams RL, Krause J, Fiorillo MA, Gheradini G. Photographic standards in plastic surgery. Plast Reconstr Surg. 1998;102(2):559–68.
4. Muraco L. Improved medical photography: key tips for creating images of lasting value. JAMA Dermatol. 2020;156(2):121–3.

5. Lester JC, Clark L Jr, Linos E, Daneshjou R. Clinical photography in skin of colour: tips and best practices. Br J Dermatol. 2021;184(6):1177–9.
6. Robinson JK, Bhatia AC, Callen JP. Protection of patients' right to privacy in clinical photographs, video, and detailed case descriptions. JAMA Dermatol. 2014;150(1):14–6.
7. Faccioli N, Perandini S, Comai A, D'Onofrio M, Pozzi MR. Proper use of common image file formats in handling radiological images. Radiol Med (Torino). 2009;114(3):484–95.
8. Richard H, Wiggins I, Davidson HC, Harnsberger HR, Lauman JR, Goede PA. Image file formats: past, present, and future. Radiographics. 2001;21(3):789–98.
9. Kabachinski J. TIFF, GIF, and PNG: get the picture? Biomed Instrum Technol. 2007;41(4):297–300.
10. Burian PK. Mastering digital photography and imaging. Alameda, UNITED STATES: Wiley, Incorporated; 2004.
11. van Geel N, Hamzavi I, Kohli I, Wolkerstorfer A, Lim HW, Bae JM, et al. Standardizing serial photography for assessing and monitoring vitiligo: a core set of international recommendations for essential clinical and technical specifications. J Am Acad Dermatol. 2020;83(6):1639–46.
12. Gombrich EH. The story of art: Phaidon Press Ltd; 1995.
13. Thomas VA, Rugeley PB, Lau FH. Digital photograph security: what plastic surgeons need to know. Plast Reconstr Surg. 2015;136(5):1120–6.
14. HIPAA restricts some photography, but not all. Hospital access management. 2018;37(3).
15. Jothishankar B, Stein SL. Impact of skin color and ethnicity. Clin Dermatol. 2019;37(5):418–29.
16. McLaurin CI. Unusual patterns of common dermatoses in blacks. Cutis. 1983;32(4):352–5.
17. Taylor SC. Skin of color biology structure function and implications for dermatologic disease. J Am Acad Dermatol. 2002;46(2):S41-62.
18. Berardesca E, Maibach H. Ethnic skin: overview of structure and function. J Am Acad Dermatol. 2003;48(6 Suppl):S139–42.
19. Kurtti A, Austin E, Jagdeo J. Representation of skin color in dermatology-related google image searches. J Am Acad Dermatol. 2022;86(3):705–8.
20. Hereford B, Kim Y, Zaenglein AL, Hollins LC. Photographic representation of skin tones in three dermatology journals. Pediatric Dermatol. 2021;38:146–8.
21. Reilley-Luther J, Cline A, Zimmerly A, Azinge S, Moy J. Representation of Fitzpatrick skin type in dermatology textbooks compared with national percentiles. Dermatol Online J. 2020;26(12):1.
22. Lester JC, Taylor SC, Chren M-M. Under-representation of skin of colour in dermatology images: not just an educational issue. Br J Dermatol. 2019;180(6):1521–2.

Teledermoscopy

Shelley Uppal, Akhil Gupta, and Giovanni Pellacani

Abstract Teledermoscopy is a novel for the diagnosis and management of skin disease when face-to-face assessment (FTF) is limited by logistical, geographical, or resource-limiting constraints. Teledermoscopy has been shown to be effective in the diagnosis of pigmented and nonpigmented lesions, with diagnostic accuracy comparable to that of FTF diagnosis. Inclusion of clinical and dermoscopic images improves the diagnostic accuracy of teledermatology services, thereby reducing unnecessary specialist referrals and costly treatments, time to intervention or management, and overall healthcare costs. Mobile teledermoscopy is an economically viable option for patients, as inexpensive mobile dermatoscopes have emerged on the market to reduce consumer out-of-pocket costs. The utility of teledermoscopy is limited in special settings, such as skin cancer screening and the diagnosis of complex lesions in high-risk patients. Further research is recommended to investigate the role of dermoscopic expertise on the accuracy of telediagnosis and artificial intelligence on the evaluation of teledermoscopic images.

Keywords Teledermatology · Teledermoscopy · Artificial intelligence · Telemedicine

1 Introduction

Teledermatology involves the transfer of medical information from a patient to a remote dermatologist either through virtual or telecommunication [1]. The visual character of dermatology makes it well-suited for teledermatology, as the color and

S. Uppal (✉)
Albany Medical College, Albany, NY, USA
e-mail: drskuppal@gmail.com

A. Gupta
Advanced Dermatology and Cosmetic Surgery, Margate, FL, USA

G. Pellacani
Department of Dermatology, University of Modena and Reggio Emilia, Modena, Italy

K. Nouri (ed.), *Telemedicine and Technological Advances in Dermatology*,
https://doi.org/10.1007/978-3-031-69091-4_17

distribution of skin lesions provide indications and clues in accurately diagnosing lesions and xanthems [2]. Teledermatology has been used for over two decades to provide improved access to care, especially to underserved communities, while simultaneously reducing health care costs [3]. Teledermatology has also proven to be comparable in accuracy rates compared to in-person or face-to-face (FTF) care in regards to diagnosis, management, and clinical outcomes [2].

Teledermoscopy refers to the acquisition of dermoscopic images from a remote site through digital platforms (i.e. mobile or digital teledermoscopy) for improving the remote assessment of pigmented and non-pigmented lesions. While FTF care remains the gold standard for diagnosing pigmented lesions, direct visualization of these lesions is difficult in settings with high patient volumes or in situations where logistical barriers prevent direct FTF assessments [4]. Teledermoscopy is an effective tool that providers can utilize to ameliorate barriers to FTF care and improve the remote assessment of pigmented and non-pigmented lesions [1]. This chapter will review the digital platforms used for the teledermoscopic evaluation of skin lesions and discuss the advantages, limitations, and special considerations for teledermoscopy in the clinical setting.

2 Digital Platforms for Teledermoscopy

Mobile devices (mobile teledermoscopy) and non-mobile digital devices (digital teledermoscopy) are frequently used to acquire and transmit digital dermoscopic images. Images acquired through mobile or digital devices can be adapted to the clinical setting and used for sequential monitoring, machine learning, and teledermoscopy [1, 5]. Sequential digital dermoscopy (SDDI) is the capture and storage of dermoscopic images, which allows for the monitoring of skin lesions over time for changes [5]. By comparing 2 images of a lesion taken at different time points, SDDI analyzes for specific dynamic criteria that infers the biologic behavior of a pigmented skin lesion [6]. Early studies have shown that SDDI allows for early detection of melanomas and reduces the number of unnecessary excisions [5, 6].

Machine learning is a type of artificial intelligence (AI) that uses computational algorithms (i.e., neural networks) through computer programs to analyze large data sets and improve accuracy. In dermatology, machine learning has been used to train computers to identify cancerous skin lesions, through the analysis of large image databases of cancerous lesions [5]. In 2017, Esteva et al. demonstrated an artificially intelligent algorithm, a convolutional neural network (CNN), that was able to classify skin lesions with comparable accuracy to a group of 21 dermatologists after learning from a curated database of nearly 130,000 images [5, 7, 8]. Similarly, the International Skin Imaging Collaboration (ISIC) published results of a study that demonstrated that a machine learning fusion algorithm utilizing predictions from 16 algorithms exceeded the performance of most dermatologists in the classification of 100 dermoscopic images of melanomas and melanocytic nevi [5, 9]. Machine learning is limited by data sets that do not have a full spectrum of skin lesions or less common lesions (i.e. pigmented seborrheic keratoses, amelanotic melanomas). Furthermore, for machine algorithms to improve, they require access to standardized, high-quality digital dermoscopic image databases [5]. Machine learning represents a harbinger of what is to come with the future of medicine and dermatology. Harnessing its potential can benefit practicing physicians, irrespective of any physicians' experience, and can revolutionize the way we deliver care and improve patient outcomes.

Teledermoscopy is mainly practiced through 2 models: live-interactive video consultation (synchronous telemedicine) or storage of images for future consultation ("store-and-forward" or asynchronous telemedicine) [1, 5]. Synchronous telemedicine involves the use of live, real-time, and collaborative telecommunications technology (audio and/or video) to facilitate a physician–patient encounter [3]. Asynchronous telemedicine uses store-and-forward (SAF) technologies, such as secure text, email, and internal or external SAF systems, to facilitate patient visits [3, 10]. Hybridization involves the use of asynchronous and synchronous modalities simultaneously [3]. Among active teledermatology programs in the United States, 72% of programs utilize store-and-forward teledermatology only, in contrast to 45% and 35% using live-interactive only and a hybrid of the two modalities, respectively [11]. Furthermore, store-and-forward teledermatology alone is the most popular approach compared to simultaneous use of store-and-forward and live-interactive modalities during patient encounters [11]. As part of asynchronous telemedicine, internal SAF systems offer many advantages over external SAF systems, including maintenance of records within one system, ability to capture other telemedicine benchmark data, and better continuity of care due to improved access to patient medical records [10]. In contrast, external SAF teledermatology systems operate independently from the primary electronic medical or health record and have many limitations, including fragmentation of care, communication lapses among clinicians of an interdisciplinary team, and privacy and security concerns [10]. One study that utilized an Epic-based internal SAF teledermatology system for dermatologic care in an urban city found that it improved access to dermatologic care by decreasing wait times and time to treatment or intervention and increasing referral rates by primary care physicians. Among 79 cases, diagnostic concordance between 2 teledermatologists was at least partially concordant (level 1[a] and level 2[b]) in 79 of 79 cases (100%), similar to previously published studies [10]. Epic-based SAF teledermatology has the potential to reduce the burden on safety-net hospital dermatology clinics by allowing for the effective management of cases remotely. In addition, it facilitates the monitoring of clinical outcomes and implementation of recommendations by referring clinicians [10]

3 Digital Teledermoscopy

With digital teledermoscopy, either a digital dermatoscope with image capturing capabilities or a digital camera interfaced with a dermatoscope is utilized to electronically send clinical images to remote providers via a secure web-based teledermoscopy platform [1]. Like mobile teledermatology, digital teledermoscopy affords high levels of diagnostic accuracy. However due to the ease of use and accessibility of smartphones, research efforts have been directed to optimize mobile teledermoscopy use in the clinical setting.

The disadvantages of digital teledermoscopy are difficulty of use and varying image quality. After each set of images is captured, most digital cameras require a manual transfer of the images to a computer using a data transfer cable or a memory card reader [12]. The images must then be imported into an electronic medical record or proprietary Internet application for reading [12]. While the process to uploading, transferring, and storing information via digital teledermoscopy is tedious, new solutions are emerging to add wireless transfer functionality to existing digital cameras, such as the *microDERM® wireless* software [12].

4 Mobile Teledermoscopy

Mobile teledermoscopy is a newer application of teledermoscopy where mobile devices (i.e. smartphones, tablets) are used to capture and deliver clinical and dermoscopic images [1, 13]. It is a digital alternative to conventional FTF consultation that integrates the photographic and telecommunicative features of mobile devices with those of an adaptor capable of functioning as a magnifying device. With the addition of mobile applications and secure web-based teledermoscopy platforms, mobile teledermoscopy allows for enhanced skin self-examination (SSE) [1, 14, 15].

Massone et al. in 2008, carried out the first teledermoscopy study using mobile phones for image capture, storage, and as referral platforms for two teledermatologists. The study found that, in the diagnosis of pigmented lesions, diagnostic concordance was 89% and 94% compared to FTF examination. In 2011, Kroemer used cell phones, without a special dermatoscope adaptor, to capture clinical and dermatoscopic images of 80 patients (104 lesions). The study found that clinical and dermoscopic tele-evaluation had a concordance rate of 85% and 79%, respectively, compared to FTF examination [13].

A major benefit of mobile teledermoscopy is that medical personnel can use apps provided by electronic health records, such as the Epic Canto app, to directly upload images into the electronic medical record (EMR) in such a way to maintain HIPAA standards for the use and disclosure of patient health information (PHI) [12]. Given that mobile dermatoscope attachments are also relatively inexpensive compared to other teledermoscopic solutions, mobile dermoscopy has the potential to expand the reach of teledermoscopy to the average consumer [12]. Mobile teledermoscopy is also easy-to-use and lightweight, and allows for the rapid acquisition of images [16]. Images can also be stored in a digital archive for follow-up, dermoscopic-pathologic correlation, educational purposes, or sent to colleagues for second opinions [16]. Use of mobile teledermoscopy for the purpose of triaging patients has been shown to be both feasible and economically viable [1, 17]. While there a variety of popular devices (Dermlite, Canfield) available on the market that can be attached to smart-phones for effective dermoscopy, the main disadvantage of these devices is their high cost, as many start at approximately 700 USD [1]. Nonetheless, more affordable dermatoscopes have emerged for the average consumer. The economical mobile dermatoscopes include the DermLite DL1 (285.00 USD), DermLite HUD (99.95 USD), dyplens (29.95 USD), MedicMind Skin Scope (75.00 USD), Molescope (99.00 USD), and Molescope II (299.00 USD) [1].

The disadvantage of mobile teledermoscopy is that the camera quality of older smartphones is typically inferior to digital cameras [12]. However, the newer generation of cellular phones do not have the limitations in image quality as seen in optical systems presented with older devices. Furthermore, in-built cameras seen with the new generation of mobile smartphones have improved image quality [12]. A comprehensive list of commercially available dermatoscopes is presented in Table 1.

5 The Rise of Teledermatology and Teledermoscopy During the COVID-19 Pandemic

With the growth of digital health in recent years, teledermoscopy has become an increasingly popular platform for providers that has been used to supplement teledermatology visits [1]. The COVID-19 pandemic has stimulated great advances in the application and use of various telehealth services, and dermatology has been in the forefront of such developments [18]. Given that dermatologists and other healthcare providers, alike, are exposed to patients through high-volume clinics and that asymptomatic carriers are able to shed viral particles, hospital-based dermatology departments and private clinics were closed to non-emergent, routine, in-person clinic visits [18, 19]. Screening patients and canceling appointments only for those patients with fevers or symptoms did not suffice given the risk for asymptomatic viral transmission and a prolonged incubation period [19]. Instead, teledermatology and teledermoscopy were and continue to be used as vital methods for delivering care remotely to patients as the COVID-19 pandemic wanes [20]. Furthermore, a hybrid of teledermatology and in-person visits may be most ideal in future pandemics to reduce contact and potential transmission while also ensuring timely diagnosis and treatment of urgent skin conditions. [21].

During the COVID-19 pandemic, there was a significant increase in utilization of teledermatology services worldwide [20]. A systematic review by Loh et al. analyzed

Table 1 A list of the commercially available digital dermatoscopes for teledermoscopy

Digital dermatoscope	Interfacing device (mobile device or camera)	Requires separate image-capturing device? (Y/N)
Dermlite Cam*	N/A	N
Dermlite DL1	Mobile device[a]	Y
Dermlite DL200 (HR and Hybrid)	Mobile device or digital camera	Y
Dermlite DL4/DL3N	Mobile device or digital camera	Y
Dermlite FOTO X/X Plus	Mobile device or DSLR[b] camera	Y
Dermlite Foto II Pro	Any Nikon or Canon full-frame or 2/3 frame DSLR camera	Y
DermLite HUD	Mobile device	Y
Dermlite handyscope with Handyscope 2 app/FotoFinder Hub	Mobile device	Y
Dyplens/Firstcheck app	Mobile device	Y
VEOS DS3	Apple mobile devices	Y
Canfield VEOS HD1/VEOS HD2	Apple mobile devices	Y
Canfield VEOS SLR	Canon SLR camera	Y
MoleMax HD	Built-in video or image capturing device in dermatoscope	N
DermoGenius II	Digital camera	Y
DermoGenius ultra	Built-in video or image capturing device in dermatoscope	N
Dynamify Wireless Dermatoscope	Built-in video or image capturing device in dermatoscope	N
Illuco IDS-1100 Dermatoscope	Mobile device or digital camera	Y
DE300 Polarizing Dermatoscope/Dermascope	Built-in video or image capturing device in dermatoscope	N
DE350 Wireless Polarizing Dermatoscope/Dermascope	Built-in video or image capturing device in dermatoscope	N
FotoFinder Medicam 1000	Built-in video or image capturing device in dermatoscope	N

(continued)

Table 1 (continued)

Digital dermatoscope	Interfacing device (mobile device or camera)	Requires separate image-capturing device? (Y/N)
Heine NC2 Dermatoscope/iC1 app	Apple mobile device	Y
Heine DELTA 20 T Dermatoscope	DSLR camera	Y
Heine iC1 Dermatoscope/iC1 app	Apple mobile device	Y
Molescope/Molescope II/ Molescope app	Mobile device	Y
Microderm Luminis	Digital camera	Y
MedicMind Skin Scope	Mobile device	Y

27 studies that utilized either asynchronous teledermatology, synchronous teledermatology, or a hybrid in the remote analysis of skin lesions [20]. Synchronous teledermatology was utilized most to diagnose synchronous acne, psoriasis, eczema, nonspecific dermatitis, and dermatophytosis [20]. Asynchronous teledermatology was found to be effective in evaluating acne, psoriasis, oncodermatology cases, hair disorders, infantile hemangiomas, tinea, eczema, intertrigo, photodermatitis, pityriasis rosea, and pyogenic granuloma [20]. Given that clinical photographs are essential to asynchronous teledermatology, dermoscopic images can significantly improve diagnosis in the remote assessment of lesions. One study assessed the impact of dermoscopy on decision-making by dermatologists, including confidence, diagnostic accuracy, and triaging urgency, during the COVID-19 pandemic [22]. The study found that dermoscopy increased diagnostic accuracy to 53.6% compared to 45.3% with the use of clinical images alone [22]. The greatest increase in diagnostic accuracy was seen with malignant neoplasms (54% vs 31%; $p = 0.0007$) [22]. In addition, dermoscopy significantly reduced triage urgency scores for both non-neoplastic (mean 1.2 vs 1.6; $p < 0.001$) and benign neoplastic (mean 1.35 vs 1.43; $p = 0.01$) pathologies, and increased urgency scores for malignant neoplasms (mean 1.64 vs 1.47; $p = 0.01$) [22]. Furthermore, inclusion of dermoscopic assessment increased providers' confidence in their management decisions by 7.6% ($p < 0.0001$) [22].

6 Advantages of Teledermoscopy

In the clinical setting, teledermoscopy is not only useful for diagnosing skin disease, but also for monitoring disease course and treatment response [22]. In addition to single patient encounters, teledermoscopy has been successful in mass screening events and reaching underserved areas that are remote from local dermatologists [4, 15, 23]. Inclusion of clinical and dermoscopic images to a teledermatology visit has been shown to improve the diagnostic accuracy by approximately 15% while adding only 1–2 min to consultation time [4, 15]. Studies agree that incorporating dermoscopic images in a teleconsultation can improve the sensitivity and specificity of telediagnosis [24]. Studies have found that interobserver concordance between FTF and teledermoscopic diagnosis is excellent, particularly in assisting with teledermatological management of pigmented and non-pigmented lesions [24–26]. Kromer et al. compared the intraobserver diagnostic concordance in clinical and mobile teledermoscopic diagnosis of skin lesions among two teledermatologists and found a 85% and 79% concordance rate, respectively [27]. Not only does teledermoscopy increase diagnostic concordance, but also improves triaging and reduces treatment delay for more malignant tumors [26]. However, teledermoscopy is limited in diagnosing and managing very difficult lesions, such as melanoma in situ [24, 26]. Similarly, the management concordance between mobile teledermoscopy and FTF assessment is generally positive, with 81–91% full or partial diagnostic concordance between both modalities [1, 4, 28]. With the transition of care from FTF to telemedicine appointments, more research in teledermoscopy is underway to elucidate its benefits in the clinical setting.

Another advantage of SAF teledermoscopy is that it can improve accessibility to specialists while reducing healthcare costs, the number of "no-shows" at FTF clinics, and surgery waiting times compared to paper referrals [1, 4, 17]. A study by Börve et al. found that smartphone teledermoscopy referrals could be assessed within 24 h, reducing the median time to diagnosis and treatment for all skin cancer types and allowing for more efficient management (such as surgical treatment when required) in skin cancer patients on their FTF visit [17]. Smartphone teledermoscopy referrals were also found to reduce waiting times for first-time FTF visits with dermatologists and for primary treatment of melanoma, melanoma in situ, squamous cell carcinoma, squamous cell carcinoma in situ, and basal cell carcinoma [17]. Similarly, Lim et al. demonstrated that teledermoscopy reduced the mean waiting time for a first assessment by a dermatologist was reduced from 114 to 39 days [17].

Teledermoscopy also reduces the number of inaccurately triaged referrals and frees up time for more urgent cases involving potentially life-threatening cancers [15, 17]. The IMAGE IT trial by Tan et al. found that teledermoscopy approximated 100% sensitivity and 90% specificity for detecting melanoma and nonmelanoma skin cancers [28] of significance, 74% of lesions were able to be managed by the general practitioner (GP) without the need to follow-up with a dermatologist [28]. As a triage and monitoring instrument, teledermoscopy has also been shown to reduce the number of unnecessary and urgent referrals, wait times, and overall healthcare cost [1, 4, 17]. A similar study involving a Virtual Lesion Clinic (VLC) by Congalton et al. found that the teledermoscopy had a positive predictive value of 63% in the diagnosis of melanomas [29]. In addition, VLC operation for 1 year resulted in cost reductions in excess of $364,000 (or $1174/patient) [29].

Another major advantage of teledermoscopy is that it can allow for consultation with specialists in remote or medically undersupplied locations, which is especially helpful in locations where there are shortages in dermatologists [4]. Teledermatology can also be a useful educational tool for dermatologists and other health care providers, the latter who can send an image of a difficult rash or lesion to a more experienced colleague for diagnosis and management [4]. It is also useful for monitoring patients with chronic conditions that require frequent follow-up and changes for treatment optimization [1, 4]. Despite reduced FTF interaction with providers, especially with SAF or asynchronous teledermoscopy, patients report satisfaction with mobile teledermatology services, citing improved waiting times, convenience, reassurance, and privacy [1, 4, 28, 30]. One study found that patients had a positive perception of mobile teledermoscopy and believed it would improve their skin self-examination and surveillance for cancer and motivate them to check their skin more often [1, 4]. Most importantly, patients reported feeling comfortable and competent with taking dermoscopic images with only minimal instructions. Similarly, parents of young patients also expressed willingness to use a pediatric teledermatology service if it was available [1, 4].

7 Teledermoscopy in Skin of Color Patients

Individuals of African descent or skin of color (SOC) patients have brown-black skin and eyes, and rarely get sunburned when exposed to sunlight. Furthermore, they are classified as skin types V and VI, according to the Fitzpatrick scale [31]. Dermoscopic patterns of skin lesions (i.e. pigment and vascular network) often differ depending on a patient's Fitzpatrick skin type [1, 31]. In skin types V and VI, acquired melanocytic nevi are dermoscopically defined by a reticular pattern with a tendency toward central hyperpigmentation and high frequency of gray and black [1, 31]. Nevi in skin types V and VI also show similar characteristics to melanocytic lesions exposed to sunlight, with the following structures: black dots, pigment blotches, prominent network, and decreased areas of hypopigmentation [32]. In contrast, patients with skin types I and II, and often skin types III, have a tendency towards lighter brown color with uniform distribution, and multifocal hyperpigmentation and hypopigmentation [1, 31, 33]. Despite differences in dermoscopic features, diagnostic accuracy in light and dark skin populations is similar, since darker skin does not interfere with the identification of single dermoscopic features [1, 32]. The use of new-generation dermatoscopes with sufficient light-emitting diode illumination is helpful in difficult cases where use of a strong light source is needed to evaluate lesions in SOC patients, as darker skin absorbs larger amounts of UV-light than lighter skin [1, 32]. Nonetheless, presentation of diseases in patients of SOC is underrepresented in current digital resources, stressing the need for educational resources to comprehensively illustrate pathology across all skin tones [34]. Additional research also needs to be performed in areas of diagnostics and surveillance so as to optimize evaluation of lesions in SOC patients [34].

8 Disadvantages of Teledermoscopy

While teledermoscopy is efficacious in the assessment of most lesions, it is limited in cases involving complex melanocytic and hypo- or nonpigmented lesions, and in the setting skin cancer screening. In addition, teledermoscopy brings out about ethical issues regarding the safe and confidential transfer of patient information. Limitations of teledermoscopy in the clinical setting will be discussed below.

8.1 Complex Melanocytic and Hypo- or Nonpigmented Lesions

In 2016, de Giorgi et al. assessed the efficacy of teledermoscopy in evaluating complex melanocytic lesions by having 10 different teledermatologists analyzing 10 challenging pigmented lesions via telemedicine or in-person [1, 13, 35]. The interobserver agreement (K^1) between teledermatology and FTF assessment was 0.38 and 0.60, respectively, indicating that was final histopathological diagnosis compared with final histopathological diagnosis, teledermatology was significantly inferior to FTF dermatology [1, 35]. Interestingly, in this study, the diagnostic concordance of telediagnosis decreased after teledermoscopic observation [35]. The researchers attributed the low interobserver concordance to the complexity of select cases that were evaluated during the study, such as Spitzoid proliferation and atypical melanocytic nevi of the elderly, which represent potential diagnostic failures due to their complicated dermatoscopic characteristics [1, 13, 35]. Histopathologically, Spitzoid lesions exhibit peripheral, irregular radial streaks and pseudopods, while atypical melanocytic nevi of the elderly exhibit widespread regression [35]. In atypical melanocytic nevi of the elderly, widespread regression is a significant confounding dermoscopic parameter because it tends to cover or destroy other parameters, thereby preventing an accurate diagnosis [13, 35]. These dermoscopic features are especially confounding and can justify the low diagnostic concordance between telediagnosis and histopathology in this study.

In another study, Fabbrocini et al. assessed the reliability of teledermoscopy for diagnosing rare and atypical lesions. Many of the lesions were characterized by poor and/or absent pigmentation, the absence of regular network, and a diameter < 5 mm [1, 13, 36]. The study demonstrated that certain dermoscopic elements are identified with more or less ease through teledermoscopy compared to FTF diagnosis. Dermoscopic features, such as leaf structures, pseudocysts, comedo-like openings, “blue-white structures”, and “blotches”, are detected with the same frequency in FTF assessment and teledermoscopy [1, 35]. However, other dermoscopic features, such as pigment network, regression structures, and diffuse pigmentation, are more easily visualized in teledermoscopic versus FTF observation, whereas vascular pattern, radiated streaks, and spots/globules are less frequently detected [1, 13, 36]. The study also underlined the ineffectiveness of SAF teledermoscopy in evaluating scarcely pigmented lesions (52%) compared to FTF assessment (66%), although both modalities demonstrate poor concordance with histopathological diagnosis ($p < 0.05$) [36].

8.2 *Skin Cancer Screening*

Most skin cancers, especially melanomas, are initially detected by either patients or their families [14]. In the absence of population-based skin cancer screening programs, naked-eye skin self-examination has become the recommended method for skin cancer prevention and early detection by cancer agencies [14].

Previous studies have approximated the sensitivity of skin self-examination to vary widely from 25 to 93% [14]. While dermoscopy has improved the sensitivity for diagnosing skin cancers, in addition to most melanocytic and nonmelanocytic lesions in FTF encounters [12], evidence for use in the setting of skin self-examination is contradicting. In one study, the efficacy of mobile teledermoscopy was assessed in comparison to skin self-examination (control). Although mobile teledermoscopy had a high sensitivity ($\geq$75%) for identifying skin cancers (pigmented and nonpigmented), more cancers were missed with mobile teledermoscopy ($n = 17$) than control ($n = 7$) [1, 14]. In this study, participants utilizing mobile teledermoscopy more commonly missed basal cell carcinomas (44%) than did participants in the control group (21%), indicating that instructions for digitally capturing basal cell carcinomas require further improvement [1, 14]. It is thought that decreased detection of skin cancers may also be due to lower rates of whole-body skin self-examination with mobile teledermoscopy [1, 14]. With fewer numbers of FTF appointments, there is an increased risk of so-called "unimaged melanomas" which are incidentally discovered by the dermatologist as part of the FTF examination but often overlooked by referring PCPs. Furthermore, loss of direct patient-physician encounters carries the risk of diagnostic and treatment delays given that there are fewer earlier or incidentally diagnosed melanomas [1, 37].

Monitoring of atypical lesions concerning for malignancy, instead of screening for new lesions, through mobile teledermoscopy has been proposed as an effective method for skin cancer prevention [38]. On the basis that melanomas change significantly over time, digital follow-up of atypical melanocytic lesions has been a proposed strategy to recognize melanomas that may lack distinct dermatoscopic features at baseline but gradually evolve overtime [38]. There is increasing evidence that the two-step method of digital follow-up, digital dermoscopy with total-body photography (TBP), can also aid in early detection of melanoma in high-risk patients (Breslow thickness, body site location, histological subtype, history of prior melanomas) [25, 39]. It is well documented that subsequent melanomas in patients with a history of primary melanomas tend to be thinner at diagnosis than the patient's first melanoma [39]. Body site location of melanomas in high-risk populations also shows a pattern of body site distribution (primarily on the limbs in women and trunk in men) and histological subtype (superficial spreading melanoma and melanoma in situ) [39]. The combination of SDDI and TBP also has been shown to improve the diagnosis of clinically featureless and de novo melanomas overlooked by dermoscopy alone, and has been proposed as a more sensitive strategy in melanoma screening in high-risk patients [39].

Mobile teledermoscopy has very high cancer detection rates for patients presenting with specific skin lesions, especially in high-prevalence settings [40]. The primary categorical diagnostic concordance rate between mobile teledermoscopy and in-person assessment is 82% (95% confidence interval 0.73–0.89), with a Kappa coefficient of 0.62 indicating good agreement [41]. Lesion directed teledermatological assessments, especially lesion directed SAF procedures, are time-efficient and have similar detection rates as in-person lesion directed assessments [40]. In several studies, the reliability of teledermatology based management recommendations has been shown to be comparable to FTF consultations. Feasibility and reliability for cancer detection, in addition, has already been shown in high prevalence settings [40]. Store and forward mobile teledermatology can be utilized for skin cancer screening for lesions of concern but precaution is advised when evaluating high-risk patients requiring full-body examination or patients with morphologically complex and pigmented lesions [1].

8.3 Other Limitations

Teledermoscopy limitations include technological challenges in elderly populations and ethical concerns regarding the confidential and secure exchange of data [1, 37]. Concerns regarding confidentiality of data can be addressed by encrypting data through the medical-related smart-phone apps, use of anonymity, or transfer of data to encrypted platforms [1, 37]. Another limitation concerns the standardization of image quality and regulation of smartphone apps [37]. Some apps have a low diagnostic sensitivity that may induce false negatives, erroneously reassuring patients to not seek specialist care [37]. While many of these apps are certified by regulatory bodies, certification does not guarantee effective application function and diagnostic performance [37, 42]. Therefore, greater control of these smartphone apps by federal authorities, including the US Food and Drug Administration (FDA), is necessary to guarantee mobile applications are safe for patients to use [20, 37, 42]. Similarly, standardization of image and service equipment is required for adequate functioning of a teledermoscopy service. Practical guidelines from the American Telemedicine Association (ATA) advised display systems have at least 24 bit-color depth in 2008 and an image resolution of 800×600 pixels and 1024×768, preferably, in 2012 [13]. Other standardization features include techniques such as ambient conditions (illumination, background, and camera position), patient pose, patient consent, privacy, and confidentiality [13]. Altogether, these features can alter the appearance of the lesion, emphasizing a need for standardization to allow for the consistent use of valid and reliable instrumentation that maximizes image quality and accurate diagnosis [13]. Once standardization techniques are implemented, image acquisition could be utilized for broader population-based screening [13]. Future advances in mobile teledermatology may address these concerns and increase the accuracy of self-skin examinations.

Another anticipated difficulty with teledermoscopy is the omission of specific areas that are either difficult to access, such as hair (i.e. apical melanocytic lesions), the back, or the ear, or those considered sensitive (i.e. genitalia), which could interfere with the lesion identification [1, 37].

9 Conclusion

Teledermoscopy is an effective platform for the prevention, diagnosis, and treatment of skin disease in situations, especially when specialized dermatological assistance is not available. It is an effective triage and monitoring tool that can be utilized in the educational and clinical setting, and for the effective diagnosis of uncomplicated pigmented and nonpigmented lesions in low-risk patients with similar diagnostic accuracy to FTF diagnosis. Future research is needed to identify the elaborate the role of teledermoscopy in managing complex lesions in adults, with special emphasis on complex pigmented or hypopigmented lesions and lesions in high-risk patients with a history of skin cancer. In addition, further investigation is recommended to assess the role of dermoscopic expertise on the accuracy of telediagnosis and the role of artificial intelligence (AI) and neuronal networks in teledermoscopy.

10 Key Points

- Teledermoscopy is an evolving tool that has comparable accuracy to face-to-face (FTF) assessment and has been shown decrease overall healthcare costs.
- Teledermoscopy is an effective triage and monitoring tool that increases access to dermatologists and allows for remote assessment of skin lesions in underserved areas.
- Teledermoscopy is limited in selecting settings involving high risk patients and ambiguous lesions, such as morphologically complex pigmented or non-pigmented lesions.

Conflicts of Interest The authors have no conflicts of interest to declare.

References

1. Uppal SK, Beer J, Hadeler E, Gitlow H, Nouri K. The clinical utility of teledermoscopy in the era of telemedicine. Dermatol Ther. 2021;34(2):e14766.
2. Tensen E, van der Heijden JP, Jaspers MW, Witkamp L. Two decades of teledermatology: current status and integration in national healthcare systems. Curr Dermatol Rep. 2016;5:96–104.
3. Kazi R, Evankovich MR, Liu R, Liu A, Moorhead A, Ferris LK, Falo LD Jr, English JC III. Utilization of asynchronous and synchronous teledermatology in a large health care system during the COVID-19 pandemic. Telemed e-Health. 2021;27(7):771–7.
4. Lee K, Finnane A, Soyer P. Recent trends in teledermatology and teledermoscopy. Dermatol Pract Concept. 2018;8:214–23.
5. Bleicher B, Levine A, Markowitz O. Going digital with dermoscopy. Cutis. 2018;102(2):102–5.
6. Tschandl P. Sequential digital dermatoscopic imaging of patients with multiple atypical nevi. Dermatol Pract Concept. 2018;8(3):231–7.
7. Esteva A, Kuprel B, Novoa RA, et al. Dermatologist-level classification of skin cancer with deep neural networks. Nature. 2017;542(7639):115–8.
8. Park AJ, Ko JM, Swerlick RA. Crowdsourcing dermatology: dataderm, big data analytics, and machine learning technology. J Am Acad Dermatol. 2018;78(3):643–4.
9. Marchetti MA, Codella NCF, Dusza SW, et al. Results of the 2016 international skin imaging collaboration international symposium on biomedical imaging challenge: comparison of the accuracy of computer algorithms to dermatologists for the diagnosis of melanoma from dermoscopic images. J Am Acad Dermatol. 2018;78(2):270-277.e271.
10. Carter ZA, Goldman S, Anderson K, et al. Creation of an internal teledermatology store-and-forward system in an existing electronic health record: a pilot study in a safety-net public health and hospital system. JAMA Dermatol. 2017;153(7):644–50.
11. Yim KM, Florek AG, Oh DH, McKoy K, Armstrong AW. Teledermatology in the United States: an update in a dynamic era. Telemed e-Health. 2018;24(9):691–7.
12. Singh SR, Meka AP, Nguyen G, Tejasvi T. Teledermoscopy for teledermatology. Curr Dermatol Rep. 2016;5(2):71–6.
13. Barcaui CB, Lima PMO. Application of teledermoscopy in the diagnosis of pigmented lesions. Int J Telemed Appl. 2018;2018:1624073–1624073.
14. Janda M, Horsham C, Vagenas D, et al. Accuracy of mobile digital teledermoscopy for skin self-examinations in adults at high risk of skin cancer: an open-label, randomised controlled trial. Lancet Digit Health. 2020;2(3):e129–37.
15. Lee KJ, Soyer HP. Future developments in teledermoscopy and total body photography. Int J Dermatol Venereol. 2019;2(1):15–8.
16. Massone C, Brunasso AM, Campbell TM, Soyer HP. Mobile teledermoscopy–melanoma diagnosis by one click? Semin Cutan Med Surg. 2009;28(3):203–5.
17. Börve A, Dahlén Gyllencreutz J, Terstappen K, et al. Smartphone teledermoscopy referrals: a novel process for improved triage of skin cancer patients. Acta Derm Venereol. 2015;95(2):186–90.
18. BT19: the use of a novel teledermatology/teledermoscopy service to maintain a dermatology cancer service in the midst of the COVID-19 pandemic. *Br J Dermatol.* 2021;185(S1):184.
19. Kwatra SG, Sweren RJ, Grossberg AL. Dermatology practices as vectors for COVID-19 transmission: a call for immediate cessation of nonemergent dermatology visits. J Am Acad Dermatol. 2020;82(5):e179–80.
20. Loh CH, Chong Tam SY, Oh CC. Teledermatology in the COVID-19 pandemic: a systematic review. JAAD Int. 2021;5:54–64.
21. Sun Q, McMahon DE, Ugwu-Dike PO, et al. How coronavirus disease 2019 changed dermatology practice in 1 year around the world: perspectives from 11 countries. Dermatol Clin. 2021;39(4):639–51.

22. McCrary MR, Rogers T, Yeung H, Krueger L, Chen SC. Abstract PO-042: would dermoscopic photographs help triage teledermatology consults in the COVID-19 era. Clin Cancer Res. 2020;26(18 Supplement):PO-042.
23. Naka F, Lu J, Porto A, Villagra J, Wu ZH, Anderson D. Impact of dermatology eConsults on access to care and skin cancer screening in underserved populations: a model for teledermatology services in community health centers. J Am Acad Dermatol. 2018;78(2):293–302.
24. Lowe A, Atwan A, Mills C. Teledermoscopy as a community based diagnostic test in the era of COVID-19? Clin Exp Dermatol. 2021;46(1):173–4.
25. Arzberger E, Curiel-Lewandrowski C, Blum A, et al. Teledermoscopy in high-risk melanoma patients: a comparative study of face-to-face and teledermatology visits. Acta Derm Venereol. 2016;96(6):779–83.
26. Dahlén Gyllencreutz J, Paoli J, Bjellerup M, et al. Diagnostic agreement and interobserver concordance with teledermoscopy referrals. J Eur Acad Dermatol Venereol. 2017;31(5):898–903.
27. Kroemer S, Fruehauf J, Campbell TM, et al. Mobile teledermatology for skin tumour screening: diagnostic accuracy of clinical and dermoscopic image tele-evaluation using cellular phones. Br J Dermatol. 2011;164:973–9.
28. Tan E, Yung A, Jameson M, Oakley A, Rademaker M. Successful triage of patients referred to a skin lesion clinic using teledermoscopy (IMAGE IT trial). Br J Dermatol. 2010;162(4):803–11.
29. Congalton AT, Oakley AM, Rademaker M, Bramley D, Martin RCW. Successful melanoma triage by a virtual lesion clinic (teledermatoscopy). J Eur Acad Dermatol Venereol. 2015;29(12):2423–8.
30. Hadeler E, Gitlow H, Nouri K. Definitions, survey methods, and findings of patient satisfaction studies in teledermatology: a systematic review. Arch Dermatol Res. 2020;313(4):205–15.
31. Tuma B, Yamada S, Atallah ÁN, Araujo FM, Hirata SH. Dermoscopy of black skin: a cross-sectional study of clinical and dermoscopic features of melanocytic lesions in individuals with type V/VI skin compared to those with type I/II skin. J Am Acad Dermatol. 2015;73(1):114–9.
32. de Giorgi V, Trez E, Salvini C, et al. Dermoscopy in black people. Br J Dermatol. 2006;155(4):695–9.
33. Zalaudek I, Argenziano G, Mordente I, et al. Nevus type in dermoscopy is related to skin type in white persons. Arch Dermatol. 2007;143(3):351–6.
34. Hadeler E, Beer J, Uppal S, Nouri K. Identifying areas for improvement in remote skin cancer management: surveillance, diagnostics, and skin of color. J Drugs Dermatol. 2021;20(7):792–3.
35. de Giorgi V, Gori A, Savarese I, et al. Teledermoscopy in doubtful melanocytic lesions: is it really useful? Int J Dermatol. 2016;55(10):1119–23.
36. Fabbrocini G, Balato A, Rescigno O, Mariano M, Scalvenzi M, Brunetti B. Telediagnosis and face-to-face diagnosis reliability for melanocytic and non-melanocytic 'pink' lesions. J Eur Acad Dermatol Venereol. 2008;22(2):229–34.
37. Rat C, Hild S, Rault Sérandour J, et al. Use of smartphones for early detection of melanoma: systematic review. J Med Internet Res. 2018;20(4):e135–e135.
38. Salerni G, Carrera C, Lovatto L, et al. Characterization of 1152 lesions excised over 10 years using total-body photography and digital dermatoscopy in the surveillance of patients at high risk for melanoma. J Am Acad Dermatol. 2012;67(5):836–45.
39. Moloney FJ, Guitera P, Coates E, et al. Detection of primary melanoma in individuals at extreme high risk: a prospective 5-year follow-up study. JAMA Dermatol. 2014;150(8):819–27.
40. Markun S, Scherz N, Rosemann T, Tandjung R, Braun RP. Mobile teledermatology for skin cancer screening: a diagnostic accuracy study. Medicine (Baltimore). 2017;96(10):e6278–e6278.
41. Lamel SA, Haldeman KM, Ely H, Kovarik CL, Pak H, Armstrong AW. Application of mobile teledermatology for skin cancer screening. J Am Acad Dermatol. 2012;67(4):576–81.
42. Thissen M, Udrea A, Hacking M, von Braunmuehl T, Ruzicka T. MHealth app for risk assessment of pigmented and nonpigmented skin lesions-a study on sensitivity and specificity in detecting malignancy. Telemed J E Health. 2017;23(12):948–54.

Optical Coherence Tomography in Dermatology

Charlotte Gust, Cristel Ruini, Fabia Daxenberger, Sandra Schuh, Elke Sattler, and Julia Welzel

Abstract Non-invasive imaging techniques opened new horizons in the dermatological daily practice. Besides reflectance confocal microscopy, optical coherence tomography (OCT) and line-field confocal OCT have been used in the diagnosis, grading and follow-up of non-melanoma skin cancers and other non-neoplastic dermatological conditions such as mite infections and inflammatory skin diseases. OCT and dynamic OCT reach the deeper dermis and provide an overview of the blood vessel morphology and density, allowing semi-automated objective measurements of blood flow but also of skin thickness, roughness, and the attenuation coefficient. LC-OCT can count on lower penetration depth than OCT but higher resolution and can therefore be compared intuitively with histology. Both devices can potentially be used in artificial intelligence guided diagnostic studies.

Keywords Optical coherence tomography · Line-field-confocal optical coherence tomography · Dynamic optical coherence tomography · Non-invasive imaging · Skin cancer · Inflammatory skin diseases

1 Brief Introduction

Non-invasive imaging devices have become a valuable part of the clinical practice in dermatology for the bedside diagnosis of numerous skin pathologies, especially skin cancer [1–4]. The latter belongs to the most frequently occurring cancers in humans and has shown an increased incidence in the last few decades worldwide [5, 6].

C. Gust · C. Ruini · F. Daxenberger · E. Sattler
Department of Dermatology and Allergy, University Hospital, LMU, Munich, Germany

C. Ruini
School in Clinical and Experimental Medicine, University of Modena and Reggio Emilia, Modena, Italy

S. Schuh · J. Welzel (✉)
Department of Dermatology and Allergy, University Hospital, Augsburg, Germany
e-mail: Julia.Welzel@uk-augsburg.de

K. Nouri (ed.), *Telemedicine and Technological Advances in Dermatology*,
https://doi.org/10.1007/978-3-031-69091-4_18

Whereas malignant melanomas are known to have the highest skin cancer mortality, skin cancer arising from keratinocytic cells like basal cell carcinomas (BCC) and squamous cell carcinomas (SCC) are more common [5, 6].

Optical coherence tomography (OCT) is a non-invasive imaging modality that generates transversal and en-face images of the skin up to a depth of 1.5–2 mm. The commercially distributed device called Vivosight® (Michelson Diagnostics Ltd, Maidstone, Kent, UK) is a multibeam Fourier domain OCT using a swept-wavelength diode laser operating at a centre wavelength of 1305 nm. Its dynamic mode (D-OCT) enables the visualisation of blood flow whilst displaying the morphologic features of the tissue [7]. The use of OCT is not limited to skin cancer but plays an important role in the diagnosis and treatment of inflammatory and infectious diseases as well [8–10].

The new Line-field Confocal OCT (LC-OCT) enables skin imaging with a higher resolution than OCT (nearly cellular), albeit having a lower detection depth up to the mid dermis. The LC-OCT device deepLive™ (DAMAE Medical, Paris) is based on a two-beam interference microscope and offers three imaging modes (vertical, en-face and 3D) by using line illumination [11, 12]. LC-OCT has been applied to the non-invasive characterization of healthy skin, keratinocyte skin cancer, mites infestations, bullous autoimmune diseases, preliminary study of melanocytic lesions while more applications fields are yet to be explored [13–19].

The following chapter will offer an insight into the most frequent skin conditions OCT is confronted with in the daily practice.

2 Technique

2.1 OCT

2.1.1 Principle

OCT, an interferometric optical imaging modality, has been used in ophthalmology for decades before being introduced into the clinical field of dermatology in the late 1990s [20]. Through detection of the reflected light from the skin tissue, it allows a non-invasive, real-time and cross-sectional imaging of the skin. The cross-sectional images of the skin are generated with a lateral optical resolution of <7.5 μm and an axial resolution of 5–10 μm. OCT allows 6 mm × 6 mm imaging of skin layers into a depth of 1.5–2 mm, therefore it is helpful to analyze morphological features of the epidermis and dermis. Nevertheless, the imaging or analysis of small individual cells is not possible. OCT images can be horizontal or vertical, with a higher resolution, but lower penetration depth than sonography.

2.1.2 Device

The commercially available OCT device (VivoSight®; Michelson Diagnostics, Kent, UK) is a multibeam Fourier domain technique based on a swept-wavelength diode laser (Axsun, Billerica, USA) operating at a centre wavelength of 1305 nm. It belongs to the class 1 laser devices and can be therefore used without protection.

The OCT device consists of a central unit connected to a handheld probe and a monitor, with a keyboard and mouse. It is provided with a wheeled cart, to be easily moved towards the patient. The flexible hand piece allows measurements of any skin region. The device is provided with a series of plastic tools to adjust the contact to different skin sites based on their thickness. The image acquisition is reproduced on the connected monitor in real time in different scales of gray and red when acquiring D-OCT images. It takes only 15 s for a structural 3D-scan. A single cross-sectional image is displayed in real time.

2.2 D-OCT

2.2.1 Principle

Whereas healthy skin usually shows a homogenous vascular pattern, multiple skin conditions, for instance inflammatory diseases and skin tumors, are associated with a change of the cutaneous microcirculation and vascular pattern. Additionally, as compared to conventional OCT, D-OCT is able to image capillary blood flow and to visualize deep dermal vessels. The device detects the motion of blood cells during multiple, fast OCT scans of the same skin area; moving blood components can therefore be differentiated from static tissue up to a depth of 0.5 mm. Conventionally, blood vessels are displayed in red color in contrast to the surrounding skin appearing in different shades of gray. Vessels can be studied in transversal and horizontal sections.

2.2.2 Device

Further development of the Vivosight device as described above has led to the addition of the so-called dynamic mode with the ability to visualize blood flow in vessels. It takes about 30 s for a combined structural and vascular 3D-scan. While acquisition and interpretation of images is operator dependent, the additional software tool "VivoTools®" consents the standardized measurement of objective parameters, including: epidermal thickness (ET), optical attenuation coefficient (AC), skin surface roughness (SR), vascular plexus profile including vessel diameter, density and depth. D-OCT allows the in-vivo study of physiological and pathological changes of skin blood circulation ranging from temperature and positional related vasoconstriction, to tumoral neoangiogenesis, and to local effects of selective $\alpha 2$ adrenal receptor agonist or vascular lasers.

2.3 *LC-OCT*

2.3.1 Principle

LC-OCT is a non-invasive imaging modality, which offers the simultaneous display of horizontal and vertical images with a higher resolution than conventional OCT yet to the price of a lower penetration depth. It combines the principle of OCT interferometry with reflectance confocal microscopy (RCM) spatial filtering. Its system is based on a two-beam interference microscope with line illumination, line detection, a light source and a line-scan camera. The microscope uses a broadband spatially coherent light source, classified as a class 1 supercontinuum laser with a central wavelength of 800 nm. LC-OCT analyses the time of flight and amplitude of light backscattered from the tissue microstructures and collects multiple, parallel A-scans from the skin surface to a depth of $\sim$ 500 μm [11, 21].

Like conventional OCT, LC-OCT allows a real-time examination of the skin without causing pain or tissue damage, allowing an application on children or pregnant women as well. It is a class 1 laser device.

2.3.2 Device

The LC-OCT device consists of a central unit connected with a handheld probe and a monitor. It is propped on a wheeled cart, making acquisition at bedside possible. Immersion oil is applied between the glass window of the probe and the skin surface for index matching.

The LC-OCT device (DAMAE Medical, Paris) offers three different imaging modalities. The vertical or en-coupe mode allows direct comparison with OCT and histology. The horizontal or en-face mode on the other hand can be compared with RCM. In both modes, short movies and stacks can be acquired from the surface into the depth. The 3D stack makes a three-dimensional reconstruction possible and can either be used in vertical or horizontal mode. The device features an axial resolution of 1.1 μm, a lateral resolution of 1.3 μm, a field of view of 1.2×0.5 mm^2 (en-coupe) and 0.5×1.2 mm^2 (en-face) up into a scanning depth of 500 μm. The line-scan camera allows an orientation in the lesion during the acquisition of the scans. The acquisition speed of 10 images/s (2D) and 15 s per 3D stack allows a live acquisition and imaging evaluation concurrently. The acquired images are displayed in a grey scale. Both single captures and videos can be acquired [11, 21].

2.4 *Artificial intelligence and OCT*

Artificial intelligence (AI) aims to develop software simulating intelligent human behavior and therefore assist clinical decisions. Simple machine learning programs have evolved to complex deep learning (DL) algorithms, which require however a multitude of data. Through DL, representation-learning methods with multiple levels of abstraction are conceived to process data with no manual intervention, in order to automatically recognize complex data structures stacked in a hierarchy of increasing complexity and abstraction. First interesting approaches of AI to OCT imaging have been published in the last years in regard to ophthalmology, for example in diabetic retinopathy, premature retinopathy and glaucoma [22]. In dermatology, preliminary AI applications were focused on the automatic recognition of BCC [23] and other non-melanoma skin cancer [24–28]. DL algorithms for the detection and subtyping of BCC, of the dermo-epidermal junction (DEJ) and its continuity (which plays a significant role in actinic keratosis), as well as for the classification of BCC and AKs subtypes are in course of development and might assist the clinician in the near future.

3 Indications in Dermatology

3.1 *Skin cancer*

3.1.1 Keratinocyte Skin Cancer

Basal Cell Carcinoma

BCC is the most frequently occurring type of skin cancer in the general population. Its incidence is rising worldwide every year and is expected to continue to do so in the next years [29, 30]. There is a close link between sun exposure and skin tumor development. Sun exposed areas are predestined locations for the development of BCCs. The diagnostic process of BCCs entails a skin biopsy followed by a histopathological examination [30, 31]. Recently, non-invasive imaging tools, such as OCT, [3, 32, 33] and more recently LC-OCT [17, 18], have gained a foothold in the detection process of BCCs. The following diagnostic criteria for the detection of BCCs have been established: dark ovoid basaloid cell nests with a dark hyporeflective peripheral boundary (halo), alteration of the dermo-epidermal junction, dilated vessels, palisading and a general disruption of the skin layering (Fig. 1) [32, 34–36]. Superficial BCCs are characterized by round ovoid nests in connection with the DEJ, arranged in a string of pearls pattern, while infiltrating BCCs present a shoal of fish pattern due to the presence of elongated tumor strands.

The characteristic tumor conglomerates have a similar signal-intensity compared to the epidermis. Whereas superficial tumor nests have their origin in the epidermis,

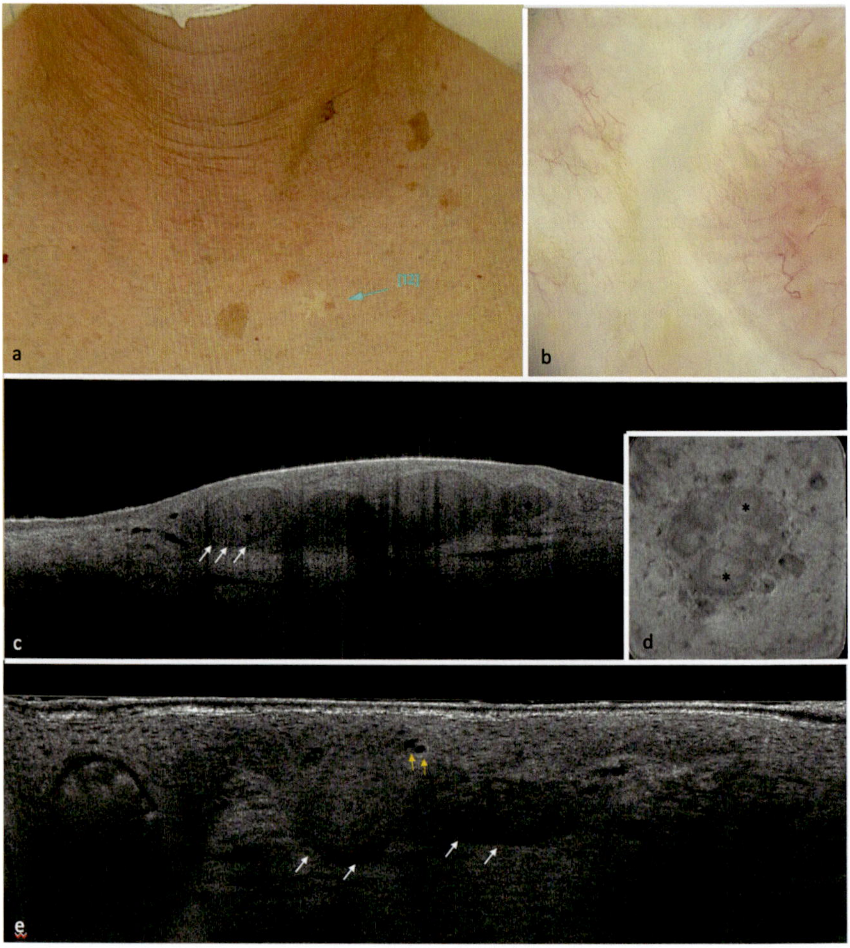

Fig. 1 a. clinical and b. dermoscopic correlates of a relapse of a nodular BCC in a 53-year-old male patient on the left parasternal chest side (blue arrow). c. The BCC is visible as sharply demarcated tumor nests indicated by black asterisks, surrounded by a dark cleft (white arrows). d. 6 mm × 6 mm en-face image of the nodular BCC. Tumor nests are also exemplarily marked by black asterisks. e. LC-OCT image of a BCC of a 74 year-old male. The cleft around the tumor nests is again indicated by white arrows. The BCC shows dark cystic structures (orange arrows) and tumor nests associated with the epidermis

deeper nests are demarcated from the dermis and surrounded by fibrous stroma. A scoring system to aid with the diagnosis of BCC is the Berlin score, it entails the presence of the following features: a dark border beneath the tumor, hyporeflective nests, ovoid structures and disruption of the DEJ. With the help of the score, an overall sensitivity of 90% and specificity of 60% for BCC diagnosis with OCT can be reached. Furthermore, the tumor thickness and subtype can be assessed with the help of OCT. The detection of serpiginous, branching vessels at a depth of 300 μm in D-OCT is an indicator for a nodular subtype and reduces the risk of a superficial BCC. Therefore, BCCs can be diagnosed and distinguished from other precancerous lesions or epithelial tumors with the help of OCT.

Keratinocyte Skin Cancer and Field Cancerization

Keratinocyte skin cancer (KC), caused through intraepithelial UV-induced damage, belongs to the most common tumors in older generations. It is especially common in fair-skinned people and immunosuppression, chronic wounds, radiation exposure or medications as for instance BRAF mutation inhibitors increase the lifetime risk. In early stages, KC appears as actinic keratosis (AK) or Bowen‘s disease (BD), however it can progress into an invasive squamous cell carcinoma (SCC) or an invasive Bowen carcinoma. SCCs can arise without a precursor lesion, remain locally invasive for a while, but have the potential to spread to regional lymph nodes and have a higher potential to metastasize than BCC, whose risk of metastasis is anecdotical. In order to prevent the transformation into an invasive SCC, early recognition and treatment is crucial. In daily practice, the diagnosis of KC relies on clinical and dermoscopic examination, followed by a biopsy, when needed. OCT has been shown to be a helpful tool for a noninvasive diagnosis of KC.

In OCT, AKs can be distinguished from normal skin through a thickened and strongly scattered stratum corneum as a result of parakeratosis. The epidermis appears thicker overall. The differentiation between epidermis and dermis is still possible (Fig. 2). Features in OCT that can appear in AK and SCC are a destruction of the epidermis and a thickened epidermal layer. A disruption of the DEJ, a disarranged epidermal pattern and atypical keratinocytes are criteria typical for SCC. One has to be aware that severe hyperkeratosis can result in a signal shadow and a more difficult analysis of the DEJ and dermis, possibly disguising an invasive tumor below. In D-OCT curved vessels are an indicator for AK, whereas blob vessels are predominantly seen in Bowen's disease. In LC-OCT, due to the higher resolution, single keratinocytes are visible and the analysis of the cellular morphology and tissue architecture is possible (Fig. 3). Most common LC-OCT findings of KC are hyperkeratosis/parakeratosis, disruption of the stratum corneum, broadened epidermis, basal and suprabasal keratinocyte atypia, dilated vessels/neoangiogenesis and elastosis/collagen alterations. The preserved DEJ is less common in SCC compared to AK and BD, while BD displays marked keratinocyte atypia involving all epidermal layers (bowenoid pattern). SCC shows ulceration, increased epidermal thickness, keratin plugs, acantholysis, not visible/interrupted DEJ and epidermal bright particles [16, 37]. The downward proliferation pattern of keratinocytes, the PRO-grading, is also evaluable with a good agreement with histology [16].

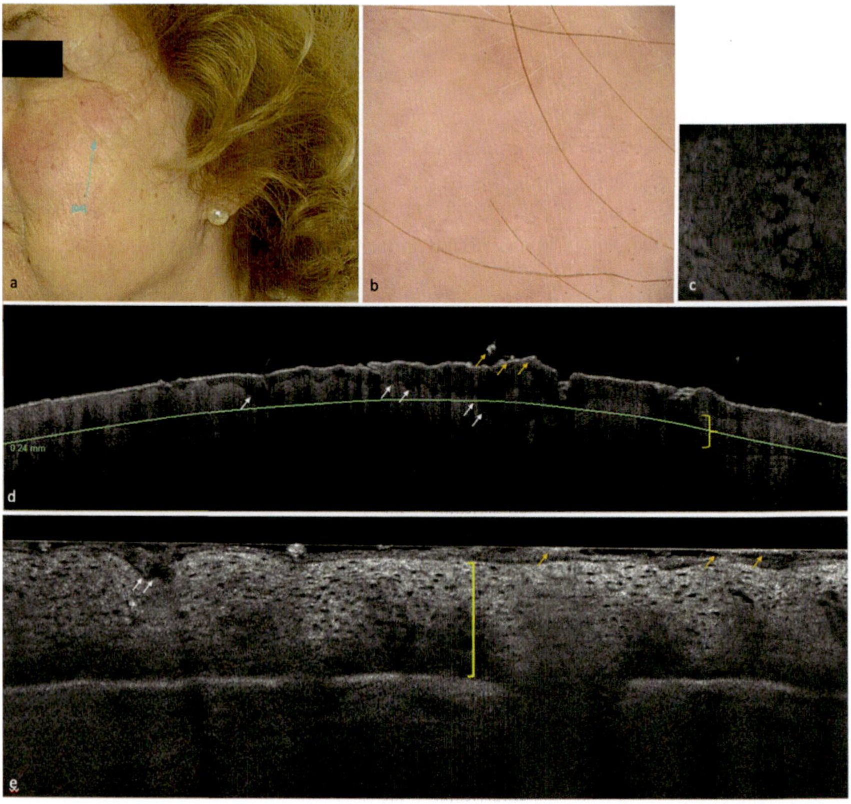

Fig. 2 a. clinical (blue arrow) and b. dermoscopic images of a histologically confirmed actinic keratosis is located on the left zygomatic arch in an 85 year-old female patient. The typical strawberry pattern can be seen. c. OCT image of the lesion in en-face mode. d. B-Scan of the actinic keratosis. The white arrows indicate the typical thickening of the epidermis with increased DEJ thickness and prominence, orange arrows point at keratosis/hyperkeratotic layering. The curly bracket shows the irregular layering of normal skin architecture. Normal skin architecture can be seen on the left side of the OCT scan. e. LC-OCT image of the same lesion. It shows hyperkeratosis and parakeratosis (orange arrows) and atypical keratinocytes (yellow bracket)

Treatment Monitoring

Treatment monitoring and therapeutic success of topical immune modulators or photodynamic therapy can be evaluated non-invasively with OCT. If a surgical excision is not the treatment of choice, a topical therapy with for example Imiquimod or 5-fluorouracil, photodynamic therapy or laser therapy can be indicated for superficial BCC, AK and BD. Since all of these options can be associated with recurrence, OCT and LC-OCT can be helpful for monitoring the treatment response. As an example, residues of BCC after Imiquimod treatment appear as cyst-like structures in OCT.

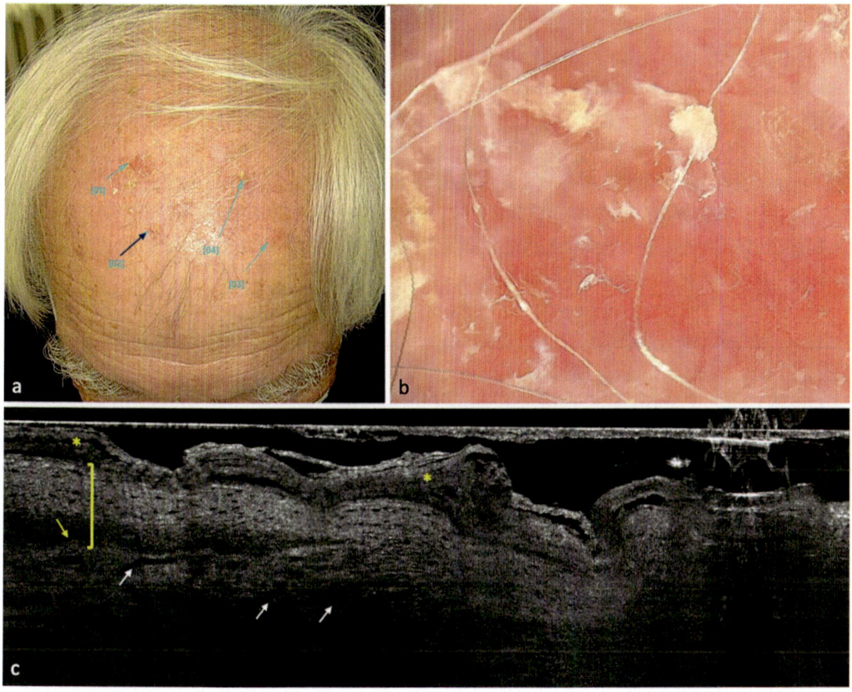

Fig. 3 a. clinical (dark blue arrow) and b. dermoscopic images of a histologically verified Bowen´s disease in an 87 year-old male patient on the right ventral scalp. c. The LC-OCT image shows a thickened spinous layer, a preserved DEJ (yellow arrow), hyperkeratosis and parakeratosis (asterisk), dilated vessels (white arrow) and atypical keratinocytes (yellow bracket)

Oral hedgehog inhibitors (HHIs), as Vismodegib and Sonidegib, have gained importance in the treatment of advanced or metastatic BCC during the last years. The efficacy of the treatment has usually been evaluated by clinical photography and radiographic scans so far. Besides the detection of BCCs in the skin, OCT has shown to be valuable to evaluate treatment progress of HHIs as well. Signs of tumor regression in OCT are coarse collagen fibers, demarcated, dark round structures and pseudocysts. Therefore, non-invasive imaging tools are a valuable option to monitor nonsurgical treatment of BCCs.

If surgery is needed, tumor margins can be defined preoperatively with OCT. Mohs Micrographic Surgery (MMS) can be supported with OCT to detect tumor margins, avoiding the need for numerous staged tumor excisions.

Melanoma

Melanoma arises from uncontrolled proliferation of melanocytes and can develop in any organ containing melanocytes, from skin and mucosal surfaces to the spinal cord and brain. The cutaneous melanoma is the most common one and can appear as a superficial spreading, nodular, acral lentiginous or lentigo maligna melanoma variant. Due to the infiltrative tumor growth of malignant melanoma, the DEJ is not detectable in OCT. It can be visible in junctional nevi but is difficult to detect or can be missing in compound nevi. Additionally, melanin causes an irregular scattering in OCT images, and no firm specific criteria to differentiate between benign pigmented lesions and malignant melanoma have been established. However, in thin melanomas the tumor thickness can be estimated, since the scattering within the melanocyte nests diverges from the surrounding collagen.

Melanoma staging depends on tumor thickness estimated by histology. The Breslow Index correlates with the outcome, thicker lesions are associated with lower survival rates. Neoangiogenesis is crucial for tumor progression and can be evaluated with D-OCT. Dotted vessels become more irregularly distributed with increasing tumor thickness. Curved vessels can be found in melanomas with a > 1 mm thickness and coiled and serpiginous vessels are an indication for a tumor thickness greater than 2 mm. However, below a depth of 500 μm the evaluation of vascular morphology is less precise.

In LC-OCT dermal nests of melanocytes in nevi have been described as wave pattern; junctional nests are also visible. The pagetoid spreading of malignant melanocytes in the epidermis and the abrupted DEJ can be identified intuitively [14].

Inflammatory Skin Diseases

Not only tumors, but also Inflammatory skin diseases and autoimmune dermatological diseases can be examined by D-OCT. This is appropriate because above-mentioned diseases are often accompanied by abnormalities of the skin vessels and the pathologies are typically localized in the upper part of the skin. An inflammatory reaction of the skin for instance, can go along with dilation of blood vessels in the upper dermis and an edema, resulting in a reduction of the light attenuation coefficient, especially in the dermis. The entrance signal appears multilayered or thickened due to the parakeratosis of the stratum corneum. Furthermore, the epidermal thickness can be measured allowing further analysis of the progress of acanthosis in the inflamed tissue. Acute contact dermatitis, for example, shows an increased input signal and epidermal thickness compared to healthy skin. Here, acute spongiosis is expressed by enlarged intercellular spaces between keratinocytes, increased microvascularization, vasodilation, increased blood flow, and, especially in severe reactions, macrovesicles and coalescing vesicles (Fig. 4). Spongiosis results in thickening of the epidermis, with both skin attenuation coefficient and blood flow correlating with the severity of the reaction at 0.2 and 0.35 mm penetration depth [38]. In eczema, particularly atopic dermatitis, D-OCT has been applied to therapy monitoring for biologics such as dupilumab. Eczematous skin was characterized at baseline by increased vesicle number and higher vascular thresholds at 150 and 300 μm depth, as well as increased epidermis thickness and lower mean collagen

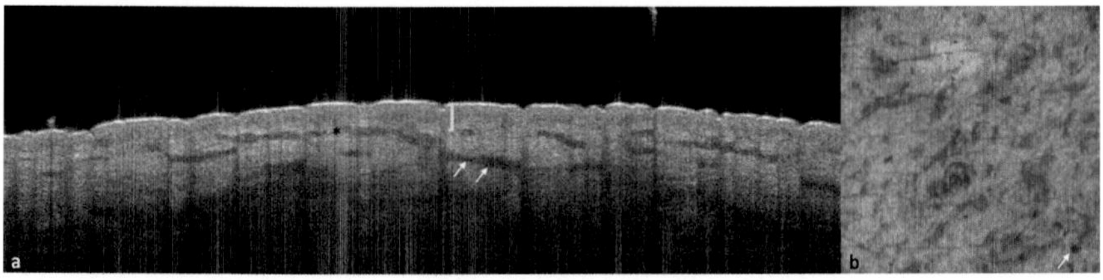

Fig. 4 a. OCT B-scan of an acute contact allergic dermatitis with a positive patch test for nickel on the back of a 37 year-old female subject. The image shows a regular epidermis (yellow bracket), a mildly positive reaction manifested by acute spongiosis (black asterisk) and dilation of blood vessels (white arrow). b. en-face OCT: The dilated blood vessels (white arrow) can also be seen in the structural horizontal OCT image

density compared to clinically healthy skin. After therapy, there was a reduction in epidermal thickness, vesicles, interrupted input signal and dermo-epidermal junction (DEJ) and vascular thresholds, and an increase in collagen density [8].

A skin condition that presents with a thickening of the epidermis, esp. the stratum corneum, is psoriasis. Psoriatic skin presents with hyperkeratosis, acanthosis and dilated capillary vessels in the papillary dermis, also referred to as spikes in D-OCT. Furthermore, a stronger entrance signal due to a more irregular skin surface, dilated blood vessels and a weakened signal intensity in the dermis can be detected in OCT scans. The lower scattering is a consequence of edema and inflammatory infiltration in the dermis. OCT can also detect abnormalities of vasculature in psoriatic nails and treatment efficacy as well as disease activity can be monitored [39].

The inflammatory skin reaction of bullous autoimmune diseases can be displayed with OCT. In order to distinguish between pemphigus and bullous pemphigoid the detection of the location of the blisters in the skin layers is essential. Intraepidermal blisters can be found in pemphigus, whereas subepidermal blisters are characteristic of bullous pemphigoid. OCT and LC-OCT can detect the depth of blistering and differentiate between bullous autoimmune diseases without a skin biopsy. Changes in inflammatory skin can be examined by measuring the signal attenuation coefficient and the thickness of skin layers. Other inflammatory dermatoses characterized with D-OCT include acne, rosacea, dermatomyositis, and scleroderma (in which the dermis has increased density with loss of skin appendages). In seborrheic dermatitis of the scalp, a transition of the vasculature from the superficial plexus (small dilated vessels, alternating with thinner branched vessels) to the deep plexus ("lava-like" dilated branched vessels, distributed in a reticular fashion) was observed [9]. In addition to increased vascular density, increased epidermal thickness and skin attenuation coefficient were also measured.

Wounds/Burns

A cutaneous injury, such as a surgical wound or a burn can result in a fibrotic disorder of the skin structure. An excessive collagen production and synthesis of vascular tissue emerges from the origin of the skin injury, leading to the formation of a hypertrophic scar. OCT is able to evaluate the changes in skin fibrosis and can help to differentiate between normal and scar tissue. Besides collagen imaging, OCT can quantify the vascularity of hypertrophic scar tissue, showing an increased proliferation of large vessels and a higher vascular density in fresh scars. Post-traumatic scars or acne scars treatment can entail laser therapy. The laser response can be monitored with OCT, evaluating potentially new synthesized collagen, inflammation and the dermal remodeling process. In conclusion, OCT is a helpful tool to identify fibrotic skin diseases and enables monitoring and quantifying skin tissue responses to treatment without the need of a biopsy.

In venous ulcers, D-OCT was able to display specific vessel patterns like coils and blobs in the center and border of the ulcer, whereas serpiginous vessels were found in dermatosclerosis surrounding the ulcer [40].

A time efficient and correct assessment of a burn is crucial for a successful treatment and avoiding the risk of infection or scarring. In a clinical setting burns are categorized in three different degrees, mainly through visual inspection and sometimes auxiliary diagnostic tools. The categorizing assessment includes the following parameters: surface morphology, blood flow and impaired skin depth. Only the superficial epidermis is damaged in a first-degree burn, whereas the lower epidermis and dermis are affected in a second-degree burn, resulting in blisters. The classification of a third-degree burn entails damage of the epidermis, dermis and the subcutaneous tissue. While most first- and third-degree burns are easy to categorize, second degree burns are more difficult to distinguish from the rest due to the ambiguity of the burn boundary. In order to improve the accuracy of a burn diagnosis, OCT has been used to objectively evaluate burn injuries [41]. OCT allows visualizing of superficial burns into a depth of 2 mm. Changes in skin structure and collagen can be quantified. Moreover, blood flow changes due to thermal damage and edema characteristics can be assessed with D-OCT. Edema, vessel and tissue destruction depth estimated with OCT are viable analyzation criteria for tissue burns and could be helpful criteria in the burn assessment protocol in the future.

Infectious Skin Diseases

Parasites such as scabies mites or larva migrans affecting humans are a widespread health issue. Scabies is caused by an ectoparasite, Sarcoptes scabiei var. hominis, and can cause a progressive rash or inflammatory excoriated papules in humans with strong pruritus. Diagnosis is based on clinical examination, dermoscopy and the presence of the previously mentioned characteristic clinical features. OCT can be used to non-invasively detect scabies infestations. In OCT a scabies mite impresses as signal strong structure beneath the stratum corneum [42]. In LC-OCT the exact location of the mite and its burrow can be recreated with the 3D mode [43]. The higher, almost cellular, resolution enables the detection of eggs and skybala of the mites and even the different body parts of the mite can be displayed. Both devices offer a quick and painless in-vivo examination of mites with a diagnosis at bedside.

Other Indications (Allergy Testing, Cosmetic Indications)

Contact dermatitis to environmental allergens has a prevalence of 20% in the general population. Its origin can either be allergic as a cell-mediated type IV immune response or irritant/toxic. The diagnosis is based on a detailed medical history, clinical examination and a standard skin patch test. The patch test reaction is evaluated through visual inspection and palpation, taking morphological criteria as erythema, papules and vesicles into consideration. In clinically doubtful reactions, OCT offers a more objective and accurate option to grade patch tests. Spongiosis with microvesicles, macrovesicles and coalescing vesicles are indicators for an allergic reaction of the skin (Fig. 4). Increased epidermal thickness, which can be measured with the software *OCT research tools*, is a result of spongiosis and correlates with the severity grade of the acute contact allergic reaction. The operator-independent measurement of the blood flow and the AC provide additional, objective information for a more consistent patch test grading. Moreover, signs of skin aging can be evaluated with OCT. A decreased epidermal thickness and blood vessel depth is found in aged skin, whereas UV-exposure leads to a greater thickness [44]. Besides the epidermal thickness as an objective parameter for skin evaluation, the attenuation coefficient is a helpful parameter to assess aging and damage of skin tissue. Determining the light attenuated from the tissue, a high attenuation coefficient is a sign of skin tissue dense with collagen and hyaluronic acid. Scar tissue and sun damaged skin show a decreased attenuation coefficient. Semi-automatic measurement of the skin roughness also proves to be helpful in the field of aesthetic dermatology e.g., in the evaluation of the effectiveness of methods as skin rejuvenation and scar treatment (Fig. 5) [45, 46].

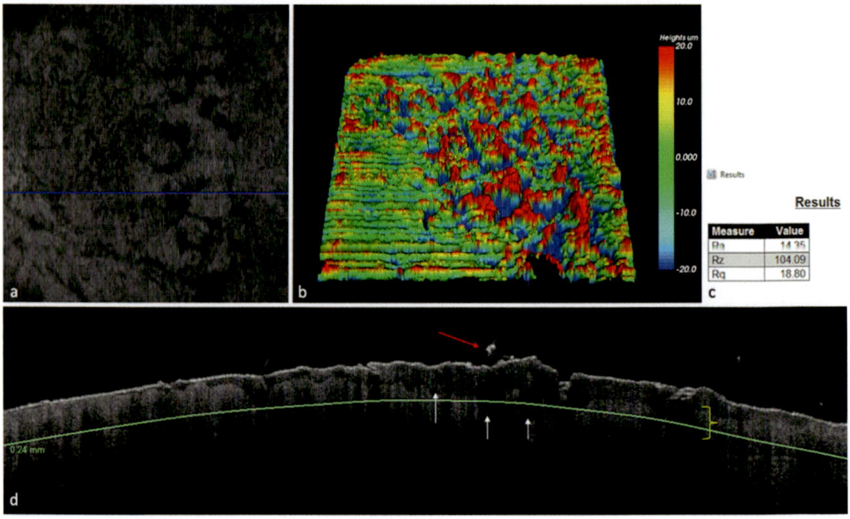

Fig. 5 a. 6 mm × 6 mm en-face image of an OCT scan. b. Semi-automatic measurement of objective skin parameters using VivoTools. 3D representation of the skin roughness on the left cheek of an 85 year-old female with actinic keratosis. The 3D surface profile is represented via a heat map with colors ranging from blue (low surface) to red (high surface). c. the associated Ra, Rz and Rq values. d. corresponding B-Scan of the histologically confirmed actinic keratosis. White arrows indicate a thickened epidermis. The irregular layering of normal skin architecture is indicated by the curly bracket, the red arrow shows keratosis

4 Key Points (3 Main Takeaway Points)

(1) OCT and LC-OCT are modern imaging techniques that allow the non-invasive visualization of the upper layers of the skin in real time. While OCT offers a higher penetration depth up to 1.5–2 mm, LC-OCT enables a view in the superficial layers in almost histological resolution.
(2) Main indications are skin tumors, especially non-melanoma skin cancer, but also inflammatory skin diseases and other dermatoses by the evaluation of diagnostic criteria and characteristic imaging patterns.
(3) Both techniques are suitable for the use of artificial intelligence and deep learning algorithms, for which pilot studies show very promising results.

5 Conclusion

In addition to other imaging techniques like dermoscopy and reflectance confocal microscopy, OCT and LC-OCT are two innovative modern imaging methods both with high benefit for today's patient care. They both enable us to diagnose different kinds of skin diseases non-invasively in real time, especially well established for skin tumors, with best evidence for non-melanoma skin cancers. More recent studies also show their value in the detection of other skin diseases like inflammatory and autoimmune dermatoses. Additionally, objective measurements of different parameters like epidermal thickness, attenuation coefficient and blood flow are possible.

First data show promising results for the use of artificial intelligence in both techniques, yet more data for the training of deep learning algorithms are necessary for their successful support and usage in modern imaging diagnosis.

References

1. Dinnes J, Deeks JJ, Chuchu N, et al. Reflectance confocal microscopy for diagnosing keratinocyte skin cancers in adults. Cochrane Database Syst Rev. 2018;12(12):cd013191. https://doi.org/10.1002/14651858.cd013191.
2. Dinnes J, Deeks JJ, Saleh D, et al. Reflectance confocal microscopy for diagnosing cutaneous melanoma in adults. Cochrane Database Syst Rev. 2018;12(12):cd013190. https://doi.org/10.1002/14651858.cd013190.
3. Ferrante di Ruffano L, Dinnes J, Deeks JJ, et al. Optical coherence tomography for diagnosing skin cancer in adults. Cochrane Database Syst Rev. 2018;12(12):013189. https://doi.org/10.1002/14651858.cd013189.
4. Welzel J, Schuh S. Noninvasive diagnosis in dermatology. J Dtsch Dermatol Ges. 2017;15(10):999–1016. https://doi.org/10.1111/ddg.13347.
5. Leiter U, Keim U, Garbe C. Epidemiology of skin cancer: update 2019. Adv Exp Med Biol. 2020;1268:123–39. https://doi.org/10.1007/978-3-030-46227-7_6.
6. Bolick NL, Geller AC. Epidemiology of melanoma. Hematol Oncol Clin North Am. 2021;35(1):57–72. https://doi.org/10.1016/j.hoc.2020.08.011.
7. Ulrich M, Themstrup L, de Carvalho N, et al. Dynamic optical coherence tomography in dermatology. Dermatology. 2016;232(3):298–311. https://doi.org/10.1159/000444706.
8. Manfredini M, Liberati S, Ciardo S, et al. Microscopic and functional changes observed with dynamic optical coherence tomography for severe refractory atopic dermatitis treated with dupilumab. Skin Res Technol. 2020;26(6):779–87. https://doi.org/10.1111/srt.12868.
9. Rajabi-Estarabadi A, Vasquez-Herrera NE, Martinez-Velasco MA, et al. Optical coherence tomography in diagnosis of inflammatory scalp disorders. J Eur Acad Dermatol Venereol. 2020;34(9):2147–51. https://doi.org/10.1111/jdv.16304.
10. Wan B, Ganier C, Du-Harpur X, et al. Applications and future directions for optical coherence tomography in dermatology. Br J Dermatol. 2020. https://doi.org/10.1111/bjd.19553.
11. Dubois A, Xue W, Levecq O, Bulkin P, Coutrot AL, Ogien J. Mirau-based line-field confocal optical coherence tomography. Opt Express. 2020;28(6):7918–27. https://doi.org/10.1364/OE.389637.
12. Ogien J, Levecq O, Azimani H, Dubois A. Dual-mode line-field confocal optical coherence tomography for ultrahigh-resolution vertical and horizontal section imaging of human skin. Biomed Opt Express. 2020;11(3):1327–35. https://doi.org/10.1364/BOE.385303.
13. Ruini C, Schuh S, Hartmann D, French L, Welzel J, Sattler E. Noninvasive real-time imaging of mite skin infestations with line-field confocal optical coherence tomography. Br J Dermatol. 2021;184(1):e3. https://doi.org/10.1111/bjd.19318.
14. Ruini C, Schuh S, Sattler E, Welzel J. Line-field confocal optical coherence tomography-practical applications in dermatology and comparison with established imaging methods. Skin Res Technol. 2021;27(3):340–52. https://doi.org/10.1111/srt.12949.
15. Lacarrubba F, Verzi AE, Puglisi DF, Broggi G, Caltabiano R, Micali G. Line-field confocal optical coherence tomography of xanthogranuloma: correlation with vertical and horizontal histopathology. J Cutan Pathol. 2021. https://doi.org/10.1111/cup.14067.

16. Ruini C, Schuh S, Gust C, et al. In-vivo LC-OCT evaluation of the downward proliferation pattern of keratinocytes in actinic keratosis in comparison with histology: first impressions from a pilot study. Cancers (Basel). 2021;13(12):2856. https://doi.org/10.3390/cancers13122856.
17. Ruini C, Schuh S, Gust C, et al. Line-field optical coherence tomography: in vivo diagnosis of basal cell carcinoma subtypes compared to histopathology. Clin Exp Dermatol. 2021. https://doi.org/10.1111/ced.14762.
18. Suppa M, Fontaine M, Dejonckheere G, et al. Line-field confocal optical coherence tomography of basal cell carcinoma: a descriptive study. J Eur Acad Dermatol Venereol. 2021;35(5):1099–110. https://doi.org/10.1111/jdv.17078.
19. Tognetti L, Cinotti E, Suppa M, et al. Line field confocal optical coherence tomography: an adjunctive tool in the diagnosis of autoimmune bullous diseases. J Biophotonics. 2021;14(5):e202000449. https://doi.org/10.1002/jbio.202000449.
20. Welzel J, Lankenau E, Birngruber R, Engelhardt R. Optical coherence tomography of the human skin. J Am Acad Dermatol. 1997;37(6):958–63. https://doi.org/10.1016/s0190-9622(97)70072-0.
21. Ogien J, Levecq O, Azimani H, Dubois A. Dual-mode line-field confocal optical coherence tomography for ultrahigh-resolution vertical and horizontal section imaging of human skin in vivo. Biomed Opt Express. 2020;11(3):1327–35. https://doi.org/10.1364/BOE.385303.
22. Ting DSW, Pasquale LR, Peng L, et al. Artificial intelligence and deep learning in ophthalmology. Br J Ophthalmol. 2019;103(2):167–75. https://doi.org/10.1136/bjophthalmol-2018-313173.
23. Marvdashti T, Duan L, Aasi SZ, Tang JY, Ellerbee Bowden AK. Classification of basal cell carcinoma in human skin using machine learning and quantitative features captured by polarization sensitive optical coherence tomography. Biomed Opt Express. 2016;7(9):3721–35. https://doi.org/10.1364/BOE.7.003721.
24. Jørgensen TM, Tycho A, Mogensen M, Bjerring P, Jemec GB. Machine-learning classification of non-melanoma skin cancers from image features obtained by optical coherence tomography. Skin Res Technol. 2008;14(3):364–9. https://doi.org/10.1111/j.1600-0846.2008.00304.x.
25. Roffman D, Hart G, Girardi M, Ko CJ, Deng J. Predicting non-melanoma skin cancer via a multi-parameterized artificial neural network. Sci Rep. 2018;8(1):1701. https://doi.org/10.1038/s41598-018-19907-9.
26. Sharma AN, Shwe S, Mesinkovska NA. Current state of machine learning for non-melanoma skin cancer. Arch Dermatol Res. 2021. https://doi.org/10.1007/s00403-021-02236-9.
27. Tschandl P, Rosendahl C, Akay BN, et al. Expert-level diagnosis of nonpigmented skin cancer by combined convolutional neural networks. JAMA Dermatol. 2019;155(1):58–65. https://doi.org/10.1001/jamadermatol.2018.4378.
28. Young AT, Xiong M, Pfau J, Keiser MJ, Wei ML. Artificial intelligence in dermatology: a primer. J Invest Dermatol. 2020;140(8):1504–12. https://doi.org/10.1016/j.jid.2020.02.026.
29. Lang BM, Balermpas P, Bauer A, et al. S2k guidelines for cutaneous basal cell carcinoma—part 1: epidemiology, genetics and diagnosis. J Dtsch Dermatol Ges. 2019;17(1):94–103. https://doi.org/10.1111/ddg.13733.
30. Peris K, Fargnoli MC, Garbe C, et al. Diagnosis and treatment of basal cell carcinoma: European consensus-based interdisciplinary guidelines. Eur J Cancer. 2019;118:10–34. https://doi.org/10.1016/j.ejca.2019.06.003.
31. Lang BM, Balermpas P, Bauer A, et al. S2k guidelines for cutaneous basal cell carcinoma—part 2: treatment, prevention and follow-up. J Dtsch Dermatol Ges. 2019;17(2):214–30. https://doi.org/10.1111/ddg.13755.
32. Holmes J, von Braunmühl T, Berking C, et al. Optical coherence tomography of basal cell carcinoma: influence of location, subtype, observer variability and image quality on diagnostic performance. Br J Dermatol. 2018;178(5):1102–10. https://doi.org/10.1111/bjd.16154.
33. Sinx KAE, van Loo E, Tonk EHJ, et al. Optical coherence tomography for noninvasive diagnosis and subtyping of basal cell carcinoma: a prospective cohort study. J Invest Dermatol. 2020;140(10):1962–7. https://doi.org/10.1016/j.jid.2020.01.034.

34. Themstrup L, De Carvalho N, Nielsen SM, et al. In vivo differentiation of common basal cell carcinoma subtypes by microvascular and structural imaging using dynamic optical coherence tomography. Exp Dermatol. 2018;27(2):156–65. https://doi.org/10.1111/exd.13479.
35. Ferrante di Ruffano L, Dinnes J, Deeks JJ, et al. Optical coherence tomography for diagnosing skin cancer in adults. Cochrane Database Syst Rev. 2018;12:CD013189. https://doi.org/10.1002/14651858.CD013189.
36. Schuh S, Kaestle R, Sattler EC, Welzel J. Optical coherence tomography of actinic keratoses and basal cell carcinomas—differentiation by quantification of signal intensity and layer thickness. J Eur Acad Dermatol Venereol. 2016;30(8):1321–6. https://doi.org/10.1111/jdv.13569.
37. Ruini C, Schuh S, Gust C, et al. Line-field confocal optical coherence tomography for the in-vivo real-time diagnosis of different stages of keratinocyte skin cancer: a preliminary study. J Eur Acad Dermatol Venereol. 2021. https://doi.org/10.1111/jdv.17603.
38. Ruini C, Rahimi F, Fiocco Z, et al. Optical coherence tomography for patch test grading: a prospective study on its use for noninvasive diagnosis of allergic contact dermatitis. Contact Dermatitis. 2021;84(3):183–91. https://doi.org/10.1111/cod.13714.
39. Aldahan AS, Chen LL, Fertig RM, et al. Vascular features of nail psoriasis using dynamic optical coherence tomography. Skin Appendage Disord. 2017;2(3–4):102–8. https://doi.org/10.1159/000449230.
40. Holmes J, Schuh S, Bowling FL, Mani R, Welzel J. Dynamic optical coherence tomography is a new technique for imaging skin around lower extremity wounds. Int J Low Extrem Wounds. 2019;18(1):65–74. https://doi.org/10.1177/1534734618821015.
41. Lindert J, Tafazzoli-Lari K, Tüshaus L, et al. Optical coherence tomography provides an optical biopsy of burn wounds in children-a pilot study. J Biomed Opt. 2018;23(10):1–6. https://doi.org/10.1117/1.Jbo.23.10.106005.
42. Banzhaf CA, Themstrup L, Ring HC, Welzel J, Mogensen M, Jemec GB. In vivo imaging of sarcoptes scabiei infestation using optical coherence tomography. Case Rep Dermatol. 2013;5(2):156–62. https://doi.org/10.1159/000352066.
43. Ruini C, Schuh S, Pellacani G, French L, Welzel J, Sattler E. In vivo imaging of Sarcoptes scabiei infestation using line-field confocal optical coherence tomography. J Eur Acad Dermatol Venereol. 2020;34(12):e808–9. https://doi.org/10.1111/jdv.16671.
44. Kislevitz M, Akgul Y, Wamsley C, Hoopman J, Kenkel J. Use of optical coherence tomography (OCT) in aesthetic skin assessment-a short review. Lasers Surg Med. 2020;52(8):699–704. https://doi.org/10.1002/lsm.23219.
45. Kunzi-Rapp K, Dierickx CC, Cambier B, Drosner M. Minimally invasive skin rejuvenation with erbium: YAG laser used in thermal mode. Lasers Surg Med. 2006;38(10):899–907. https://doi.org/10.1002/lsm.20380.
46. Olesen UH, Mogensen M, Haedersdal M. Vehicle type affects filling of fractional laser-ablated channels imaged by optical coherence tomography. Lasers Med Sci. 2017;32(3):679–84. https://doi.org/10.1007/s10103-017-2168-z.

Reflectance Confocal Microscopy

Isabella Dreyfuss, Francelia J. Eckembrecher, Daphne G. Eckembrecher, and Keyvan Nouri

Abstract This chapter will discuss the technology behind reflectance confocal microscopy (RCM). RCM is a non-invasive horizontal imaging technique that illuminates the skin at a specific area or lesion of the epidermis. The confocal pinhole of the RCM focuses the reflective light on the pinhole to prevent it from focusing on any other areas of the skin. Additionally, this chapter will evaluate its applications as a form of non-invasive imaging in the diagnosis and monitoring of treatment for dermatologic conditions including skin cancer and inflammatory skin conditions. Some of these conditions include psoriasis, scarring and nonscarring alopecia, dermatitis/eczema, and parasitic skin infections with scabies. The benefits of using RCM include evaluation of free movement across the skin, in addition to challenging smaller areas, such as the periocular regions, nasal crease, concha, and interdigital web spaces. This device also allows for free movement across the skin. Physicians can assess Mohs micrographic surgery margins with RCM, as well as the effectiveness of topical treatments. In contrast, the limitations of RCM include evaluation of hyperkeratotic lesions, hair covered areas of the skin, nodular lesions, areas of fibrin, coagulated blood, and keratin aggregates, and the palms and soles. Current modalities, such as the Vivascope® 1500, have increased the imaging up to 8 × 8 mm areas and aided in the diagnosis of dermoscopy alone.

Keywords Reflectance confocal microscopy · Skin cancer · Non-invasive imaging · Inflammatory skin conditions · Papillary dermis · Dermo-epidermal junction · Melanoma · Basal cell carcinoma · Squamous cell carcinoma · Psoriasis

Key Concepts

I. Dreyfuss (✉) · F. J. Eckembrecher · D. G. Eckembrecher · K. Nouri
Dr. Phillip Frost Department of Dermatology and Cutaneous Surgery, Miller School of Medicine, University of Miami, Miami, FL, USA
e-mail: id233@mynsu.nova.edu

K. Nouri
e-mail: knouri@med.miami.edu

K. Nouri (ed.), *Telemedicine and Technological Advances in Dermatology*,
https://doi.org/10.1007/978-3-031-69091-4_19

1. RCM focuses light through an optical lens through a small pinhole and forms an image on a photodetector in a non-invasive, painless method.
2. RCM can aid in the evaluation of Mohs micrographic surgery margins.
3. Current RCM modalities, such as Vivascope® 1500, increase the ability of other clinical technologies, such as dermoscopy.

Learning Objectives

- Understand the technological advancement and design of RCM as a non-invasive imaging technique using a horizonal view of the epidermis layer.
- Evaluate the benefits of RCM to contribute to the sensitivity and specificity of clinical diagnosis of basal cell carcinoma, squamous cell carcinoma, actinic keratosis, scabies, psoriasis, and other examples of diseases.
- Rule in the benefits and limitations of RCM when applying this diagnostic modality to patients in specific circumstances.

1 Overview

1.1 Introduction

Reflectance Confocal Microscopy (RCM) is an optical imaging technique that uses a horizontal view of the skin. In dermatology, RCM is a non-invasive imaging technique that enables in vivo visualization of the epidermis down to the papillary dermis in real-time. Resolution is almost comparable to conventional histology. It has the advantage of allowing the clinician to do a "virtual biopsy" of the skin and obtain diagnostic clues while minimizing unnecessary skin biopsies [1].

RCM is clinically used to increase the specificity and sensitivity of the diagnosis of skin cancers, guide biopsy of lesions, define margins of lesions for surgical excision, and follow clinical therapeutic evolution of a skin diseases.

2 Technological Design

RCM uses the diode laser as a source of monochromatic and coherent light. The light passes through a beam splitter, a scanning and focusing optical lens and a skin contact device. The light then penetrates the skin and illuminates a small tissue spot with a focus on the same diffraction-limited spot. Light reflected from the focal point reflects back through the lens, which focuses it into a small pinhole and forms an image on a photodetector. The pinhole only allows light from a focal point to pass through (i.e. it is confocal), and prevents light from another tissue point or out-of-focus plane from getting through [2].

RCM relies on reflectance (back-scattering) of light from structures with endogenous contrast, such as melanin, hemoglobin, and some organelles. Reflectance occurs at the boundaries of two structures with different refractive indices, such as membranes, keratohyalin granules and melanosomes.

RCM features that can be seen are the stratum corneum, stratum granulosum, stratum spinosum, stratum basale, the dermo-epidermal junction, and dermis.

3 Current Modalities

The commercially available Vivascope® 1500 by Caliber I.D. uses a laser of 830 nm, as this wavelength does not cause tissue injury for the patient or injury to the eyes of the operator. This imaging machine uses an in vivo confocal tool with a low-powered laser to provide non-invasive, real-time, high-resolution images of the superficial collagen layers. The depth of penetration is 200–300 μm, which generally corresponds to the papillary dermis or upper reticular dermis. A series of horizontal images are captured in a "Z-depth" from the surface of the skin in a parallel manner. Vivascope® has the ability to image up to an 8 × 8 mm area [3]. 16 studies have concluded that Vivascope® appears to be a cost-effective diagnostic assessment of equivocal melanomas and basal cell carcinomas (BCC). There is a 100% sensitivity for dermoscopy plus Vivascope® 1500 versus 100% dermoscopy alone [3].

4 Examples

Conditions examined in both benign and malignant cases include melanoma, especially lentigo maligna, BCC, squamous cell carcinoma (SCC), and inflammatory conditions. Inflammatory conditions include psoriasis, dermatitis/eczema, and scabies.

On RCM, psoriasiform dermatitis is evaluated with RCM with the presence of high refractive round to polygonal structures inside the stratum corneum. Papillomatosis is seen as enlarged dermal papillae with thin, interpapillary epidermal spaces in plaque psoriasis. Seborrheic dermatitis will show dilated vessels horizontally around adnexal structures.

Scalp disease, such as alopecia, will show high bleeding in sensitive anatomical areas. RCM can distinguish between scarring alopecia (SA) and nonscarring alopecia (NSA) [4]. NSA is characterized by androgenic alopecia with miniaturization of the hair shaft and follicular keratosis. Comparatively, SA is defined as interface dermatitis that has the involvement of the dermo-epidermal junction. RCM will show the absence of the normal rimming and obscuration of the dermal papillae [5, 6].

Parasitic skin infections can also be evaluated for diagnosis and resulting treatment through RCM. *Sarcoptes scabiei* and *Demodex folliculorum* has shown eggs and droppings from these infections, as well as the head, upper limbs, trunk, and inferior limbs [7].

5 Case Studies (3)

A RCM study has shown that this tool can be used on a clinically negative biopsy site before Mohs micrographic surgery. In a consecutive biopsy BCC evaluation, cases were labeled RCM positive or negative after Mohs micrographic surgery had margins and a 15 μm serial vertical sections. 61 patients with a mean lesion size of 5.1 mm were 73.8% positive on RCM and under histopathologic examination. While RCM can miss the residual deep layers of tumor evaluation, RCM was shown to reduce further unnecessary Mohs surgical layer removal [8].

Additionally, prospective RCM imaging has helped with the diagnosis of SCC and actinic keratosis (AK). 38 lesions in 24 patients were assessed using RCM, showing 7 AKs, 25 SCCs in situ, 3 invasive SCCs, and 3 keratoacanthomas. RCM shows atypical honeycombing or a scattered pattern of the spinous-granular layer of the epidermis. The SCC evaluation showed round, nucleated cells with spinous-granular layers and round blood vessels in the superficial dermis [9].

Evaluation of plaque psoriasis under RCM has shown horizontal sections of the epidermis and upper dermis in 10 patients with psoriasis. While vertical section examination is the gold standard for diagnosis of psoriasis, comparative findings with RCM would help define a precise finding of psoriasis for patients [10].

6 Benefits

RCM is a hand-held device that can get into smaller areas. Caliber I.D. addresses this concern with their Vivascope 3000 model. This is a flexible, hand-held confocal imaging device that allows the operator to access small lesions and lesions in difficult locations such as the periocular regions, nasal crease, concha, and interdigital web spaces. This device also allows for free movement across the skin. The depth of imaging is 200–300 μm, correlating to the papillary dermis mainly [11].

As demonstrated through case studies, RCM can assess appropriate surgical margins ex vivo in Mohs surgery.

Furthermore, RCM can even monitor the effectiveness of imiquimod in treating AKs.

7 Limitations

RCM has limitations in evaluating certain areas of skin. For example, hyperkeratotic lesions are challenging to evaluate with a high backscattering of light due to keratin but can be treated with keratolytic ointment for evaluation. Hairy areas of the skin can also have a poor adherence of the lens and presence of air. The 3000 RCM and haircuts can aid to improve these diagnostics. Nodular lesions limit the penetration of RCM to the upper dermis. Lesions with scales can impair the visualization of the dermo-epidermal junction. Fibrin, coagulated blood, and keratin aggregates limit the examination of the patient's evaluation but focusing on the peri-ulcer or peri-crust tissue can improve this. RCM also cannot differentiate between benign spitzoid lesions from melanoma. Deep inflammatory processes can be challenging for this particular tool to evaluate as the RCM is contained to describing the upper dermis. Palms and soles are also difficult for the RCM to evaluate, as they focus on hyperkeratosis and acanthosis epidermis to reflect light.

The physical size of the RCM makes it challenging to place it into small sites of the ear and canthus. This limitation puts more emphasis on the extensive training required to interpret the small, layered images [5].

Key Points

1. RCM is a non-invasive imaging technique that is used for diagnostic methodology that can initially be an alternative to invasive biopsy techniques.
2. RCM can assess Mohs micrographic surgery margins and the effectiveness of topical treatments.
3. Vivascope® 1500 is a current RCM that increases clinical diagnostic ability if used in conjunction with dermoscopy.

8 Conclusion

In conclusion, RCM is a high-resolution, noninvasive imaging technique that is used in the evaluation of melanoma and nonmelanoma skin tumors.

Quiz Questions and Answers

1. What layer of the skin can reflectance confocal microscopy not evaluate?
    a. Stratum corneum
    b. Stratum granulosum
    c. Stratum basale
    d. Hypodermis
    e. Dermo-epidermal junction
        i. Answer: d. Hypodermis.
2. What can reflectance confocal microscopy aid in the evaluation of with other diagnostic techniques?

   a. Mohs micrographic surgery margins
   b. Treatment improvement, such as with topical Imiquimod
   c. The depth of scabies infection
   d. The depth of basal cell carcinoma invasion
   e. Both a and c
      i. Answer: e. Both a and c.
3. What is the main way that reflectance confocal microscopy technologically evaluates the skin?
   a. Horizontal imaging
   b. Invasive imaging
   c. Vertical imaging
   d. 90° angle
   e. None of the above
      i. Answer: a. Horizontal imaging.

References

1. Calzavara-Pinton PG, Rossi MT, Zanca A, Arisi M, Gonzalez S, Venturini M. Retraction: oral polypodium leucomotos increases the anti-inflammatory and melanogenic responses of the skin to different modalities of sun exposures: a pilot study. Photodermatol Photoimmunol Photomed. 2016;32(5–6):331.
2. Guida S, Pellacani G, Ciardo S, Longo C. Reflectance confocal microscopy of aging skin and skin cancer. Dermatol Pract Concept. 2021;11(3):e2021068.
3. Edwards SJ, Mavranezouli I, Osei-Assibey G, Marceniuk G, Wakefield V, Karner C. VivaScope(R) 1500 and 3000 systems for detecting and monitoring skin lesions: a systematic review and economic evaluation. Health Technol Assess. 2016;20(58):1–260.
4. Ardigo M, Agozzino M, Franceschini C, et al. Reflectance confocal microscopy for scarring and non-scarring alopecia real-time assessment. Arch Dermatol Res. 2016;308(5):309–18.
5. Franceschini C, Persechino F, Ardigo M. In vivo reflectance confocal microscopy in general dermatology: how to choose the right indication. Dermatol Pract Concept. 2020;10(2):e2020032.
6. Agozzino M, Gonzalez S, Ardigo M. Reflectance confocal microscopy for inflammatory skin diseases. Actas Dermosifiliogr. 2016;107(8):631–9.
7. Cinotti E, Perrot JL, Labeille B, Cambazard F. Reflectance confocal microscopy for cutaneous infections and infestations. J Eur Acad Dermatol Venereol. 2016;30(5):754–63.
8. Navarrete-Dechent C, Cordova M, Aleissa S, et al. Reflectance confocal microscopy confirms residual basal cell carcinoma on clinically negative biopsy sites before Mohs micrographic surgery: a prospective study. J Am Acad Dermatol. 2019;81(2):417–26.
9. Rishpon A, Kim N, Scope A, et al. Reflectance confocal microscopy criteria for squamous cell carcinomas and actinic keratoses. Arch Dermatol. 2009;145(7):766–72.
10. Verzi AE, Lacarrubba F, Caltabiano R, Broggi G, Musumeci ML, Micali G. Reflectance confocal microscopy features of plaque psoriasis overlap with horizontal histopathological sections: a case series. Am J Dermatopathol. 2019;41(5):355–7.
11. Calzavara-Pinton P, Longo C, Venturini M, Sala R, Pellacani G. Reflectance confocal microscopy for in vivo skin imaging. Photochem Photobiol. 2008;84(6):1421–30.

The Application of High-Resolution Ultrasound in Dermatology

Jalal Maghfour, Betty Nguyen, and Iltefat H. Hamzavi

Abstract High-resolution ultrasonography (HRUS), also known as high-frequency ultrasonography, is a safe, non-invasive, and rapid method of imaging the epidermis and dermis. HRUS uses high-frequency sound waves, usually in the range of 2–12 MHz, to obtain high resolution images. It is useful for not only diagnosis, but also for monitoring and treating dermatologic conditions. Applications of HRUS include assessing melanoma and non-melanoma skin cancer, inflammatory skin conditions, systemic disorders, and vascular lesions. It is also routinely used to visualize structural landmarks when performing dermatologic procedures such as fillers. In this chapter, we discuss these standard and novel applications of high-resolution ultrasonography in dermatology.

Keywords High-resolution ultrasound · HRUS · Dermatology · Inflammatory skin disorders · Hidradenitis suppurativa · Scleroderma

Learning Objectives

- To understand the basic principles of High-resolution Ultrasound
- To understand the general application of High-resolution Ultrasound in dermatology
- To appreciate the role of High-resolution ultrasound in clinical practice
- To recognize common morphologic features of skin cancer and inflammatory skin disorders (e.g., atopic dermatitis, hidradenitis suppurativa, psoriasis) on ultrasound

J. Maghfour (✉) · I. H. Hamzavi
Photobiology and Photomedicine Research Unit, Department of Dermatology, Henry Ford Health System, Detroit, MI, USA
e-mail: jmaghfo1@hfhs.org

B. Nguyen
Dr. Phillip Frost Department of Dermatology and Cutaneous Surgery, University of Miami School of Medicine, Miami, FL, USA

K. Nouri (ed.), *Telemedicine and Technological Advances in Dermatology*,
https://doi.org/10.1007/978-3-031-69091-4_20

- To recognize common morphologic features of sclerotic disorders and vascular anomalies on ultrasound
- To appreciate the application of ultrasound in cosmetic dermatology.

1 Introduction

High-resolution ultrasonography (HRUS) is a non-invasive, readily applicable imaging technique that can depict real time static and dynamic morphological information concerning various organ systems [1]. HRUS has a versatile application and due to its high diagnostic value, safety profile and low cost to patients, it is widely used in clinical medicine.

Ultrasonography relies on the use of high-frequency sound waves to generate high-resolution images. In general, the frequency used in ultrasounds is above the limit of human ear (20,000 kHz)—usually in the range of 2–12 MHz [2, 3]. In order to obtain high-resolution images, it is recommended to use the highest-frequency transducer capable of penetrating to the desired depth. A transducer is a handheld device composed of thousands of piezoelectric crystals. These crystals, when stimulated, generate sound waves that pass through tissue and are reflected back to the transducer. The sounds waves received by the transducer are converted into electrical energy and are interpreted by a monitor [4]. The monitor can display the amplitude mode (A-mode), which can be used to interpret echogenicity at various distances from the probe [1]. Echogenicity, or the ability to reflect a sound wave, is a property inherent to each tissue. In brightness mode (B-mode), an image is generated with different intensities of brightness. The monitor displays images using shades of gray (ranging from black to white). The velocity of sound waves depends on the density of the tissue, with velocity being inversely proportional to the fluid content of a tissue. These characteristics have clinical implications, as low echogenicity may indicate infiltration and/or inflammation of the tissue [1].

The application of ultrasound technology in dermatology dates back three decades ago [5]. In 1979, it was determined that ultrasonic imaging can be useful in distinguishing between healthy and diseased skin. Since then, the use of ultrasound imaging in dermatology has expanded in scope. Routine and novel applications of ultrasound in dermatology include assessing skin cancer, inflammatory skin conditions, systemic disorders, and vascular lesions. Cosmetic dermatology has also adopted ultrasound use. The aim of this chapter is to review the principles of HRUS in cutaneous imaging and its current applications in the evaluation of various dermatologic conditions.

2 Instrumentation and Examination of High-Resolution Ultrasonography in Dermatology: A Guide

The evaluation of cutaneous imaging relies on the use of high-frequency transducers (6–30 MHz) [1]. Although high-frequency ultrasound devices are unable to easily travel through tissues, they are able to produce high-resolution images of superficial structures (e.g., epidermis, dermis) [2, 6]. It is important to note that dermal thickness varies based on regional body sites. As such, different transducers of a specific frequency should be used for optimal visualization of lesions in various anatomic sites.

The epidermis strongly reflects sound waves due to its primary component of keratin, a polymer made up of type I and type II intermediate filaments. The presence of keratin makes the epidermis hyperechoic. Similar to the epidermis, the dermis is also depicted as a hyperechoic structure on ultrasonic imaging. Due to the presence of collagen, the dermal layer is less hyperechoic compared to the epidermis. On the other hand, the subcutis is hypoechoic as the presence of fat lobules interferes with transduction of sound waves [5].

There are important considerations to be aware of when interpreting echogenicity for non-disease healthy skin [7, 8]. Aging results in skin thinning, which translates into a reduced skin thickness on HRUS imaging. However, the echogenicity increases with age due to the increase in collagen production [8, 9].

To obtain high quality images, the operator should understand how to manipulate and adjust the ultrasound system [10]. In order to minimize artifact when imaging the skin, the probe should be held firmly and very close to its footprint. A generous amount of gel should be used as it decreases the motion artifact and enables a clear demarcation between the epidermis and the dermis. Direct contact of the probe with skin and/or compression should be avoided as it can result in a perceived skin thinning and may displace superficial nodules out the operator's view. When evaluating inflammatory skin conditions, the contralateral normal skin is often used as a control.

In regard to anatomic position, images are obtained using two perpendicular axes, longitudinal and transverse. Often time, images can be obtained using additional axes such as transverse-oblique and longitudinal-oblique [10, 11].

Furthermore, the assessment of vasculature, particularly for inflammatory and malignant skin conditions, is an integral component of ultrasound examination and many ultrasound devices include a Doppler analysis for characterization of blood flow and vasculature anatomy [2, 11].

HRUS is often used for various dermatologic conditions. For malignant lesions, it has been shown to be useful for evaluating detailed morphology of skin neoplasms, monitoring the course and therapeutic efficacy of inflammatory skin conditions (e.g., psoriasis, hidradenitis suppurativa), sclerotic lesions (e.g., systemic scleroderma, morphea). In the following sections, we will be discussing the clinical utility and application of HRUS in the diagnosis and management of skin neoplasm and inflammatory skin conditions.

3 Malignancy

3.1 Non-melanoma Skin Cancer

HRUS has been shown to play an essential role in the diagnosis and management of non-melanoma skin cancer (NMSC). This imaging technique is used to delineate lesion depth, thickness and borders. In addition, it is a useful modality to monitor for disease progression, treatment efficacy and recurrence [12].

Basal cell carcinoma (BCC) is the most common NMSC. Many studies have reported the clinical utility of HRUS in the management of BCC [13, 14]. On ultrasound, BCC is characterized by a hypoechoic structure with irregular borders. Doppler analysis often reveals an internal vascularity [14]. Distinct ultrasonic features of BCC include a focal hyperechoic spot in the center of the tumor [14]. This is believed to be due to the presence of keratin, seen as keratin nests on a BCC histology. This hyperechoic feature is of clinical importance as it is believed to be a distinct marker for BCC and can help differentiate a BCC from melanoma on ultrasound [15].

HRUS has been used as a preoperative tool by delineating the borders of skin tumor and treatment margins. Many studies have found that preoperative use of HRUS reduces the rate of BCC recurrence [16, 17]. Of note, certain ultrasonographic markers such as hyperechoic spots on HRUS are considered strong features of BCC subtypes (e.g., micronodular, sclerosing variant, and morpheiform) and that the number of hyperechoic spots can be predictive for local BCC recurrence [17].

3.2 Squamous Cell Carcinoma

Similar to BCC, squamous cell carcinoma (SCC) is depicted as a hypoechogenic tumor. As such, this feature is not specific to SCC. Compared to BCC, SCC does not have central hyperechoic spots [18]. On Doppler, SCC exhibits lesional low flow vessels [19].

It is important to note that some SCCs can clinically present with a severe crusting and/or hyperkeratotic scale. The excess of keratin can interfere with the accuracy of SCC testing. Therefore, it is recommended to remove the scale and/or crust. Furthermore, unlike BCC tumors, delineating the borders of SCC can be a challenge owing to the inflammation and scar tissue surrounding the lesion. For these reasons, HRUS cannot solely be used to diagnose and evaluate for SCC [20]. Instead, it is recommended to be used to complement clinical exam, dermoscopy and lesion biopsy.

3.3 *Melanoma*

Several published studies have highlighted the clinical implications of using HRUS for evaluation and management of melanoma [21–24]. Although HRUS is unable to detect the degree and amount of melanin pigment, it has been shown to be a useful modality for calculating a Breslow index in a large number of patients with cutaneous melanoma (CM) [21, 24].

Specifically, it was determined that the use of higher frequency probe (20 MHz) strongly correlates with the depth of thick melanomas but poorly correlated with thin melanomas [24].

Other studies revealed a similar pattern highlighting that ultrasound findings strongly correlate with melanoma thickness measured on histology [25]. This correlation depends on the frequency of the transducer. In general, a transducer at a frequency ranging from 10 to 15 MHz was shown to differentiate melanomas measuring up to one mm in thickness. This is of clinical utility as CM greater than 1 mm often requires a sentinel lymph node biopsy. It was also proposed that HRUS can be an alternative test to SLNB as patients with positive nodes on HRUS can undergo radical surgery with lymphadenectomy [25].

HRUS has also been shown to be more sensitive and specific than clinical examination (e.g., palpation) in the detection of metastases. Several studies have pointed to the high sensitivity of HRUS in detecting in-transit metastases (defined as metastases beyond 2 cm from primary tumor but have not reached local lymph node basin) and satellite metastases [26].

4 Inflammatory Skin Disorders

4.1 *Psoriasis*

Psoriasis is a common inflammatory skin disorder. While a dermatologic exam is often sufficient to make a diagnosis of psoriasis, imaging modalities may prove to be useful in disease management. A recent study published in 2019 evaluated the ultrasound characteristics of psoriatic lesions. Using a high frequency (20 MHz) transducer, it was shown that psoriatic lesions exhibited an increase in skin thickness relative to non-lesional skin and that skin thickness was accompanied by a hypoechoic pattern. This hypoechoic pattern refers to the subepidermal lower-echogenic band (SLEB) [27]. The latter was higher in psoriatic lesions compared to non-diseased healthy skin. However, SLEB is not specific to psoriasis and has been documented in photodamaged skin and in atopic dermatitis (AD) lesions. Nevertheless, SLEB is considered to reflect the degree of inflammation and edema [28].

4.2 Atopic Dermatitis

Similar to psoriasis, AD is also characterized by the presence of SLEB. Previous studies determined that SLEB in AD skin lesions can be used as an objective marker to assess for disease severity [29–31].

In addition, there appears to be a good correlation between skin thickness and histologic findings. A recent study revealed the negative correlation between the presence of low echogenic band thickness and the degree of inflammation noted on histology [30]. Specifically, low AD skin echogenicity correlated strongly with the degree of epidermal hyperplasia, epidermal hyperkeratosis, parakeratosis, spongiosis, and inflammatory infiltrates as well as the physician assessed Eczema Area and Severity Index (EASI) scores. HRUS is also useful to monitor treatment response. In two studies, the mean SLEB thickness was significantly reduced following completion of phototherapy and tacrolimus [31, 32].

4.3 Hidradenitis Suppurativa

Hidradenitis suppurativa is a debilitating inflammatory skin disorder. While history and dermatologic examination remain the gold standard for making a diagnosis of HS, clinical examination is limited by its precision, as it can be difficult to identify and distinguish between sinus tracts, nodules, and fistula.

In the past recent years, ultrasound has been used to characterize HS lesions and was shown to be more accurate, compared to clinical examination, for disease staging [33–37]. This is likely due to the ability of an ultrasound to detect significant, non-clinically evident, lesions and provide high quality images, which enable the differentiation between key lesion types. On ultrasound, HS lesions appear as a hypoechoic structure associated with dermal fluid collection of different sizes, numbers, and locations. HS lesions are also characterized, on ultrasound, by an increase in dermal thickness and enlargement of hair follicles in nonaffected skin of HS patients.

In one study, it was determined that clinically assessed lesions extend beyond their demarcation when they are examined on ultrasound [35]. These findings are of clinical importance, particularly during pre-operative surgical procedures. Identifying the extent of HS lesions is a key element to reduce the risk of recurrence. In addition to being an important tool to help with disease diagnosis and management, HRUS plays a critical role in surgical management of HS lesions.

In addition to routine ultrasound analysis, it is recommended to use Doppler in the assessment of HS lesions as it enhances the diagnosis and staging of the disease. In a retrospective study of 198 lesions, the majority of vascular distribution of nodules, and abscesses was peripheral. Communicating fistula tract displayed both peripheral and mixed vascular distribution. High body mass index (BMI), high sartorius score, longer disease duration positively correlated with intensity of power doppler and mixed vascular distribution.

In a multicenter study of 143 HS patients, 44.7% of patients, classified as having Hurley stage I disease, were found to have HS lesions consistent with stage III disease on ultrasound [36]. Early identification and accurate assessment of subclinical and clinically evident lesions is of clinical importance as it allows for an accurate treatment planning and can therefore alter the course of the disease and prevent the disabling complications associated with HS.

While there are many outcome measures for HS, only Hurley staging was found to have a good inter-rater reliability. However, Hurley staging does not take into account disease burden and disease impact on patients 'quality of life, and it does not adequately capture disease activity. As such, better outcome measures are needed to adequately measure disease activity. A recent study has evaluated the clinical utility of HRUS in improving inter-rater reliability for multiple outcome measures (e.g., Sartorius, Hidradenitis suppurativa clinical response [HiSCR]) [37]. Compared to pre-ultrasound, the use of ultrasound resulted in a significant improvement in the rater agreement for sartorius and HiSCR nodules and draining fistula count. The findings from this study highlight the importance of incorporating ultrasound in the clinical assessment of HS lesions.

Recently, a group of HS expert physicians (made of dermatologists and radiologists) have recommended the routine use of ultrasound in the assessment of both axilla and groin areas, irrespective of the absence of clinical lesions.

Although HRUS continues to be an important non-invasive imaging modality in HS management, a significant limitation is that current terms used to describe HS lesions clinically may not be synonymous to lesions identified on ultrasound. As such, there is a need for developing a standardized terminology that can be used interchangeably when evaluating HS lesions clinically and on ultrasound.

4.4 Scleroderma

Localized scleroderma is an inflammatory skin disorder characterized by skin thickening due to excessive collagen deposition. Dermal thickness has been used as an outcome measure in various clinical trials and was shown to be a good predictor for treatment response [38, 39].

When evaluating scleroderma on ultrasound, the use of transducers with a frequency ranging between 15 and 20 MHz provides an accurate assessment of skin thickness. Using HRUS, scleroderma is characterized by an increase in epidermal and dermal thickness. While skin thickness alone is unable to distinguish between early edematous and late fibrotic changes, echogenicity can distinguish between those two characteristics [39].

It is important to highlight that ultrasound is a dynamic imaging modality that is sensitive to detect changes following treatment course.

Localized scleroderma exhibits a dermal hypoechogenicity and thickening, which represents early edematous changes. Following treatment initiation, clinical improvement is seen as an increase in echogenicity and a reduction in dermal thickening on ultrasound [39]. Furthermore, following treatment completion, there is a reduction in the thick hyperechoic bands, which represent a bundle of collagen on histology [39].

In contrast, when evaluating late stage of scleroderma, fibrosis is depicted as dermal hyperechogenicity. Often time, hyperechoic foci in the dermis may be seen. These foci represent perivascular and periadnexal round cell infiltrates that are often seen on histology.

There is conflicting data regarding blood flow characteristics of localized scleroderma [40]. One study did not identify any changes in the arterial and venous blood flow between lesions and control. However, another study reported an increase in blood flow in lesions considered to be clinically active [41]. Hyperemia is another characteristic that can be captured using Doppler. Monitoring changes in hyperemia has clinical implications, as loss of hyperemia has been shown to be associated with clinical improvement while a return of hyperemia represents a sign of clinical deterioration. As such, hyperemia can guide treatment decisions.

4.5 *Lichen Sclerosis*

HRUS has been used to distinguish between morphea and extra-genital lichen sclerosis (LS) [42]. Some of the unique ultrasonographic features of LS include a hyperechogenic entrance echo, a normoechogenic area (representing the dermis) and a hypoechogenic zone associated with hypodermis. In addition, a polycyclic surface of the entrance echo is a distinct feature of LS [42].

4.6 *Systemic Sclerosis*

Systemic sclerosis (SSc) is a connective tissue disorder that causes progressive tissue fibrosis and may involve skin and subcutaneous tissue. HRUS has been shown to accurately measure skin thickness, texture, and disease activity in patients with SSc in small studies [43, 44]. In a study including 28 patients with diffuse cutaneous systemic sclerosis (dcSSc), Liu and colleagues (2017) independently rated skin thickness and echogenicity using an 18 MHz probe and found that skin thickness was positively correlated with increased echogenicity on ultrasonography [43]. Comparable results were observed by Li et al. [44]. In this study, it was found that the total skin thickness positively correlated with the European Scleroderma Trial and Research Disease Activity Index (EUSTAR-DAI), a validated measure of SSc activity. Skin thickness measured by ultrasound demonstrated a good agreement with histological skin thickness [45]. In 2020, Naredo and team found that ultra-high frequency ultrasound at 50 MHz precisely measured the thickness of the dermis and could discriminate differences in the texture of the dermis/hypodermis between diseased and healthy skin [46]. Collectively, these findings indicate that HRUS is a promising clinical tool for staging SSc and monitoring treatment response.

4.7 Vascular Lesions

HFUS may be a rapid diagnostic tool in evaluating vascular lesions, including port-wine stains (PWS), arteriovenous malformations (AVMs), and spider nevi. PWS may appear as hypoechoic structures in the dermis without involvement of the subcutaneous tissue [47]. The hypoechoic nature of PWS may be due to their poor vascularization with venous blood flow, in contrast to AVMs which appear hyperechoic from containing both arterial and venous blood. However, color doppler of PWS may show increased vascularity compared to normal skin [47]. Color doppler HRUS has also been used in the imaging of cutaneous AVMs. Using a linear probe with up to a frequency of 22 MHz, researchers observed dilated blood vessels in the mid to lower dermis and subcutaneous tissues with areas of increased and faster blood flow. These findings were especially seen in larger lesions with more intense red or dark pink coloring [48]. Although HRUS is not commonly used to image spider nevi, Doppler analysis of spider nevi is characterized by a high vascularity with an arterial biphasic waveform, consistent with other high-flow vascular lesions.

4.8 Cosmetic

Applications of HRUS in cosmetics include monitoring skin hydration, visualizing blood vessels during injections, and evaluating skin response to vitamin C therapy. In a study including 27 participants, treatment with topical skin moisturizers on the chin and cheeks was monitored using HRUS [49]. There was a significant difference in dermal echogenicity following a 14 day treatment course; these findings suggest that HRUS may be a novel method in monitoring treatment response to topical moisturizers [49]. HRUS is routinely used during injection and removal of fillers. Doppler ultrasonography can be used during injections to ensure that fillers are not accidentally injected into blood vessels. HRUS is able to visualize and in some cases, distinguish between different types of fillers including hyaluronic acid and silicone oil. Hyaluronic acid filler appears echogenic or hypoechoic on ultrasound [50]. Due to its ability to visualize filler material, HRUS can be used to detect, and monitor pre-existing fillers as well as guide surgical removal of fillers [51]. In another study evaluating the efficacy of topical vitamin C on skin texture, researchers used HRUS to measure thickness of the epidermis and the number of echogenic pixels before and after treatment [52]. They found that medium and high echogenic pixels, a measurement of protein synthesis, increased after treatment [52]. These novel applications of HRUS are among other ways that HRUS is used in dermatology.

5 Conclusion

As advancements in the field of ultrasonography continue, the many applications of HRUS will continue to rise. It is becoming clear that HRUS is a promising tool in the diagnostic and therapeutic management of various dermatologic conditions. Given the increasing popularity of ultrasound use, a core international task force group formed by 15 physicians from 11 countries called the DERMUS (dermatologic ultrasound) group recommends dermatologists use Doppler-capable ultrasound devices with a frequency of at least 15–22 MHz in all ultrasound examinations of the skin. As the operator's skill can influence the results and interpretation of ultrasound, it was recommended that the dermatologist functions as the operator and in order to achieve minimum competency, the ultrasound should be used 300 times per year.

Nevertheless, the ultrasound is a dynamic, cheap and a reliable tool to aid in diagnosing, monitoring, and treating dermatologic conditions by providing more objective assessment measures.

Conflict of Interest Dr. Iltefat Hamzavi is an investigator for PCORI, Incyte Corporation, L'Oréal, Beiersdorf, Estee Lauder, Unigen Inc., Ferndale Healthcare Inc., Pfizer, Allergan, UCB, Jansen and Johnson & Johnson and has served as a consultant for Pfizer, Johnson and Johnson, and Beiersdorf. None of the remaining authors have any conflict of interest to disclose.

Funding/Support No relevant funding/support to disclose.

References

1. Levy J, Barrett DL, Harris N, et al. High-frequency ultrasound in clinical dermatology: a review. Ultrasound J. 2021;13:24. https://doi.org/10.1186/s13089-021-00222-w.
2. Schneider SL, Kohli I, Hamzavi IH, Council ML, Rossi AM, Ozog DM. Emerging imaging technologies in dermatology: Part I: basic principles. J Am Acad Dermatol. 2019;80(4):1114–20. https://doi.org/10.1016/j.jaad.2018.11.042.
3. Mlosek RK, Malinowska S. Ultrasound image of the skin apparatus and imaging basics. J Ultrason. 2013;13(53):212–21. https://doi.org/10.15557/JoU.2013.0021.
4. Bhatta AK, Keyal U, Liu Y. Application of high frequency ultrasound in dermatology. Discov Med. 2018;26(145):237–42.
5. Izzetti R, Oranges T, Janowska A, Gabriele M, Graziani F, Romanelli M. The application of ultra-high-frequency ultrasound in dermatology and wound management. Int J Low Extrem Wounds. 2020;19(4):334–40. https://doi.org/10.1177/1534734620972815.
6. Jemec GB, Gniadecka M, Ulrich J. Ultrasound in dermatology. Part I. High frequency ultrasound. Eur J Dermatol. 2000;10(6):492–7.

7. Iyengar S, Makin IR, Sadhwani D, Moon E, Yanes AF, Geisler A, et al. Utility of a high-resolution superficial diagnostic ultrasound system for assessing skin thickness: a cross-sectional study. Dermatol Surg. 2018;44(6):855–64. https://doi.org/10.1097/DSS.0000000000001445.
8. de Rigal J, Escoffier C, Querleux B, Faivre B, Agache P, Leveque JL. Assessment of aging of the human skin by in vivo ultrasonic imaging. J Invest Dermatol. 1989;93(5):621–5. https://doi.org/10.1111/1523-1747.ep12319741.
9. Sandby-Moller J, Wulf HC. Ultrasonographic subepidermal low-echogenic band, dependence of age and body site. Skin Res Technol. 2004;10(1):57–63. https://doi.org/10.1111/j.1600-0846.2004.00056.x.
10. Ihnatsenka B, Boezaart AP. Ultrasound: basic understanding and learning the language. Int J Shoulder Surg. 2010;4(3):55–62. https://doi.org/10.4103/0973-6042.76960.
11. Schneider SL, Kohli I, Hamzavi IH, Council ML, Rossi AM, Ozog DM. Emerging imaging technologies in dermatology: Part II: applications and limitations. J Am Acad Dermatol. 2019;80(4):1121–31. https://doi.org/10.1016/j.jaad.2018.11.043.
12. Pilat P, Borzecki A, Jazienicki M, Gerkowicz A, Krasowska D. High-frequency ultrasound in the diagnosis of selected non-melanoma skin nodular lesions. Postepy Dermatol Alergol. 2019;36(5):572–80. https://doi.org/10.5114/ada.2019.89505.
13. Bard RL. High-frequency ultrasound examination in the diagnosis of skin cancer. Dermatol Clin. 2017;35(4):505–11. https://doi.org/10.1016/j.det.2017.06.011.
14. Khlebnikova A, Molochkov V, Selezneva E, et al. Ultrasonographic features of superficial and nodular basal cell carcinoma. Med Ultrason. 2018;20:475–9.
15. Harland CC, Kale SG, Jackson P, Mortimer PS, Bamber JC. Differentiation of common benign pigmented skin lesions from melanoma by high-resolution ultrasound. Br J Dermatol. 2000;143(2):281–9. https://doi.org/10.1046/j.1365-2133.2000.03652.x.
16. Wang SQ, Liu J, Zhu QL, et al. High-frequency ultrasound features of basal cell carcinoma and its association with histological recurrence risk. Chin Med J (Engl). 2019;132(17):2021–6. https://doi.org/10.1097/CM9.0000000000000369.
17. Wortsman X, Vergara P, Castro A, Saavedra D, Bobadilla F, Sazunic I, Zemelman V, Wortsman J. Ultrasound as predictor of histologic subtypes linked to recurrence in basal cell carcinoma of the skin. J Eur Acad Dermatol Venereol. 2015;29:702–7. https://doi.org/10.1111/jdv.12660.
18. Wortsman X. Ultrasound in dermatology: why, how, and when? Seminars in ultrasound, CT and MRI. 2013;34(3):177–95.
19. Barcaui Ede O, Carvalho AC, Lopes FP, Piñeiro-Maceira J. Barcaui CB high frequency ultrasound with color doppler in dermatology. An Bras Dermatol. 2016;91(3):262–73.
20. Jambusaria-Pahlajani A, Schmultz CD, Miller CJ. Test characteristics of high-resolution ultrasound in the preoperative assessment of margins of basal cell and squamous cell carcinoma in patients undergoing Mohs micrographic surgery. Dermatol Surg. 2009;35:9–16.
21. Pellacani G, Seidenari S. Preoperative melanoma thickness determination by 20 MHz sonography and digital videomicroscopy in combination. Arch Dermatol. 2003;139:293–8.
22. Mandava A, Ravuri PR, Konathan R. High-resolution ultrasound imaging of cutaneous lesions. Indian J Radiol Imaging. 2013;23(3):269–77. https://doi.org/10.4103/0971-3026.120272.
23. Szymanska E, Nowicki A, Mlosek K, Litniewski J, Lewandowski M, Secomski W, et al. Skin imaging with high frequency ultrasound—preliminary results. Eur J Ultrasound. 2000;12(1):9–16. https://doi.org/10.1016/s0929-8266(00)00097-5.
24. Kozarova A, Kozar M, Tonhajzerova I, Pappova T, Minarikova E. The value of high-frequency 20 MHz ultrasonography for preoperative measurement of cutaneous melanoma thickness. Acta Dermatovenerol Croat. 2018;26(1):15–20.
25. Belfiore MP, Reginelli A, Russo A, et al. Usefulness of high-frequency ultrasonography in the diagnosis of melanoma: mini review. Front Oncol. 2021;11:673026. https://doi.org/10.3389/fonc.2021.673026.
26. Czarnecka A, Czarnecki R, Witkiewicz W, Hryncewicz-Gwóźdź A. Importance of sonography of the skin and subcutaneous tissue in the early diagnosis of melanoma in-transit metastasis with the presentation of two cases. Postepy Dermatol Alergol. 2018;35(2):204–7. https://doi.org/10.5114/ada.2018.75244.

27. Şomlea MC, Boca AN, Pop AD, et al. High-frequency ultrasonography of psoriatic skin: a non-invasive technique in the evaluation of the entire skin of patients with psoriasis: a pilot study. Exp Ther Med. 2019;18(6):4981–6. https://doi.org/10.3892/etm.2019.8140.
28. Gupta AK, Turnbull DH, Harasiewicz KA, Shum DT, Watteel GN, Foster FS, Sauder DN. The use of high-frequency ultrasound as a method of assessing the severity of a plaque of psoriasis. Arch Dermatol. 1996;132(6):658–62 PMID: 8651715.
29. Sabau M, Boca AN, Ilies RF, Tataru A. Potential of high-frequency ultrasonography in the management of atopic dermatitis. Exp Ther Med. 2019;17(2):1073–7. https://doi.org/10.3892/etm.2018.6984.
30. Polanska A, Danczak-Pazdrowska A, Silny W, Wozniak A, Maksin K, Jenerowicz D, et al. Comparison between high-frequency ultrasonography (Dermascan C, version 3) and histopathology in atopic dermatitis. Skin Res Technol. 2013;19(4):432–7. https://doi.org/10.1111/srt.12064.
31. Polanska A, Silny W, Jenerowicz D, Kniola K, Molinska-Glura M, Danczak-Pazdrowska A. Monitoring of therapy in atopic dermatitis–observations with the use of high-frequency ultrasonography. Skin Res Technol. 2015;21(1):35–40. https://doi.org/10.1111/srt.12153.
32. Osmola-Mankowska A, Polanska A, Silny W, Zaba R, Adamski Z, Danczak-Pazdrowska A. Topical tacrolimus vs medium-dose ultraviolet al phototherapy in the treatment of atopic dermatitis-a preliminary study in relation to parameters of the epidermal barrier function and high-frequency ultrasonography. Eur Rev Med Pharmacol Sci. 2014;18(24):3927–34.
33. Lacarrubba F, Dini V, Napolitano M, Venturini M, Caposiena Caro DR, Molinelli E, et al. Ultrasonography in the pathway to an optimal standard of care of hidradenitis suppurativa: the italian ultrasound working group experience. J Eur Acad Dermatol Venereol. 2019;33(Suppl 6):10–4. https://doi.org/10.1111/jdv.15847.
34. Nazzaro G, Passoni E, Muratori S, Moltrasio C, Guanziroli E, Barbareschi M, et al. Comparison of clinical and sonographic scores in hidradenitis suppurativa and proposal of a novel ultrasound scoring system. G Ital Dermatol Venereol. 2018. https://doi.org/10.23736/S0392-0488.18.06196-5.
35. Wortsman X, Moreno C, Soto R, Arellano J, Pezo C, Wortsman J. Ultrasound in-depth characterization and staging of hidradenitis suppurativa. Dermatol Surg. 2013;39(12):1835–42. https://doi.org/10.1111/dsu.12329.
36. Loo CH, Tan WC, Tang JJ, Khor YH, Manikam MT, Low DE, et al. The clinical, biochemical, and ultrasonographic characteristics of patients with hidradenitis suppurativa in northern peninsular Malaysia: a multicenter study. Int J Dermatol. 2018;57(12):1454–63. https://doi.org/10.1111/ijd.14210.
37. Lyons AB, Narla S, Kohli I, Zubair R, Nahhas AF, Braunberger TL, Joseph MK, Nicholson CL, Jacobsen G, Hamzavi IH. Assessment of inter-rater reliability of clinical hidradenitis suppurativa outcome measures using ultrasonography. Clin Exp Dermatol. 2021. https://doi.org/10.1111/ced.14889.
38. Ranosz-Janicka I, Lis-Swiety A, Skrzypek-Salamon A, Brzezinska-Wcislo L. An extended high-frequency ultrasound protocol for assessing and quantifying of inflammation and fibrosis in localized scleroderma. Skin Res Technol. 2019;25(3):359–66. https://doi.org/10.1111/srt.12660.
39. Arisi M, Lorenzi L, Incardona P, Fusano M, Zanca A, Rossi MT, et al. Clinical, histological and high-frequency ultrasonographic evaluation (50 MHz) of morphea treated with ultraviolet al phototherapy. Clin Exp Dermatol. 2019;44(3):270–6. https://doi.org/10.1111/ced.13693.
40. Wortsman X, Wortsman J, Sazunic I, Carreño L. Activity assessment in morphea using color doppler ultrasound. J Am Acad Dermatol. 2011;65(5):942–8. https://doi.org/10.1016/j.jaad.2010.08.027. Epub 2011 May 7 PMID: 21550692.
41. Li SC, Liebling MS, Ramji FG, et al. Sonographic evaluation of pediatric localized scleroderma: preliminary disease assessment measures. Pediatr Rheumatol Online J. 2010;8:14. https://doi.org/10.1186/1546-0096-8-14.
42. Białynicki-Birula R, Reszke R, Szepietowski JC. High-frequency ultrasonography (HFUS) as a useful tool in differentiating between plaque morphea and extragenital lichen sclerosus lesions. Postepy Dermatol Alergol. 2017;34(5):485–9. https://doi.org/10.5114/ada.2017.71118.

43. Liu H, Hou Y, Zhu QL, Xu D, Wang L, Li JC, Jiang YX, Wang Q, Li MT, Zhang FC, Zeng XF. A preliminary study of skin ultrasound in diffuse cutaneous systemic sclerosis: does skin echogenicity matter? PLoS ONE. 2017;12(3):e0174481. https://doi.org/10.1371/journal.pone.0174481. PMID:28339492; PMCID:PMC5365121.
44. Li H, Furst DE, Jin H, Sun C, Wang X, Yang L, He J, Wang Y, Liu A. High-frequency ultrasound of the skin in systemic sclerosis: an exploratory study to examine correlation with disease activity and to define the minimally detectable difference. Arthritis Res Ther. 2018;20(1):181. https://doi.org/10.1186/s13075-018-1686-9. PMID:30115105;PMCID:PMC6097225.
45. Chen C, Cheng Y, Zhu X, Cai Y, Xue Y, Kong N, Yu Y, Xuan D, Zheng S, Yang X, Zhu Z, Zhao T, Wan W, Zou H, Liang M. Ultrasound assessment of skin thickness and stiffness: the correlation with histology and clinical score in systemic sclerosis. Arthritis Res Ther. 2020;22(1):197. https://doi.org/10.1186/s13075-020-02285-x. PMID:32843083;PMCID:PMC7448329.
46. Naredo E, Pascau J, Damjanov N, Lepri G, Gordaliza PM, Janta I, Ovalles-Bonilla JG, López-Longo FJ, Matucci-Cerinic M. Performance of ultra-high-frequency ultrasound in the evaluation of skin involvement in systemic sclerosis: a preliminary report. Rheumatology (Oxford). 2020;59(7):1671–8. https://doi.org/10.1093/rheumatology/kez439. PMID: 31665474.
47. Gong X, Yu W, Li J, Ding A, Xiong P, Lin X. High-frequency ultrasound investigation of port-wine stains: hemodynamic features revealed by 10 and 22 MHz transducers. J Ultrasound Med. 2019;38(3):641–8. https://doi.org/10.1002/jum.14732. Epub 2018 Oct 2 PMID: 30280405.
48. Rodríguez Bandera AI, Feito Rodríguez M, Chiloeches Fernández C, Stewart N, Valdivielso-Ramos M. Role of colour-doppler high-frequency ultrasonography in capillary malformation-arteriovenous malformation syndrome: a case series. Australas J Dermatol. 2020;61(4):349–52. https://doi.org/10.1111/ajd.13311. Epub 2020 May 3 PMID: 32363619.
49. Mlosek RK, Malinowska S, Sikora M, Dębowska R, Stępień A, Czekaj K, Dąbrowska A. The use of high frequency ultrasound imaging in skin moisturization measurement. Skin Res Technol. 2013;19(2):169–75. https://doi.org/10.1111/srt.12029. Epub 2013 Jan 9 PMID: 23297834.
50. Schelke LW, Decates TS, Velthuis PJ. Ultrasound to improve the safety of hyaluronic acid filler treatments. J Cosmet Dermatol. 2018;17(6):1019–24. https://doi.org/10.1111/jocd.12726. Epub 2018 Aug 6 PMID: 30084182.
51. Wortsman X, Wortsman J, Orlandi C, Cardenas G, Sazunic I, Jemec GB. Ultrasound detection and identification of cosmetic fillers in the skin. J Eur Acad Dermatol Venereol. 2012;26(3):292–301. https://doi.org/10.1111/j.1468-3083.2011.04047.x. Epub 2011 Mar 21 PMID: 21418333.
52. Crisan D, Roman I, Crisan M, Scharffetter-Kochanek K, Badea R. The role of vitamin C in pushing back the boundaries of skin aging: an ultrasonographic approach. Clin Cosmet Investig Dermatol. 2015;2(8):463–70. https://doi.org/10.2147/CCID.S84903. PMID:26366101;PMCID:PMC4562654.

AI and Tech Advances

Artificial Intelligence: Applications in Dermatology

Dennis H. Murphree, Yong-hun Kim, Michael Z. Zhang, Anirudh Choudhary, Puneet K. Bhullar, and Nneka I. Comfere

1 Introduction

Advances in the field of artificial intelligence (AI) have opened the door to new applications, including playing games, generating art, controlling phones by voice and many more. Of particular interest here, the sub-field of deep learning has made possible the processing and analysis of images and videos such that algorithms can recognize objects in an image much like a human can. Some classic contemporary examples of how we interact with image focused deep learning algorithms include security facial recognition and self-driving vehicles. This new class of algorithms, of which convolutional neural networks (CNNs) are most common, has generated excitement around the potential applications in medicine, with dermatology and dermatopathology being prime examples as more visually focused medical specialties. Other similar visually focused specialties include radiology, pathology, cardiology, and ophthalmology, among others. Furthermore, with parallel advances in pathology such as digital pathology leading to the digitization of whole slides, the fields of dermatology and dermatopathology are well-positioned for AI innovation.

This chapter will proceed to cover the landscape of AI applications in dermatology while including some key questions and concerns with regard to data processing that face every AI innovator. We also encourage the reader to consider frameworks of "augmented intelligence," in which human performance is enhanced by

D. H. Murphree (✉) · M. Z. Zhang · N. I. Comfere
Department of Dermatology, Mayo Clinic, Rochester, MN, USA
e-mail: Murphree.Dennis@mayo.edu

A. Choudhary
Department of Computer Science, University of Illinois, Urbana-Champaign, IL, USA

P. K. Bhullar
Department of Dermatology, Mayo Clinic, Scottsdale, AZ, USA

Y. Kim
Mayo Clinic Alix School of Medicine, Mayo Clinic, Rochester, MN, USA

K. Nouri (ed.), *Telemedicine and Technological Advances in Dermatology*,
https://doi.org/10.1007/978-3-031-69091-4_21

the use of AI models, rather than entirely supplanting human judgment and expertise with computers. This augmented intelligence framework is particularly appealing in healthcare applications.

Please note that a comprehensive explanation of many of the technical mentioned in this chapter is beyond a reasonable scope. Rather, we hope to guide the interested reader towards topics for further inquiry.

2 Current AI Applications in Dermatology

2.1 AI Content Review

Much like the way the choice of a statistical test (i.e., t-test, Chi-square, etc.) depends on the data category and question at hand, the choice of AI algorithms in dermatology can be determined broadly based on the input data type, the question being asked, and whether ground-truth labels are available.

Input data types can vary widely, including e.g. tabular data, imaging data, and text data. Tabular data could consist of categorical and/or continuous variables organized in a table, while text data could take the form of free text such as a pathology biopsy reports. Within dermatology, examples of imaging data would include clinical images, dermoscopic images, or digitized pathology slides—also referred to as whole-slide images (WSIs). Dermoscopic images are photos taken with a dermoscope, which is a special instrument used to provide a standardized image quality such that dermatologists may accurately and reliably assess all the relevant features of a cutaneous lesion. Meanwhile, clinical images refer to non-dermoscopic images taken by medical providers that are often different enough in quality from images taken by patients that they are considered two separate data types.

Ground-truth labels refer to the answer or solution that the AI model must replicate. For example, if an AI model is trained to identify melanoma on a dermoscopic image, then each image should be labeled whether melanoma is present. Labels can also take the form of pixel level annotations that, for example, localize specific features of melanoma on a WSI. When a model is trained with these labels available, it is referred to as supervised learning. Supervised learning is often focused on making specific predictions.

Unsupervised learning refers to model training without ground-truth labels available. This method is more often used to find similarities or relationships among unlabeled data. Commonly, this is done by forming several clusters of data points that may be used to uncover undetected patterns. Unsupervised learning might be used to e.g. find groups of similar patients, for example those who respond well to one type of medication versus another.

There is also a third type of learning known as weakly supervised learning that is gaining much interest. In the most common form of weakly supervised learning, detailed pixel-level annotations can be replaced with slide-level labels. For example, instead of needing pixel-level annotations of tissue types or anatomical structures on a WSI, all the pixels in the WSI can simply have an associated label of the diagnosis. This may be the preferred method when slide-level labels can be extracted in an automated fashion, for example from pathology reports in electronic health records and do not require manual effort. This approach comes at the cost of a significantly higher data need however.

In visually focused fields such as dermatology, common tasks that can be addressed by AI include classification and segmentation. Classification is solely concerned with identifying whether an entity is present in an image. In a binary classification model, the model is tasked with returning a prediction between two options, for example "unlikely concerning" or "follow up necessary". In a multi-class classification model, a single model is able to distinguish among multiple entities, whether they be different diseases or descriptors of an image.

Segmentation tasks require an AI model to be able to outline a particular entity if it is present, thus providing its location. More precisely, segmentation attempts to classify each pixel in an image rather than the image as a whole. Imaginably, a segmentation algorithm is more computationally expensive as there are more steps required to first recognize a particular entity in an image and then draw an outline around it. Common performance metrics that are reported for segmentation models include the Dice coefficient and Jaccard (JAC) index. Both metrics are used to compare the pixel overlap between a model's output segmentation and the ground-truth annotation. The Dice coefficient is calculated as follows:

$$\frac{2 * area\ of\ overlap\ of\ model\ segmentation\ and\ ground\ truth}{area\ of\ model\ segmentation + area\ of\ ground\ truth}$$

Meanwhile, the JAC index is calculated as follows:

$$\frac{area\ of\ overlap\ of\ model\ segmentation\ and\ ground\ truth}{area\ of\ union\ of\ model\ segmentation\ and\ ground\ truth}$$

The most common deep learning architecture currently (2022) employed in visual tasks, such as diagnosing a skin lesion in dermatology, is a CNN, which is inspired by the human visual cortex. The input to these models is numbers containing the pixel values of a portion of an image. Deep learning architectures typically feature a high number of layers with a certain number of neurons, or nodes, in each layer that connect to neurons in the preceding and subsequent layers. The most common operations performed within a CNN architecture are the convolution operator (i.e., a combination of matrix multiplication and summation over a smaller matrix called a filter) followed by feature pooling, an operation akin to averaging, to learn recognizable low-resolution features. Many of the state-of-the-art architectures used in dermatology research were originally developed by technology companies, such as the ResNet, DenseNet121, EfficientNet, and GoogLeNet.

Deep learning algorithms require significantly large amounts of training data in order to perform well. Datasets in healthcare have been limited in size compared to the massive publicly available datasets of everyday images such as ImageNet. This limitation is mostly due to the need for manual labeling or annotations, which require highly specialized knowledge and training when performed with medical images, whereas most people can easily recognize a dog or car in a photo. One approach to addressing the smaller datasets in healthcare is transfer learning, in which one starts with a model that is already trained to perform a similar task and retrains a certain number of layers on their proprietary dataset. Much of AI research in dermatology today leverages transfer learning to train deep learning models.

For a more comprehensive description of these topics specific to dermatology, please see Murphree et al. [1] and Puri et al. [2]. Next, we discuss current or recent AI applications divided by the type of task, with an additional section on dermatopathology.

2.2 *Classification*

Although dermatology as a field addresses a wide variety of skin conditions and concerns, in the AI realm the majority of applications have focused on diagnosing cancerous lesions.

Algorithmic approaches range from those of classical computer vision, often using handcrafted features, to state of the art CNN-centric deep learning. CNNs have achieved robust performance in skin lesion analysis, including showing superior performance to dermatologists in distinguishing between pigmented and non-pigmented skin lesions across several studies. Esteva et al. [3] had an early study developing a CNN model that could identify epidermal and melanocytic lesions, then comparing its performance to 21 board-certified dermatologists on two specific tasks: distinguishing squamous cell carcinomas (SCC) from benign seborrheic keratoses (SK) and malignant melanomas from benign nevi. Using a biopsy-proven validation set of 111 melanocytic dermatoscopic images and 135 epidermal plus 130 melanocytic non-dermatoscopic images, dermatologists were asked whether to biopsy, treat the lesion, or reassure the patient without biopsy. Esteva's CNN was then used to simultaneously classify the same lesions. In each case the network outperformed the average performance of the dermatologists. Although they did not compare via rigorous statistics, the authors concluded by graphical inspection that the CNN's performance was comparable to that of the board-certified dermatologists. Brinker et al. [4] also employed a CNN architecture for skin lesion classification, on a much larger dataset of 12,378 images. Utilizing a test set of 100 exemplar images they compared their network's performance to that of 157 dermatologists across 12 university hospitals in Germany. Here the AI system also outperformed the dermatologists' average, albeit only on certain metrics. Using a ResNet-based CNN, Han et al. [5] were able to classify 12 different skin disorders at a level comparable to the average of 16 dermatologists. Their study was enhanced in terms of interpretability by highlighting portions of interest in the images using gradient-based activation maps

(Grad-CAM), determining coarse and irregular portions of the lesion as important features for malignant tumors.

Haenssle et al. [6] similarly trained a CNN to classify lesions in dermatoscopic photographs as melanoma. They compared this network's performance to that of fifty eight dermatologists from various countries and with varying levels of experience (29% beginner, 19% skilled, and 52% expert). Lesions were classified by the human participants in two stages: (I) using dermoscopy alone and (II) using dermoscopy alongside clinical images and additional clinical information. Although human performance improved significantly with the stage II additional information, the AI approach (which was trained only on images) outperformed dermatologists across all experience levels in both stages. Interesting other aspects of this study include emphasizing the importance of a large cohort of human reviewers, ideally with varying levels of experience, as well as emphasizing diversity of anatomic site and variety of histologic type for optimal network training.

There are many more studies that focus less on comparison to humans and instead seek to maximize superio lesion identification. These studies often include special consideration for generalizability and avoiding dataset biases by sampling a diverse representation of ethnicities and Fitzpatrick skin types. For example, Han et al. [7] demonstrated that a deep neural network trained on images from Caucasian patients performed poorly on Asian patients and vice-versa. Gessert et al. [8] used a search strategy for skin lesion classification by employing an ensemble of deep learning models including EfficientNets, SENet, and ResNeXt WSL. Maron et al. [9] used artificial noise-based corruption and image perturbations on lesion images to develop a benchmark for detecting out-of-distribution melanoma, observing that DenseNet121 [10] was most resistant to noise-based corruption and that AlexNet was least affected by image perturbations. To address the ever-present concern of class imbalance, Sayed et al. [11] used random over-sampling followed by data augmentation to achieve state-of-the-art accuracy using SqueezeNet [12] on the International Skin Imaging Collaboration (ISIC) challenge datasets [13].

Though there have been numerous CNNs published that demonstrate comparative or superior performance to that of a dermatologist, there appears to be only a single prospective clinical trial [14] for AI applications in dermatology. We look forward to seeing similar trials conducted in the future such that AI may be introduced in clinical practice for the benefit of patients.

2.3 *Segmentation*

Deep learning has also achieved promising success in skin lesion segmentation, particularly with melanoma. Here, traditional computer vision techniques such as region-based active contouring, clustering, and simple or complex thresholds are particularly underperformant due to complexities both inherent, such as heterogeneity in regions of interest, and components of image capture, such as color variation by camera or the presence of hair. The capacity for deep neural networks to autonomously identify informative features allows them to more effectively distinguish pathological conditions from normal skin. An encoder-decoder network architecture is popular amongst AI-driven segmentation models, consisting of an "encoder" network that serves as a feature extractor for the input image followed by a "decoder" network that creates the final segmentation map.

Recent examples include the following: Goyal et al. [15] used Fully Convolutional Networks (FCN) to create segmentation maps for three distinct forms of skin lesions: benign nevi, melanoma, and seborrheic keratoses. Yuan and Lo [16] incorporated information from different colorspaces of dermatoscopic lesions, then trained a 19-layer convolutional-deconvolutional segmentation network, winning the ISIC 2017 Challenge with a Jaccard (JAC) index of 76.5%.

U-Net [17] is easily one of the most popular architectures for skin lesion segmentation. U-Net is based on Fully Convolutional Network (FCN) for natural object detection, and features a U-shaped architecture that concatenates the feature maps from the encoder layer with corresponding up-sampled decoder feature maps using "skip-connections", thus allowing it to retain fine-grained details required for segmentation.

Lin et al. [18] found U-Net-based histogram equalization to be superior to C-means clustering (dice coefficient of 77% vs. 61%) for skin lesion segmentation. U-Net is also frequently combined with additional CNN architectures in the search for better performance. Zafar et al. [19] combined U-Net with ResNet to achieve an average JAC Index of 77.2% on the ISIC-2017 dataset. More recently, Ashraf et al. [20] have achieved a state-of-the-art 80.73% JAC on the same challenge dataset by employing a combination of U-Net, ResUNet, and ResUNet++. Key to their performance was a pre-processing pipeline that included inpainting of hair structures along with image augmentation as well as a conditional random field in postprocessing. This serves as an important reminder that the choice of network is secondary to appropriate data pre- and post-processing.

2.4 *Dermatopathology*

In dermatopathology, deep learning can be applied to traditional pathology slides that have been scanned by a special optical scanner, a process called whole slide imaging (WSI). WSI provides important morphological, spatial, and architectural features that can be used as cellular-level biomarkers for deep learning algorithms.

Because of their large file sizes, digitized whole slide images require special techniques to make them more manageable for deep learning. Commonly, whole slide images are divided into smaller patches of tissue according to the accepted input size for a neural network architecture. This neural network functions as a tissue classifier, which makes predictions on the divided sections of tissue without knowing the context of the whole slide. Subsequently, a slide-level classifier is then used to make predictions based on the whole slide using the tissue-level predictions as input and the slide labels as output. The slide-level classifier is a model such as logistic regression, which is chosen to avoid overfitting, a common pitfall limiting model generalizability.

Like other applications of ML in healthcare, deep learning of WSIs is particularly prone to artifactual learning biases in the dataset rather than true physiology. For example, when the model is inadvertently trained with WSIs obtained on different scanner types, it will start to use the features based on scanner type to guide its final prediction. This bias can create misclassifications when one pathology has greater representation on a particular scanner model, which is commonly encountered in multicenter studies. This bias can also be seen if different staining protocols or scanning parameters are used.

Currently, most applications of AI in dermatopathology have used traditional formalin-fixed paraffin embedded tissue, which is the most common type of slide of dermatopathology. However, there is increased interest in using the fresh frozen tissue obtained during dermatologic surgery.

Several studies of AI in dermatopathology have aimed to extract features from WSI for diagnostic purposes such as cancer grading or subtyping. Olsen et al. [21] used 450 WSIs to train a CNN to classify basal cell carcinomas, dermal nevi, and seborrheic keratoses. Using a Visual Geometry Group (VGG) network, they obtained high AUC of basal cell carcinomas (0.99), dermal nevi (0.97), and seborrheic keratoses (0.99). Hart et al. [22] used 100 curated WSIs to develop a CNN to differentiate between Spitz and conventional melanocytic lesions on histopathology. Their model demonstrated 99% accuracy when used on curated image sections. Subsequently, they tested the model's performance on noncurated image patches of the entire slide, which only achieved a significantly lower accuracy (52.3%). Hekler et al. [23] created a CNN using 695 WSIs to classify melanocytic lesions as either melanoma or benign nevi. They compared the performance of the CNN against dermatopathologists on cropped 10× magnification sections. The CNN obtained an accuracy (68%), sensitivity (76%), and specificity (60%), while the 11 dermatopathologists obtained an accuracy (59.2%), sensitivity (51.8%), and specificity (66.5%). However, a major limitation of this study is that in the normal clinical setting, pathologists use the entire slide to determine malignancy and are not restricted to partial segments. Sankarapandian et al. [24] created a triaging system, which classified melanocytic specimens into low (MPATH I-II), Intermediate (MPATH III), or High (MPATH IV-V) categories, which enabled triage of melanoma cases. By using a pretrained ResNet50 network, the authors used transfer learning to extract patch-level features from WSI. They then used tissue-level labels to formulate the classification problem in a weakly-supervised multiple instance paradigm. By combining patch features using max-pooling, they triaged suspected melanomas without needing pixel-level annotations. This tool could be used to directly triage likely melanomas directly to subspecialists, which would reduce turnaround time and time to diagnosis. Thomas et al. [25] proposed an interpretable deep learning system to classify basal cell, squamous cell, and intraepidermal carcinoma using WSI. With manual labelling, they classified the tissue into 12 distinct classes in addition to identifying the stratified layers of the skin. Afterwards, they trained a classifier to classify the sub-regions of WSI into the 12 classes, which represents the WSI with a segmentation map. By using this segmentation map and analysing the tissue context, the authors achieved a high accuracy of WSI classification and ensured interpretability. Moreno-Andrés et al. [26] created a diagnostic tool using 59 WSIs to identify mitotic cells within tumour regions, achieving a diagnostic accuracy of 83%. This tool could be used to highlight areas of the slide with the greatest density of mitotic figures and could reduce the need for the immunohistochemical stains.

While much of the existing research has focused on classifying lesions as benign or malignant, there are limited studies in the literature that predicts patient outcomes and response to therapy based on the morphological WSIs. While researchers have tried to correlate pathological features (tumour grade/subtype) to patient prognosis, no studies have demonstrated a direct correlation between pathology images with multi-scale features and genetic profiles with survival outcomes and treatment response for adjuvant/neoadjuvant therapy.

3 Datasets and Challenges

As evidenced by some of the aforementioned studies, adequate model training relies on a sufficiently large dataset with a minimal risk of bias propagation (i.e., diverse Fitzpatrick skin types, ethnicities, etc.). Some authors may make their full datasets publicly accessible for others to build and test their AI models. Fortunately, in dermatology a few large public datasets are made available by the ISIC Archive [13] as well as The Cancer Imaging Archive (TCIA) [27]. The ISIC also hosts annual competitions for computer scientists to compare their model performance to that of others.

4 Ethical Considerations

4.1 Bias

Bias is a major concern for AI applications in healthcare. There are many examples of AI in healthcare that reflect societal biases, which further exacerbate those issues [28]. An algorithm's output is directly correlated with the quality of the input data; thus, attention must be given to the sources of the preprocessed data. For example, if an algorithm is built with primarily examples of low Fitzpatrick skin types, the generalizability of the algorithm to higher Fitzpatrick skin types would not be effective. Another real-world concern of AI is the potential for an overreliance on AI outputs, so-called "automation complacency." These biases may continue to be overlooked once models are deployed in the real world [29]. While the AI-powered tools in dermatology may bring significant benefit, care must be taken to ensure that biases are not exacerbated, which in turn could widen healthcare disparities even further.

4.2 *Explainability*

Another concern for AI deployment in clinical practice is to consider is whether the tools need to be easily explainable ("explainability") in their design. The purpose is to have the technology more easily understood by the patients and clinicians. Many models, such as CNNs, function as a "black box", in which the user provides a sample input and obtain an output prediction without understanding how the model forms its prediction. This poses a large issue if the AI model offers an incorrect diagnosis, as it would be difficult for the provider to explain to a patient how this error occurred. This should be an important consideration for AI scientists as they develop novel solutions to be deployed in clinical practice.

5 Conclusion

Dermatology is one of the most visually reliant fields of medicine due to its clinical, dermatoscopic, and histopathologic images that providers use every single day to make clinical decisions. Thus, there are numerous potential applications of AI in dermatology. Many current studies have been published on the applications of AI in dermatologic malignancies such as melanoma. However, the field extends beyond skin cancer with potentially thousands of different dermatologic diseases that affect one-third of the world's population [28–30]. We hope that improvement in AI models and discovering new applications of AI in dermatology will advance the field and our understanding of dermatology.

References

1. Murphree DH, Puri P, Shamim H, Bezalel SA, Drage LA, Wang M, Pittelkow MR, Carter RE, Davis MDP, Bridges AG, Mangold AR, Yiannias JA, Tollefson MM, Lehman JS, Meves A, Otley CC, Sokumbi O, Hall MR, Comfere N. Deep learning for dermatologists: Part I. Fundamental concepts. J Am Acad Dermatol. 2022;87(6):1343–51. https://doi.org/10.1016/j.jaad.2020.05.056.
2. Puri P, Comfere N, Drage LA, Shamim H, Bezalel SA, Pittelkow MR, Davis MDP, Wang M, Mangold AR, Tollefson MM, Lehman JS, Meves A, Yiannias JA, Otley CC, Carter RE, Sokumbi O, Hall MR, Bridges AG, Murphree DH. Deep learning for dermatologists: Part II. Current applications. J Am Acad Dermatol 2022;87(6):1352–60. https://doi.org/10.1016/j.jaad.2020.05.053.
3. Esteva A, Kuprel B, Novoa RA, Ko J, Swetter SM, Blau HM, Thrun S. Dermatologist-level classification of skin cancer with deep neural networks. Nature. 2017;542(7639):115–8. https://doi.org/10.1038/nature21056.
4. Brinker TJ, Hekler A, Enk AH, von Kalle C. Enhanced classifier training to improve precision of a convolutional neural network to identify images of skin lesions. PLoS ONE. 2019;14(6):e0218713. https://doi.org/10.1371/journal.pone.0218713.
5. Han SS, Park GH, Lim W, Kim MS, Na JI, Park I, Chang SE. Deep neural networks show an equivalent and often superior performance to dermatologists in onychomycosis diagnosis:

automatic construction of onychomycosis datasets by region-based convolutional deep neural network. PLoS ONE. 2018;13(1):e0191493. https://doi.org/10.1371/journal.pone.0191493.
6. Haenssle HA, Fink C, Schneiderbauer R, Toberer F, Buhl T, Blum A, Kalloo A, Ben Hadj Hassen A, Thomas L, Enk A, Uhlmann L, Reader Study Level-I and Level-II Groups, Alt C, Arenbergerova M, Bakos R, Baltzer A, Bertlich I, Blum A, Bokor-Billmann T, Bowling J, Braghiroli N, Braun R, Buder-Bakhaya K, Buhl T, Cabo H, Cabrijan L, Cevic N, Classen A, Deltgen D, Fink C, Georgieva I, Hakim-Meibodi L-E, Hanner S, Hartmann F, Hartmann J, Haus G, Hoxha E, Karls R, Koga H, Kreusch J, Lallas A, Majenka P, Marghoob A, Massone C, Mekokishvili L, Mestel D, Meyer V, Neuberger A, Nielsen K, Oliviero M, Pampena R, Paoli J, Pawlik E, Rao B, Rendon A, Russo T, Sadek A, Samhaber K, Schneiderbauer R, Schweizer A, Toberer F, Trennheuser L, Vlahova L, Wald A, Winkler J, Wölbing P, Zalaudek I. Man against machine: diagnostic performance of a deep learning convolutional neural network for dermoscopic melanoma recognition in comparison to 58 dermatologists. Ann Oncol Official J Eur Soc Med Oncol 2018;29(8):1836–42. https://doi.org/10.1093/annonc/mdy166.
7. Han SS, Kim MS, Lim W, Park GH, Park I, Chang SE. Classification of the clinical images for benign and malignant cutaneous tumors using a deep learning algorithm. J Investig Dermatol. 2018;138(7):1529–38. https://doi.org/10.1016/j.jid.2018.01.028.
8. Gessert N, Nielsen M, Shaikh M, Werner R, Schlaefer A. Skin lesion classification using ensembles of multi-resolution EfficientNets with meta data. MethodsX. 2020;7:100864. https://doi.org/10.1016/j.mex.2020.100864.
9. Maron RC, Schlager JG, Haggenmüller S, von Kalle C, Utikal JS, Meier F, Gellrich FF, Hobelsberger S, Hauschild A, French L, Heinzerling L, Schlaak M, Ghoreschi K, Hilke FJ, Poch G, Heppt MV, Berking C, Haferkamp S, Sondermann W, Schadendorf D, Schilling B, Goebeler M, Krieghoff-Henning E, Hekler A, Fröhling S, Lipka DB, Kather JN, Brinker TJ. A benchmark for neural network robustness in skin cancer classification. Eur J Cancer. 2021;155:191–9. https://doi.org/10.1016/j.ejca.2021.06.047.
10. Huang G, Liu Z, Van Der Maaten L, Weinberger KQ. Densely connected convolutional networks. In Proceedings of the IEEE conference on computer vision and pattern recognition, p. 4700–08.
11. Sayed GI, Soliman MM, Hassanien AE. A novel melanoma prediction model for imbalanced data using optimized SqueezeNet by bald eagle search optimization. Comput Biol Med. 2021;136: 104712. https://doi.org/10.1016/j.compbiomed.2021.104712.
12. Iandola FN, Han S, Moskewicz MW, Ashraf K, Dally WJ, Keutzer K. SqueezeNet: AlexNet-level accuracy with 50x fewer parameters and< 0.5 MB model size. 2016. arXiv preprint arXiv: 1602.07360.
13. ISIC Challenge. Retrieved January 2, 2023 from https://challenge.isic-archive.com/.
14. Han SS, Kim YJ, Moon IJ, Jung JM, Lee MY, Lee WJ, Won CH, Lee MW, Kim SH, Navarrete-Dechent C, Chang SE. Evaluation of artificial intelligence-assisted diagnosis of skin neoplasms: a single-center, paralleled, unmasked, randomized controlled trial. J Investig Dermatol. 2022;142(9):2353–2362.e2. https://doi.org/10.1016/j.jid.2022.02.003.
15. Goyal M, Yap MH, Hassanpour S. Multi-class semantic segmentation of skin lesions via fully convolutional networks. 2017. arXiv preprint arXiv:1711.10449.
16. Yuan Y, Lo Y-C. Improving dermoscopic image segmentation with enhanced convolutional-deconvolutional networks. IEEE J Biomed Health Inform. 2019;23(2):519–26. https://doi.org/10.1109/JBHI.2017.2787487.
17. Ronneberger O, Fischer P, Brox T. U-Net: convolutional networks for biomedical image segmentation. In: Medical image computing and computer-assisted intervention—MICCAI 2015 (Lecture notes in computer science); 2015. p. 234–41. https://doi.org/10.1007/978-3-319-24574-4_28.
18. Lin BS, Michael K, Kalra S, Tizhoosh HR. Skin lesion segmentation: U-nets versus clustering. In: 2017 IEEE symposium series on computational intelligence (SSCI); 2017. p. 1–7.
19. Zafar K, Gilani SO, Waris A, Ahmed A, Jamil M, Khan MN, Kashif AS. Skin lesion segmentation from dermoscopic images using convolutional neural network. Sensors. 2020;20(6):1601. https://doi.org/10.3390/s20061601.

20. Ashraf H, Waris A, Ghafoor MF, Gilani SO, Niazi IK. Melanoma segmentation using deep learning with test-time augmentations and conditional random fields. Sci Rep. 2022;12(1):3948. https://doi.org/10.1038/s41598-022-07885-y.
21. Olsen TG, Hunter Jackson B, Feeser TA, Kent MN, Moad JC, Krishnamurthy S, Lunsford DD, Soans RE. Diagnostic performance of deep learning algorithms applied to three common diagnoses in dermatopathology. J Pathol Inf. 2018;9(1):32. https://doi.org/10.4103/jpi.jpi_31_18.
22. Hart SN, Flotte W, Norgan AF, Shah KK, Buchan ZR, Mounajjed T, Flotte TJ. Classification of melanocytic lesions in selected and whole-slide images via convolutional neural networks. J Pathol Inf 2019;10(1):5. https://doi.org/10.4103/jpi.jpi_32_18
23. Hekler A, Utikal JS, Enk AH, Solass W, Schmitt M, Klode J, Schadendorf D, Sondermann W, Franklin C, Bestvater F, Flaig MJ, Krahl D, von Kalle C, Fröhling S, Brinker TJ. Deep learning outperformed 11 pathologists in the classification of histopathological melanoma images. Eur J Cancer. 2019;118:91–6. https://doi.org/10.1016/j.ejca.2019.06.012.
24. Sankarapandian S, Kohn S, Spurrier V, Grullon S, Soans RE, Ayyagari KD, Chamarthi RV, Motaparthi K, Lee JB, Shon W. A pathology deep learning system capable of triage of melanoma specimens utilizing dermatopathologist consensus as ground truth. In: Proceedings of the IEEE/CVF international conference on computer vision; 2021. p. 629–38.
25. Thomas SM, Lefevre JG, Baxter G, Hamilton NA. Interpretable deep learning systems for multi-class segmentation and classification of non-melanoma skin cancer. Med Image Anal. 2021;68: 101915. https://doi.org/10.1016/j.media.2020.101915.
26. Moreno-Andrés D, Bhattacharyya A, Scheufen A, Stegmaier J. LiveCellMiner: a new tool to analyze mitotic progression. PLoS ONE. 2022;17(7): e0270923. https://doi.org/10.1371/journal.pone.0270923.
27. Clark K, Vendt B, Smith K, Freymann J, Kirby J, Koppel P, Moore S, Phillips S, Maffitt D, Pringle M, Tarbox L, Prior F. The cancer imaging archive (TCIA): maintaining and operating a public information repository. J Digit Imaging. 2013;26(6):1045–57. https://doi.org/10.1007/s10278-013-9622-7.
28. Gianfrancesco MA, Tamang S, Yazdany J, Schmajuk G. Potential biases in machine learning algorithms using electronic health record data. JAMA Intern Med. 2018;178(11):1544–7. https://doi.org/10.1001/jamainternmed.2018.3763.
29. Parikh RB, Teeple S, Navathe AS. Addressing bias in artificial intelligence in health care. JAMA. 2019;322(24):2377–8. https://doi.org/10.1001/jama.2019.18058.
30. Bickers DR, Lim HW, Margolis D, Weinstock MA, Goodman C, Faulkner E, Gould C, Gemmen E, Dall T. The burden of skin diseases: 2004: a joint project of the American Academy of Dermatology Association and the Society for Investigative Dermatology. J Am Acad Dermatol. 2006;55(3):490–500. https://doi.org/10.1016/j.jaad.2006.05.048.

Ethical, Legal, and Social Issues in Digital Dermatology

Carlo Botrugno, Bonnie Kaplan, and Gabrielle DiBartolomeo

Abstract Telemedicine and artificial intelligence (AI) are expected to revolutionize healthcare. These digital healthcare services can contribute to increased access to quality services and improve accuracy of diagnosis and treatment. However, as in other domains of care, technological innovation can have profound implications and reveal new scenarios that deserve ethical, legal, and social scrutiny. In this chapter we identify and analyze some of the most important ethical, legal, and social issues related to the deployment of these innovations in dermatology. We assess risks that these services can pose to the doctor-patient relationship and consider their impact on healthcare accessibility. We then focus on the risks of bias intrinsic to AI predictions, particularly with regard to patients' skin color. Then we summarize the most important policies, current at the time of this writing in 2021, regarding telehealth, digital medicine, and the field of AI by the European Commission in the European Union and the Food and Drug Administration in the United States. We also present professional organization guidelines issued by late 2021 by the World Health Organization, World Medical Association, American Medical Association, and the American Academy of Dermatology. We conclude with suggestions for how dermatologists can assess ethical, legal, and social issues raised by teledermatology and AI.

Keywords Telehealth · Telemedicine · Teledermatology · Artificial intelligence · Machine learning · Digital health · Data privacy and protection · Medical devices · Ethical · Legal · Social issues

C. Botrugno (✉)
Department of Legal Sciences, University of Florence, Florence, Italy
e-mail: carlo.botrugno@unifi.it

B. Kaplan
Department of Biostatistics (Health Informatics), Bioethics Center, Information Society Project, Solomon Center for Health Law and Policy, Yale University, 238 Prospect Street, CT, 06511 New Haven, USA
e-mail: bonnie.kaplan@yale.edu

G. DiBartolomeo
Internal Medicine, Cleveland Clinic Florida, Weston, USA
e-mail: gabrielle.dibartolomeo@gmail.com

K. Nouri (ed.), *Telemedicine and Technological Advances in Dermatology*,
https://doi.org/10.1007/978-3-031-69091-4_22

Learning Objectives

- Analyze the most important ethical, legal and social issues in teledermatology and artificial intelligence (AI).
- Summarize the most important policies regarding telehealth, digital medicine, and the field of AI adopted by the European Commission (EC) in the European Union and by the Food and Drug Administration (FDA) in the United States.
- Summarize the guidelines from the World Health Organization (WHO), World Medical Association (WMA), American Medical Association (AMA), and the American Academy of Dermatology (AAD) on teledermatology, AI, and data privacy and security.

1 Introduction

Teledermatology is among the most developed domains within the wider landscape of telemedicine today [1], while AI applications show promise for improving dermatology diagnosis and treatment [2]. Dermatologists can use these digital healthcare services (DHSs) to enhance quality of treatment and to help patients manage and reduce the discomfort associated with dermatological problems [3].

DHSs, which include both telemedicine and artificial intelligence (AI) applications, have long been expected to improve care in multiple ways. DHSs promise to revolutionize medical care and the organization of healthcare delivery by improving accuracy of diagnostic processes and efficiency of treatment decisions. Their use is expected to reduce practice variability by applying the latest knowledge and protocols. They can increase access to quality services and reach the underserved at lower costs. In short, they can make care more equitable and available.

At the same time, the spread of DHSs can have profound implications for medical epistemology insofar as it strengthens the need to rely on quantitative technical standards that can be detrimental to each physician's unique, subjective experience which ultimately finds its main form of expression in the doctor-patient relationship. When looking at DHSs as a whole, it is clear that they have an enormous potential to reshape the features, the ethics, and even the aesthetics of dermatological practice.

As in other domains, the growth of the internet, digital approaches, telehealth, and AI is seen as both changing society and challenging long-standing assumptions concerning people and technologies, including epistemological and structural underpinnings of Western medicine and healthcare delivery. Scholars acknowledge that the increasing reliance on DHSs is part of an on-going wider shift from:

> less reliance on the haptic (touch) and the concept of medicine as an "art" to a focus on generating and using data on the human body, on the part of both medical practitioners and of patients [4].

Such a transition towards the digital—though not only in dermatology—deserves careful ethical, legal, and social scrutiny. Legal and regulatory categories may not adequately reflect how these services work and how they are used by both healthcare professionals and patients. There are, then, significant ethical, legal, and social issues to consider for clinicians, patients, institutions, professional organizations, and governments, and for the relationships between and among them. Addressing these issues in a timely fashion could be fundamental to enabling the delivery of high-quality (digital) dermatological care that is "sensitive to patient values and preferences" [5] and to professional values.

In light of this, in this chapter we identify and analyze some of the important ethical, legal, and social issues (ELSI) related to the deployment of these innovations in routine dermatological practice. Our analysis will mostly focus on ELSI in AI and teledermatology, including their potential convergence, which could increasingly contribute to the emergence of a "digital dermatology." After briefly tracing the state of the art of telemedicine and AI in dermatology, we discuss the impact of DHSs and assess risks these innovations can pose to the doctor-patient relationship, potentially leading to dehumanized care. We consider the impact of DHSs on healthcare accessibility and highlight the burden of digital divides. We then focus on the risks of biases intrinsic in AI predictions, particularly with regard to patients' skin color. Then we summarize the most important policies, as of the time of this writing in 2021, regarding telehealth, digital medicine, and the field of AI, focusing on medical device and on privacy regulation in the European Commission (EC) in the European Union (EU) and the Food and Drug Administration (FDA) in the United States. We also present professional guidelines issued by the World Health Organization (WHO), World Medical Association (WMA), American Medical Association (AMA), and the American Academy of Dermatology (AAD). We conclude with suggestions for how dermatologists can assess ethical, legal, and social issues raised by teledermatology and AI.

2 A Brief Overview on Teledermatology and AI for Dermatology

2.1 Telemedicine and Telehealth

The terms telehealth and telemedicine may often be used interchangeably; nonetheless, their definitions differ primarily based on their scope. Telehealth is a broad, umbrella term encompassing the utilization of electronic and telecommunications technology within the healthcare field. Telemedicine, on the other hand, is considered a subdivision of telehealth. The World Health Organization (WHO) broadly defines it as:

> the delivery of healthcare services, where distance is a critical factor, by all healthcare professionals using information and communication technologies for the exchange of valid information for diagnosis, treatment and prevention of disease and injuries, research and evaluation, and for the continuing education of healthcare providers, all in the interests of advancing the health of individuals and their communities [6].

Since the 1950s, telemedicine's prevalence, use, and limitations have shifted as technology advanced. From its inception in the early 1950s, it was seen as a way to reduce disparities and bring care to those without ready access, including people in remote locations ranging from space stations to rural isolated communities, as well as in underserved areas of inner cities [7, 8]. Telemedicine was envisioned to reduce travel time for both patients and clinicians, lower costs, and increase quality through the ability to access more timely and accurate data at any time or place. It would facilitate seamless and continuous care on a more equitable basis by allowing inter-organizational cooperation and ready flow of information between wherever patients and providers were. The result would broaden the scope of healthcare delivery, leading to improving healthcare not only locally, but also worldwide [9].

As technology advanced, so did telemedicine. However, it was during the COVID-19 pandemic where the demand for telemedicine grew exponentially [10, 11]. Due to hesitancy of patients to seek in-person care because of exposure risk [12] coupled with the temporary closure of non-essential outpatient and ambulatory clinics, healthcare professionals and patients turned to telemedicine. The Centers for Disease Control and Prevention (CDC) reported a 154% increase in telemedicine visits in the United States in March 2020 when compared to the previous year [13]. With its utilization proven efficient and an increase in both patient and physician satisfaction [14], it is safe to say that telemedicine has cemented its place in modern healthcare and its use will only continue to expand.

2.2 *Teledermatology*

As in telemedicine as a whole, teledermatology—the use of telemedicine in the practice of dermatology—has seen a resurgence of interest and utility as a result of the COVID-19 pandemic. Teledermatology is subdivided into three visit classifications [15]. The first is synchronous or real-time teledermatology, wherein a physician and patient meet via a live-video conferencing platform or telephone consultation. This is most analogous to an in-person clinic visit. The second classification and the most commonly used is asynchronous or store-and-forward teledermatology, wherein photography and/or videography is transmitted from patient to physician, with diagnosis, treatment, and management provided at a later time. The third and last classification is a hybrid of the two aforementioned subtypes and is known as mixed synchronous and asynchronous teledermatology.

Currently, teledermatology is used for all types of clinic visits including, but not limited to, evaluation of skin lesions, management of chronic skin conditions, and medication optimization [16]. The ability to accurately evaluate and diagnose skin conditions via teledermatology is what is most controversial and most critical. Its adequacy depends on a number of factors, including the purpose of the visit and the skin condition involved. Identifying and monitoring dermatological conditions often require the physician to use his or her senses to closely examine the skin: noting differences in color; palpating changes in temperature, texture, and elevation; and smelling exudates. Each of these is easier to do in person than via telemedicine. Where the technology available does not allow for physicians to use all their senses, diagnosis and treatment could be severely impaired.

For other conditions, teledermatology is a valuable alternative to in-person visits. Follow-up visits for chronic skin conditions such as eczema, psoriasis, and acne, as well as medication management visits can be easily doneusing telemedicine. Among the advantages of teledermatology are a high concordance of medical management between teledermatology and in-person visits, reduced waiting times for evaluation and diagnosis which result in earlier treatment, and comparable or higher patient and physician satisfaction [17–19].

2.3 AI in Dermatology

AI can be generally defined as technology formulated to mimic human cognition in the analysis of complex data [20]. Artificial intelligence within the field of dermatology has been primarily focused on improving rates of accurate diagnosis regardless of visit type—in-person or teledermatology [20]. Adoption of this technology can be traced to the increased incidence of malignant melanoma in the 1980s, which motivated the need for early diagnosis for optimal treatment and outcome [21]. Distinguishing malignant from benign pigmented skin lesions is one of the most crucial differentials in dermatology, and as such has been the primary focus for AI development [22]. Multiple studies have shown that when provided an image of a pigmented skin lesion, AI was able to correctly diagnose whether the lesion was a benign nevus or skin cancer at either a comparable or higher rate than board-certified dermatologists [21, 23–26]. AI also performed similarly to dermatology residents in identifying and distinguishing malignancy from 134 different skin diseases and then providing treatment options [27]. Transmitting images of skin conditions for automated diagnosis combines teledermatology with artificial intelligence and can make diagnosis more accurate. Although not widely adopted in clinical dermatology practices presently (2021), the future use of AI within the field of dermatology is promising [28].

The discussion thus far has largely focused on AI to identify and diagnose malignant versus benign skin findings. It should be noted that AI also is being developed for chronic skin conditions. For example, AI has been developed to not only diagnosis and assess the severity of psoriasis, but to also evaluate treatment response earlier than typical clinical evaluation [21]. AI has been developed to diagnosis other common dermatologic conditions such as atopic dermatitis, onychomycosis, and rosacea as well [29]. Although diagnosing malignant skin lesions via telemedicine has proven its worth [30], the performance of AI systems for these other conditions is suboptimal; the poor performance may be due to the heterogeneity of these cutaneous presentations [31]. A systemic review of these current skin screening smartphone applications showed variable results [32]. Further, though the AI may perform well in general, it may not for populations underrepresented in the datasets on which they are based, as when datasets used for detecting skin cancer are missing samples of darker skin types, and Google image searches for "healthy skin" return light-skinned women. Consequently, as also highlighted below (Sect. 3.3), such AI may be less accurate in detecting skin lesions when skin is dark [2, 33].

Wearables, too, with or without AI, can aid dermatologists and patients with dermatological conditions. One example is the potential convergence of digital data tracks from wrist-worn actigraphy devices that monitor scratching, sleep patterns, and heart rate frequency, which could provide new, vital information about aggravating factors such as temperature, medications, locations, and real-time insights into responses to treatment and dermatological patients' quality of life [3].

Because of AI's broad reach, in this chapter we focus mostly on machine learning (ML), a specific subset of AI that involves algorithmic program learning from a provided dataset. ML itself can be subdivided into two classifications: supervised and unsupervised. The main difference between the two involves the dataset initially provided. In supervised machine learning, which is the most commonly used form of AI in dermatology, the provided dataset is labeled and defined, most often by dermatopathologists [29]. Therefore, the program classifies new data based on these provided classifications. In unsupervised ML, the provided dataset is not labeled or defined. The AI system itself is responsible for identifying similarities, differences, and trends within the given dataset. Other AI approaches involving neural networks allow for identifying patterns from images [20, 21, 34].

It should be noted that every step of developing AI algorithms has the potential for problems: what datasets are used and how accurate and representative they are, how data are classified and labeled, how systems are trained to increase correct outputs (and what is considered "correct"), and how these systems are deployed and used. With these considerations in mind, AI can be a powerful tool in enhancing care, but clinical judgment is needed. Diagnosis and treatment were optimized when board-certified dermatologists and residents used AI in conjunction with their clinical judgment [27], which is generally recommended for artificial intelligence and clinical decision support systems in medicine. Depending on which approach and what technologies are used, some different clinical and ethical issues should be considered.

3 Teledermatology, AI, and ELSI

As the above discussion suggests, development, deployment, and use of these technologies involve professional and societal values, and therefore intersect with multiple ethical, legal, social, and policy considerations. Drawing on Kaplan's ELSI discussion [35–37], we highlight four professional values in medicine and their relationship to ELSI concerning these technologies. In discussing some of the issues—we selected the doctor-patient relationship (Sect. 3.1), digital inequalities (Sect. 3.2), biases and discrimination risk (Sect. 3.3), privacy and data protection (Sect. 4), and professional responsibility (Sect. 6) as illustrative—we take a sociotechnical perspective, i.e., a theoretical and analytical approach that focuses on the mutual interactions between humans and technological innovations [38]. Accordingly, assessing ELSI regarding digital innovations in healthcare involves understanding that they cannot be looked at as mere value-free technical artifacts at the disposal of physicians and nurses.

3.1 The Dehumanization Risk: Does Digital Dermatology Undermine the Doctor-Patient Relationship?

As argued by Deborah Lupton, medical technologies:

> represent transformations in how bodies are conceptualised, touched, managed and visually displayed. Rather than simply neutrally mirroring key aspects of a pre-given natural body, technologies as they operate in medicine and healthcare configure and reconfigure the body in certain ways, enacting how they are understood and treated [4].

This observation highlights the question of whether technology is dehumanizing, which involves interrelationships between the professional clinical values of quality of care, professional autonomy, the doctor-patient relationship, and medicine as an art/medicine as a science [35].

Since the time of Hippocrates, the evolution of the biomedical paradigm has striven for objectivity, which can also be seen as an attempt to divorce medical knowledge from the physician's and patient's subjective experience of disease [39, 40]. At least on paper, this would lead to medical knowledge that is verifiable, generalizable, and not least, easily transmissible. The pursuit of objectivity in medicine is tied to the goal of making medicine a science, to be achieved through standardized practice. This pursuit has stimulated countless sociological, philosophical, and legal debates [41–43]. Professional norms and values, such as autonomy, have been seen to thwart this goal and contribute to "high levels of variability in the practice of medicine" and an "idiosyncratic" lack of consensus on standards [44].

New ways of visualizing internal disease processes were among the technological innovations conceived as a means to increase objectivity and standardization in medicine. First dissection, then x-rays, and more recently, medical imaging, marked the birth of a new and complex "cartography of the body and of the disease" [45]. Different from anatomical paintings, however, this cartography allowed getting "self-evident maps," which, at least in theory, are deemed to be irrefutable; because they are the result of a technological representation, therefore they are thought objective. The power of seeing, in comparison to other human senses, rests upon the assumption that it does not leave room for ambiguity in interpretation, i.e., in the (human) process of attributing meaning to physical objects. Yet, using an image ultimately provides data which cannot be used except in relation to its reading. As has been argued in this regard, the "observer contributes to the variability of visual imagery" [46].

Despite the sense of objectivity, reading medical images is an interpretive process and involves negotiation among different practitioners concerning the relevance of the images together with other clinical findings and impressions [47].

The same is true for teledermatology and for AI processing of dermatological images. Interaction among patients, clinicians, and data—sensory, measurements, personal impressions and relationships—affect diagnosis and treatment. These technologies contribute to different modes of those interactions and ways of conceptualizing human bodies and illness. They challenge the importance of the physical presence of patients and physicians and how each of them experiences their relationship and the illness. Telemedicine necessarily eliminates cues that could be noticed only in person [37, 48]. Voice-only telemedicine removes more of these cues. Simply transmitting images eliminates even spoken interaction.

In the case of AI, the presence of a doctor behind the screen cannot be taken for granted [40]. Yet, as has been argued:

> At some point, the machine must analyze the patient, and the doctor must analyze the machine's analysis, i.e., the images, but we face the possibility that never the two shall meet [49].

Both telemedicine and AI, then, raise the issue of virtualization of doctor-patient interaction. Digitalized medical practice removes the need for patients and physicians to physically and simultaneously interact in the same material space. In this context, the accuracy gained due to the AI's expertise must be balanced with the reduction of cues and clues associated with a lack of conventional doctor-patient interaction.

Since the emergence of AI in healthcare, it has been warned that the deployment of DHSs could detract from the humanity intrinsic to a quality doctor patient interaction and pave the way for mechanized care in which professionals will be replaced by AI applications. However, scholarly consensus is that this is an unrealistic scenario in dermatology, at least in the near future [50, 51]. This opinion mostly rests on the fact that AI algorithms only provide for:

> a probability score of various diagnoses [and] not a diagnosis, and certainly not management of the patient [51].

From this perspective, it is clear that AI applications cannot replace the intrinsic value of the doctor-patient relationship, which is based on intimacy, proximity, and mutual trust [50]. It is worth remembering that trust and empathy are among the fundamental factors for fostering patients' compliance with medical prescriptions—though not only in dermatology—as well as for stimulating patient satisfaction and positive therapeutic outcomes. Consequently, it is no wonder that the evidence suggests that, when integrating AI into dermatology, medicine will remain an art requiring the human touch, listening ear, getting the patient to comply with recommendations, and compassion, also important to reaching the correct diagnosis and making it less likely that doctors soon will be replaced by AI [52, 53]. This art vs. science trade-off is among the long-standing topics in discussing medical technologies, including information technologies like telemedicine and AI. It reflects the on-going concerns of whether automation, or indeed, the introduction of a technology, is dehumanizing in general and whether it creates distance between doctor and patient in particular [35, 54].

Another concern is the increasing commercialization of healthcare. One area of development is AI applications that can provide triage services in primary care rather than directly serving (or replacing) dermatologists. Such services could potentially shift full body screening to primary care, improving earlier detection of skin cancers and increasing appropriate referrals [51]. Today's commercial smartphone applications for assessing dermatological conditions, together with clinical systems to identify skin lesions and pathologies, could augment this possibility. Wearables, as described in Sect. 2.2, are another example of technologies that can provide data potentially useful for monitoring dermatological conditions. Commercial applications that can be used by anyone to monitor themselves and their behaviors, and to get advice based on those data, also may lead to earlier treatment, or may lead to undue worries and actions by people trying to treat themselves.

Commercial telemedicine services are part of the increasing influence of corporatization and commercialization. Managerial models and logics of efficiency and rationality are features directly derived from the organization of commercial enterprises [55, 56]. As has been widely acknowledged, the permeation of these models into the healthcare systems of industrialized countries has turned the doctor-patient relationship into a provider-user one [57, 58]. As a result, healthcare systems seem to be losing much of the richness and complexity intrinsic to the ideal doctor-patient relationship as directly derived from the Hippocratic heritage. In such a context, it is possible to argue that the reductionist orientation of DHSs simply:

> overlap the reductionism of the biomedical paradigm and thus reflect its main ambivalence, which derives from the vocation to select, filter and thus to reduce the potential sources of knowledge available for doctors in carrying out a diagnosis and elaborating a therapy [40].

At the same time, the commercial and corporate perspectives have helped the market for telemedicine and AI flourish and provided smartphone and wearables users with attractive numerous healthcare applications. Commercialization, however, also has contributed to the shift away from the early public service motivations for telemedicine that included addressing what is now seen as a digital divide in healthcare access, delivery, and technological availability [8]. Furthermore, commercialization has implications for privacy, at least in the US, as discussed below (Sect. 4.1.3).

3.2 *Digital Health and Digital Divides*

One of the major challenges since the advent of the pandemic is the protection of the most vulnerable groups. The severe pressure faced by healthcare systems led to significant restrictions of hospital admissions to increase capacity to treat COVID patients while also reducing physical contact between other patients and healthcare professionals in order to contain infection risk [59]. As a consequence, many countries have implemented strategies aimed at digitizing healthcare delivery [60]. Those countries that promoted the use of DHSs before the pandemic outbreak were significantly advantaged in channeling the benefits of remote healthcare, while others were forced to adopt emergency measures. Regardless of whether these attempts have been effective [61], it is undeniable that the pandemic accelerated this digital transition and contributed to the birth of new awareness about the benefits of DHSs [62]. In the meantime, however, this transition made (digital) healthcare inequalities more apparent and widened the gap between those who are well acquainted with the functioning of the healthcare system and those who suffer from inequalities [63].

In all countries gravely affected by COVID-19, detainees, undocumented migrants, homeless people, people with disabilities, people housed in residences for the elderly, and other vulnerable groups were exposed to higher physical and psychological harm than any other population. This can be explained by significant, sometimes extreme, reduction of the autonomy experienced by most of these people, which often made it difficult, if not impossible, to take basic precautions against infection risk, such as maintaining social distancing, sanitizing hands frequently, and using personal protective equipment [64–66].

They, like people in remote areas, also often did not have ready access to telemedicine services and AI applications. Material access to the internet and related technologies (computer, tablet, smartphones, and other connected devices) still represents the primary digital divide [67, 68]. Disparities in the kinds of care available, together with differences in familiarity with and knowledge of both the healthcare system and digital technologies, affect deployment and use of telemedicine, further exacerbating digital divides [69, 70].

In light of these considerations, digital exclusion must be analyzed as an emerging form of social exclusion, as it contributes to worsening individuals' material and social deprivation in a "digital vicious cycle" [71]. Policy promoting using telemedicine or smartphone applications clearly helped many people from the outset of the pandemic and will continue to do so. Still, the choice of deploying these technologies instead of increasing access to care in other ways or improving conditions conducive to better health are policy choices with ethical and social implications [72]. Combined with biases in AI, the current direction risks further disadvantaging those already disadvantaged.

3.3 AI Automation, Biases, and the Risks of Discrimination

Of increasing concern related to the deployment of AI in healthcare is the possibility for bias [73]. Excessive reliance on AI results can replicate, or even amplify, human biases, leading to inadequate care. Despite assumptions and hopes that AI will free healthcare of biases due to its scientific basis, ML and some other forms of AI are based on pattern recognition built from existing banks of data. Results will be affected by whether the application's design or data on which it is based included representation from the range of communities where it is to be used. How this data are collected and organized also matters, as existing bias can be reflected in the way an algorithm weighs certain variables [74]. Bias can be introduced by those who design or train the algorithm.

Therefore, despite the promise of AI to improve care, potential gaps between real-world data and AI-training data must be acknowledged and taken into account [75]. AI algorithms may be poorly calibrated when quantifying risk in individual patients [76]. AI systems also:

> can be poor at recognising a relevant change in context or data, and this results in the system confidently continuing to make erroneous predictions based on "out-of-sample" inputs [77].

ML algorithms increase their accuracy by continuously fine-tuning their parameters and rules [78] to the point where their workings are not really known. This could lead to increased opacity (black-box), thereby compromising transparency, explainability, interpretability, testability, understandability, identifiability of inherent biases or outright errors, correctability, and accountability—all of which are considered fundamental to the trustworthiness of AI and fundamental to human rights (e.g., the EU's General Data Protection Regulation (GDPR) [79, 80]). Physicians and patients are more likely to accept AI results integrated into their care pathways where transparency and patient disclosure of their use occurs. Such disclosure is also relevant to the patient's consent for treatment. (Some have suggested that where an algorithm has proven its worth, consent should be obtained to not use it). The inherent opaqueness of ML leads to the question: Should "we demand a right to an explanation in all cases even at the expense of innovations that can be shown to improve care?" [81]. Furthermore, when considering possible biases in AI, there is also the risk of "loopthink," i.e., that automated services can be programmed to "exclude outliers and reduce abstract or even ethical thinking on the part of an AI program" [82].

Studies already have shown that these potential biases occur. As previously mentioned, skin color is particularly relevant for dermatology. In the US, patients with darker skin tones may not have access to care or be treated as other patients are [83, 84], leading them to "present with more-advanced disease and have lower survival rates than fair-skinned patients" [2]. AI may exacerbate this problem. Previous algorithms have been shown to discriminate against darker skin, as happened in 2015, when a Google photo-categorization service miscategorized black individuals as gorillas [74]. Thus, algorithmic biases can impair proper care and exacerbate racial disparities, particularly if "images of skin disease manifesting in darker skin types are not sufficiently included in training algorithms," if they are misidentified in the dataset, or if individuals training the algorithms are themselves biased [2]. This also could make algorithms developed in Western societies based on data from Western populations unsuitable to be used for non-Western patients.

It is also important to take into account the human bias either toward or against AI. One bias is the propensity for people to believe the pronouncements of a computer, potentially leading physicians and patients to, unintentionally or not, comply with automated results. The risk intrinsic to this "automation bias" is that physicians could:

> accept the guidance of an automated system and cease searching for confirmatory evidence, perhaps transferring responsibility for decision-making onto the machine [77].

People biased in the other direction may judge AI more severely when mistakes are made, even if the application performs as well as, or better than, human experts. Here the risk is in not using a helpful AI application.

Realistically speaking, dermatologists may not know how well AI algorithms work, let alone their efficacy in patient populations with varying skin colors and conditions. They may not know how safe and effective the algorithms are and how they were vetted, or understand the privacy risks of telemedicine. Much of this opaqueness results from the legal and regulatory environment, which we discuss next, for it raises questions about whether and why physicians, patients, and those making decisions for healthcare institutions and healthcare delivery should have to educate themselves about these issues. For now, they do because the burden to appropriately and prudently use AI currently is placed on physicians and their patients.

4 Governmental Policy and Regulation

Considerable legal scholarship addresses policy proposals to enhance both the deployment of telemedicine and of AI both in healthcare and more generally. Relevant concerns involve whether and how authorities deploy broadband technologies, professional regulation (reimbursement, licensure, liability, requirements for in-person visits), privacy and data protection, AI and device regulation, and intellectual property regimes.

As mentioned above, availability of internet and telephone services affect access to telemedicine care. Physicians need to be aware of how virtual visits are shaped by the technologies used. If video is present, the teleconsultation differs from voice-only. In either case, it differs from in-person, and both patients and physicians need to make appropriate adjustments.

Local requirements concerning reimbursement when telemedicine or devices are employed also affect practice. Whether clinicians are authorized or licensed to treat patients using telemedicine from other jurisdictions affects access to care as well. Similarly, different localities have different requirements for whether the patient must first have an in-person visit with that clinician. As discussed further below, liability for either following or discounting AI diagnoses or recommendations depends upon applicable standards of practice [52, 85]. Additionally, different privacy, data sharing, and data protections are governed by different political units. All these affect the uptake of telemedicine and the use of AI.

We will next discuss the legal and regulatory environment at the time of writing (2021) by focusing on the US and in the EU because they both affect governmental and commercial developments world-wide. After that, we briefly retrace the main orientations and guidelines adopted at the international and national levels by some of the influential healthcare organizations: the World Medical Association (WMA), the

World Health Organization (WHO), the American Medical Association (AMA), and the American Academy of Dermatology (AAD) current by 2021. Their principles should be carefully considered in analyzing ELSI in telemedicine and AI.

4.1 Policy and Regulation of AI and Telemedicine in the United States

4.1.1 US Telemedicine Policy

At the outset of the COVID pandemic, the US relaxed regulations regarding telemedicine reimbursement, data sharing, and licensure. This enabled the explosive growth of telemedicine services. Yet, it should be noted that the lack of broadband hindered access in underserved regions. In the wake of the pandemic, both federal and state governments have been deciding future policy.

4.1.2 US Device and AI Software Regulation

AI and device regulation affect their integration into clinical practice. In the US, the Food and Drug Administration (FDA) regulates the safety and efficacy of medical devices, i.e., devices intended for medical use, both before approval and through post-market surveillance. The FDA developed and is seeking comment on a categorization scheme for approving AI software as a medical device (SaMD) thus SaMD regulation is in flux at the time of this writing [86–89]. Additionally, the way "medical device" is defined precludes many popular smartphone applications and internet services. Consequently, they are not vetted by the FDA and there is no way to know, aside from market reputation and independent studies, how well they perform. Moreover, even for FDA-approved devices and software, intellectual property protections make it nearly impossible to examine the algorithms they use [90]. There is also no requirement for manufacturers to disclose gender, racial, or geographic data for patient data used to test their products, or even how many patients' data went into testing devices [91]. Consequently, care is needed when considering following AI recommendations because physicians are liable for their decisions.

4.1.3 US Privacy and Data Protection Regulation

Privacy is another way the FDA regulations are relevant. The Health Insurance and Portability Act (HIPAA) protects only clinical data. Therefore, data collected or transmitted by commercial devices, applications, or websites, i.e., technologies not regulated by the FDA, generally are not HIPAA protected. Instead, end-user license agreements (EULAs) allow data to be used for whatever the manufacturer or vendor desires, including selling data that may be combined with other datasets for purposes ranging from research to marketing to credit scores and employment and insurance decisions. HIPPA data privacy requirements commonly are implemented by stripping personal identifying information from the data. However, de-identified data may be re-identified when combined with enough identifiable information available from non-clinical sources. Telemedicine services, too, when provided by commercial vendors, have required patients to agree to EULAs in order to receive care through the service. EULAs are known for their lengthy, vague, and complex language, with the privacy policy, if any, difficult to find or understand. Not surprisingly, people just click through and accept them, thereby often unknowingly giving up privacy [90]. Other aspects of the telemedicine encounter, such as physician or prescription data, also may not be protected. Data security, or data protection, also is governed differently by HIPAA and by the Federal Trade Commission (FTC). The FTC enforces EULAs as part of their consumer protection function. Unlike in the EU, there is no omnibus data protection.

4.2 Policy and Regulation of AI and Telemedicine in the European Union

4.2.1 EU Telemedicine Policy

Despite the significant efforts of the European Commission to support the digital transition in EU healthcare systems, to date (2021), the EU lacks a regulatory framework unique to telemedicine [92]. During the pandemic, European governments have adopted different emergency measures aimed at fostering the spread of DHSs to curb the virus outbreak [61]. Nevertheless, there are important EU legislative acts that apply to the delivery of telemedicine and the use of AI applications in healthcare. They include the General Data Protection Regulation (GDPR) (Regulation 2016/675/EU), and the Medical Devices Regulation (MDR) (Regulation 2017/745/EU).

4.2.2 EU Data Privacy and Protection Regulation

The GDPR aims to protect "natural persons" (as opposed to "legal persons," i.e., societies) with regard to the processing of personal data as well as to the free movement of such data. The GDPR is relevant for DHSs because it applies to the processing of personal data whether or not carried out by automated means (Art. 3). To be compliant with the GDPR, data processing must be lawful, transparent, and accurate. Data should be elicited and stored only for the purposes allowed, and only for the time necessary to fulfill those purposes. Lastly, data must be conserved in their integrity and protected against unauthorized access. In the GDPR, health data are considered sensitive information and thus included among the "special categories" of data (Art. 9). This implies that particular rules apply to their collection, treatment, and circulation. Therefore, any potential use or activity (referred to as "treating") of health data, requires that the data-subject (the person the data represents) gives consent, and/or is justified by reasons of public interest, among which are preventive or occupational medicine, medical diagnosis, provision of health or social care, reacting to public health threats, and ensuring quality and safety of services, devices, and medicaments (Art. 9).

The GDPR also has privacy "by design and by default" as a key requirement (Art. 25). This entails that, from its conception, every system and process, including DHSs, must integrate data protection measures.

4.2.3 EU Device and AI Software Regulation

As for medical devices, MDR provisions are pivotal for the deployment of DHSs in the EU. The MDR is an exhaustive regulation aimed at covering all the phases of development, authorization, and marketing of medical devices, including implantable devices. Under the MDR, a medical device is a device intended to be used for medical purposes (MDR 2017). All medical devices must comply with the Regulation's safety and performance requirements and post-market surveillance regime. The MDR also established a European Database of Medical Devices (briefly known as "Eudamed"), which is meant to inform users about the main features of purchasable medical devices, their purposes, and their conformity with EU legislation.

The inclusion of a device in the scope of the MDR has always been a challenging task, particularly in the case of direct-to-consumer devices that integrate entertainment functions with the collection of health information, as the most popular wearable devices do. To help stakeholders address this issue, the MDR established an ad hoc working group that releases guidance documents that should help to establish whether devices fall within the MDR based on their intended purpose.

With regard to AI, as this is being written, the EU is developing AI regulation [93]. In 2018 the European Commission launched its "Strategy for Artificial Intelligence" [94, 95]. It is meant to trace a path for the consistent development of AI applications in all the EU Member States. The strategy includes the "Ethics Guidelines for Trustworthy AI," adopted in 2019 by the High-Level Expert Group on Artificial Intelligence [96]. They take a "human-centric approach" based on human dignity. Accordingly, the deployment of AI must be consistent with four ethical principles: respect for human autonomy, prevention of harm, fairness, and explicability (elsewhere called "explainability"). To achieve this objective, AI applications should meet seven key requirements: (1) human agency and oversight; (2) technical robustness and safety; (3) privacy and data governance; (4) transparency; (5) diversity, non-discrimination, and fairness; (6) environmental and societal well-being; and (7) accountability. The Guidelines particularly emphasize children, the disabled, and other vulnerable populations, citing power asymmetries that can put people at risk. They acknowledge that AI applications can bring both expected benefits as well as pose potential risks and negative impacts. They recommend robust measures to mitigate these risks [96].

4.2.4 Comparison of US and EU Regulation

The EU and US, then, differ in orientation and approach. There are clearly similarities, but also important differences. The EU's fundamental rights approach is different from the US legal and regulatory environment. As it has been with the GDPR, the forthcoming EU Regulation on AI could have a "Brussels effect" in influencing future developments outside the EU. The GDPR also is relevant for the deployment of DHSs at the international level because it applies to data processing activities carried outside the EU if data-subjects are within the EU (Art. 3).

Although the GDPR is much more expansive than HIPAA as it regulates all personal data, neither address one additional privacy consideration important for teledermatology. People other than the patient may be present during telemedicine visits. That can affect not only the patient's and clinician's privacy, but also the privacy of those in the vicinity. Everyone's discretion, not regulation, is the only safeguard. Further, dermatologists need to be aware of how the presence of others can influence sensitive clinical conversations and examinations.

5 Professional Organizations' Guidelines

5.1 World Health Organization (WHO) and World Medical Association (WMA)

Both the WHO and WMA have issued telemedicine and AI guidelines.

5.1.1 AI

The WHO ethics and AI guidelines are similar to the EU's. They note that in order for AI to be able to improve patient care and to inform the decisions of health policy makers or allocate resources within health systems, several challenges must be addressed. Healthcare workers and system decision-makers need to be educated about the contexts in which such systems can function safely and effectively, the conditions necessary to ensure reliable and appropriate use, and the mechanisms for continuous auditing and assessment of system performance. To empower patients and communities to control their own healthcare, they need to be assured that commercial interests will not infringe on their rights and instead keep their dignity and autonomy at the center of health decision-making. Further, these systems should be appropriate to different local settings and communities and avoid biases [97].

The 2019 WMA "Statement on Augmented Intelligence in Medical Care" recognizes the potential of AI and highlights challenges to its integration into routine care. The Statement supports the deployment of AI algorithms in healthcare provided they "conform to the principles of medical ethics, confidentiality of patient data, and non-discrimination" [98]. To achieve this goal, they recommend fostering medical education in order to promote a greater awareness of the implications of AI. They also solicit WMA member organizations to find viable solutions in order to take into account physicians' perspectives in the "development, design, validation and implementation of healthcare AI." They propose that AI applications be transparent, reproducible, and trusted by both healthcare providers and patients, and that their development should not be detrimental to the primacy of the patient-physician relationship [98].

5.1.2 Telemedicine

The WMA telemedicine guidelines also focus on the physician–patient relationship, including physician and patient responsibilities similar to those in face-to-face care. They address quality of care, informed consent, confidentiality and security, appropriate authorizations to practice, use of and access to technologies, and quality metrics to assess these. They advise on physicians' relationships with other physicians involved with patient care, telemedicine training, and assessing telemedicine [99].

The WMA further states that physicians using telemedicine should keep detailed records of the information on which advice was based to ensure traceability and responsibility. More generally, the WMA articulates a precautionary principle for physicians to keep in mind. The precautionary principle in bioethics is based on the Hippocratic mandate "to do no harm." In one manifestation of this principle, in addition to the other guidance, the WMA warned about telemedicine solely for cost-cutting [99].

5.1.3 Data Privacy, Security, and Legal Issues

The WHO assessed the level of deployment of telemedicine and mobile health technologies in a 2009 survey of member states. The results of the survey were published in two reports [6, 100]. They flagged data security as needing attention and began a collaboration with the International Telecommunication Union (ITU), the United Nations specialized agency for information and communication technologies, to provide guidance on the content and scope of data privacy and security policy for mobile telecommunications in health [100]. They also emphasized that the legal uncertainty surrounding the field of telemedicine delivery is among the biggest barriers for the spread of remote healthcare services [6]. Even though survey results are outdated, particularly after the significant spread of DHSs due to COVID-19, the lack of legal clarity still significantly hinders the development of telemedicine, especially at the international level [92].

5.2 *American Medical Association (AMA)*

5.2.1 AI

The AMA issued their first policy recommendations on what they call "augmented intelligence," a less common name for AI, in 2018 [101]. They say they plan to improve patient outcomes and physician satisfaction by integrating physicians' perspectives into developing and deploying AI that meets standards similar to those of other organizations and regulations [102, 103]. Additionally, they promote dialogue among the various stakeholders involved in the deployment of AI in routine care [104]. They encourage everyone to become educated about the promises and limitations of AI in healthcare. They will explore legal implications related to liability and intellectual property. To leverage the organization's engagement with digital health, they promote best practices in design, meeting users' needs, usability, and testing by representative end-users. Not surprisingly, they advocate reducing bias and healthcare disparities, improving care, and combining AI with human clinicians to the benefit of patients, physicians, and the broader community [102, 105].

5.2.2 Telemedicine

The AMA stresses that physicians' ethical responsibilities do not change during teleconsultations and that patients need to be able to trust that physicians honor each patient's best interests, tailor services to each patient, and inform patients of telehealth's limitations and positive and negative consequences [106]. They note some newer responsibilities, including: ensuring that information is accurate, and that protocols are sufficient to prevent unauthorized access, protect the security and integrity of patient information, and authenticate the patient's identity; and recognizing technology's limitations, and therefore, also of themselves when relying on technology. Additionally, they express concern about trust and conflict of interest surrounding direct-to-consumer telemedicine providers' influence in commercializing both the market and overseeing it [105, 107, 108].

5.3 American Academy of Dermatology (AAD)

5.3.1 AI

The AAD, too, addresses AI in familiar terms intended to uphold quality. Their 2019 position statement recognizes the potential held by AI applications to transform skin care by fostering the quadruple aims of enhancing patient experience, improving population health, reducing costs, and improving the professional fulfillment of care teams. It acknowledges the need for these technologies to be developed and used within an ethical framework. They echo the centrality of the patient and quality of the doctor-patient relationship, emphasizing that patients should feel well cared for even when interacting with software. To this end:

> Clinicians should spend time conducting work appropriate for their skills and training, while being able to delegate algorithmic tasks to machines, with the goal of enhancing patient care [109].

Meeting this goal requires education and awareness, for both patients and professionals, to address the use of these technologies for improving healthcare delivery.

They underscore the need for transparency in "how their medical information is gathered, utilized, and stored and when, what, and how [AI] technologies are utilized." They endorse the need for demonstrated effectiveness before using this technology for clinical decision making. They also warn against potentially exacerbating healthcare disparities, particularly among vulnerable populations, that arise from lack of representation in the data and the design or deployment of AI. Finally, they clarify that AI tools are not meant to "establish a legal or medical standard of care." Therefore, they advise dermatologists to use their personal and professional autonomy when referring to the recommendations provided by AI [109].

5.3.2 Telemedicine

As of this writing, the AAD has not issued guidelines for telemedicine aside from reimbursement and coding for remote visits made possible by policy changes due to COVID-19. However, the AAD has provided "tips" for potential teledermatology users. They include information to explain to patients what telemedicine (in dermatology) is, what to expect from it, and how to prepare for a remote consultation [110].

6 Conclusions: Ethics and Professional Responsibility

As is evident in the above professional organizations' guidelines, it is incumbent upon dermatologists, indeed upon all healthcare professionals, to be attentive to ethical issues related to telemedicine and artificial intelligence. Concerns similar to those expressed in the professional guidelines and regulatory regimes also have been expressed by ethicists over the past several decades [9, 36].

6.1 Liability and Standards of Care

Also evident from the above are legal issues to take into account. The implementation of AI applications in dermatological practices could open new scenarios with regard to professionals' liability. As explained above, ML algorithms can have human supervision or be fully automated (unsupervised). The presence of human oversight over AI is the most likely scenario, especially in this first phase of deployment of these applications. The presence of a physician who interprets the AI results is still an unavoidable element of the doctor-patient relationship as well as a guarantee of overall quality of healthcare delivery. However, in the future this could very well change. As AI applications become more accurate and safe, patients and physicians alike could request an AI diagnosis and advice without suitable professional (human) oversight. As Mattessich et al. [52] observe:

> An argument could be made that when an AI-provided diagnosis is superior to that of a dermatologist, deferring to AI would become best practice [52].

As this occurs, when and how to combine human and AI expertise raise a fundamental question: To what extent will dermatologists be able to override AI-based results? Given the lack of a regulatory framework for ML applications, it is possible to speculate that at least three scenarios could occur: (i) dermatologists are required to comply with AI results, (ii) dermatologists see AI as supplementary tools, or (iii) dermatologists are left free to decide whether or not to use AI. Each of these scenarios presents different potential legal consequences: in (i), dermatologists cannot be charged with the consequence of inaccuracies or mistakes made by the algorithm; in (ii), dermatologists can be asked to assume the consequences of serious mistakes and harms suffered by their patients for relying on AI; in (iii), dermatologists would be directly responsible for their choices. Which of these hypothetical scenarios would occur will depend upon myriad circumstances of a concrete case. Whether or not physicians are held liable for malpractice when their care deviates from accepted standards to the point of negligence, as they are in the US, dermatologists would be wise to learn more about the technologies and keep current as they and the legal and regulatory environment rapidly change.

6.2 Digital Dermatology and ELSI

The management of digital dermatology poses opportunities and challenges when integrated into the routine work of dermatologists and raises fundamental ethical, legal, and social issues. This chapter highlighted such issues concerning AI and telemedicine by especially focusing on doctor-patient relationships, quality of care, and fair and equitable treatment for all. We discussed these issues in terms of how both telemedicine and AI may dehumanize or enhance care, contribute to disparities and intersect with digital divides, relate to discrimination and bias, and be influenced by the legal and regulatory environment. We considered how medical professional values of autonomy, quality of care, the art and science of medicine, and the importance of the doctor-patient relationship intersect with these issues. We briefly traced applicable policy and regulatory provisions in the US and the EU and summarized guidelines provided by influential organizations.

We noted some of the ethical, legal, and social issues, drawing on ELSI discussions in various literatures, including medicine, bioethics, law, computer science, policy, social science, and health informatics. Quality of care, access, consent, and privacy are primary ongoing issues. Other, newer ethical issues related to digital innovation in healthcare include: usability, tailoring services to each patient, curriculum and training, implementation, commercialization, and licensing and liability. Interoperability, data availability, cybersecurity, and informatics infrastructure also have become more apparent policy issues. There is a continuing need to integrate ethics, informatics, medical, legal, and other scholarship to address ELSI concerns and proposed frameworks for ELSI analysis [36].

Digital dermatology presents impressive opportunities for improving quality of care and widening accessibility. While teledermatology already has spread significantly into routine practice, the integration of AI is still in its infancy and research is warranted in order to trace what its impact will be. It is important to avoid either of the two common overreactions to information technologies: Just as AI bias can skew responses toward believing AI is more accurate or attractive than it is, care also need be taken to not overly generalize against AI applications.

Dermatologists have an opportunity to shape how AI and telemedicine are introduced into their practices. The relationship between doctor and patient should not be overshadowed by technological hubris or seduction, or by fear of technology. Better care can be achieved when AI serves the doctor-patient relationship and leaves intact the unique, non-quantifiable value of physicians' practical experience and maintains the professional responsibilities of physicians to their patients. In partnership with doctors and patients, both AI and telemedicine can enhance care when developed with a view toward inclusiveness by improving accessibility for groups affected by health inequalities and digital divides, and by not reproducing social biases and discrimination.

For this, AI should meet commonly accepted ethical criteria of transparency, explicability, fairness, accuracy, interpretability, testability, understandability, identifiability of inherent biases or outright errors, correctability, accountability, and human-centeredness. All these should be part of the development and implementation processes, from initial conception to data collection for the application to the AI's use. AI applications should be based on a solid scientific foundation, reflect understanding of the applicable clinical domain, address the kinds of questions for which physicians and patients might want assistance, and deliver their results respectfully [110]. Like other uses of information technologies in clinical care, both telemedicine and AI should be designed in ways that facilitate clinical workflow and that incorporate principles of ethical design and the participation of those intended to use it. They should be deployed with the goals of facilitating patient-clinician relationships; constructing, nurturing, and developing patient-clinician communication; protecting data protection and privacy in ways specifically designed for these kinds of applications; maintaining the fiduciary relationship between the patient and the clinician; and serving a range of health systems and populations that vary in age, cultures, and ethnicities [111]. Their use should be monitored to evaluate how well they meet both ethical and clinical standards so that corrections can be made as needed [36]. Guidelines also should be re-evaluated periodically to encompass ELSI considerations that new technologies bring to light [37, 112].

Dermatologists should ask themselves, their institutions, and their organizations how deploying these technologies can affect their relationships with and care of patients, patients' families, their communities, and other healthcare professionals. They should assess how quality of care may be affected, and assess how they can minimize the negative effects of employing the technologies while capitalizing on the advantages. They should not only educate themselves on how their practice can benefit, but also should be able to advise their patients on how they can benefit from these technologies. To do this, it is important that dermatologists ask penetrating questions to evaluate these technologies [36, 72]. Our hope is that the background and discussion we presented will help dermatologists navigate the ethical use of these technologies for the benefit of their patients and the profession as a whole.

7 Multiple Choice Questions

1. Which of the following statements regarding artificial intelligence is TRUE?

a. AI algorithms are objective and free of bias.
b. Every step of developing, implementing, and using an AI algorithm should consider ethical, legal and social implications.
c. Diagnosis and treatment is optimized when physicians rely on AI alone.
d. Currently, unsupervised machine learning is the most commonly used AI within dermatology.

Correct answer: (b) Every step of developing AI algorithms should incorporate ELSI analysis, including what datasets are used, how data are classified and labeled, how systems are trained to increase correct outputs (and what is considered "correct"), and how they are used. Each of these steps can have significant ethical, legal and social implications.

Incorrect answers: (a) All algorithms have the potential to perpetuate biases depending on how they are programmed. (c) Research shows that diagnosis and treatment is optimized when physicians use AI in conjunction with their own clinical judgement. (d) Supervised machine learning, in which the dataset on which the AI is trained and is labeled and defined by an expert, is the most commonly used AI within dermatology.

2. Which one of the following patient encounters would be the best choice for using teledermatology?

a. New patient concerned about chronic lesions on her lower extremities.
b. New patient concerned about a growing, asymmetrical, pigmented lesion on his back.
c. Established patient following up regarding medication management of his psoriasis.
d. Established patient following up for a newly developed rash in his inner groin.
e. Established patient who is habitually late to appointments.

Correct answer: (c) The patient is known to the physician and the visit involves discussion of their medication management, which can easily be performed via teledermatology.

Incorrect answers: (a) and (b) Establishing care with a new patient via teledermatology is more challenging than following-up with an established patient, especially if the patient may have a lesion requiring a biopsy. (d) Not all follow-up appointments may be ideal for teledermatology visits, especially if the patient presents with an acute condition in a sensitive area. (e) Teledermatology visits should not be used merely to save time or increase productivity. Patients' health and safety should be the first priority, and because there is no additional information about this patient, this answer is not the best choice.

3. Considering the ethical, legal, and social issues associated with teledermatology and AI, which of the following statements is FALSE?

a. Teledermatology in and of itself can be used to close the "digital divide."
b. AI may contribute to the digitalization of medicine and negatively impact the patient-physician relationship.
c. A risk of adopting AI is "automation bias" wherein physicians blindly accept results from AI without requiring further investigation.
d. The implementation of AI applications in dermatological practices could open new scenarios with regard to professionals' liability.
e. In the US, data collected or transmitted by commercial devices, applications, or websites are not HIPAA protected.

Correct answer: (a) Material access to the internet and related technologies (computer, tablet, smartphones, and other connected devices) still represents the primary digital divide. As per text, all other answer choices are correct statements.

References

1. Lee JJ, English JC 3rd. Teledermatology: a review and update. Am J Clin Dermatol. 2018;19(2):253–60. https://doi.org/10.1007/s40257-017-0317-6.
2. Adamson AS, Smith A. Machine learning and health care disparities in dermatology. JAMA Dermatol. 2018;154(11):1247–8. https://doi.org/10.1001/jamadermatol.2018.2348.
3. Spinazze P, Bottle A, Car J. Digital health sensing for personalized dermatology. Sensors (Basel). 2019;19(15):3426. https://doi.org/10.3390/s19153426.
4. Lupton D. The digitally engaged patient: self-monitoring and self-care in the digital health era. Soc Theory Health. 2013;11(3):256–70. https://doi.org/10.1057/sth.2013.10.
5. Kovarik CL. Patient perspectives on the use of artificial intelligence. JAMA Dermatol. 2020;156(5):493–4. https://doi.org/10.1001/jamadermatol.2019.5014.
6. World Health Organization. Telemedicine: opportunities and developments in member states: report on the second global survey on eHealth. 2009. Geneva: WHO Press, World Health Organization. 2010. https://www.who.int/goe/publications/goe_telemedicine_2010.pdf. Accessed 7 Dec 2021.
7. Freiburger G, Holcomb M, Piper D. The STARPAHC collection: part of an archive of the history of telemedicine. J Telemed Telecare. 2007;13(5):221–3. https://doi.org/10.1258/135763307781458949.
8. Greene JA. As telemedicine surges, will community health suffer? Boston Rev [updated April 20, 2020]. https://bostonreview.net/articles/jeremy-greene-telemedicine-and-new-infrastructure-care/. Accessed 24 Nov 2021.
9. Kaplan B, Litewka S. Ethical challenges of telemedicine and telehealth. Camb Q Healthc Eth. 2008;17(4):401–16. https://doi.org/10.1017/S0963180108080535.
10. Botrugno C. Working on a right to health for the digital era. Glob Commun Yearbk Int Law Jurispru. 2020;20(1):137–56.
11. Samson L, Tarazi W, Turrini G, Sheingold S. Medicare beneficiaries' use of telehealth services in 2020—trends by beneficiary characteristics and location (Issue Brief No. HP-2021–27). Office of the Assistant Secretary for Planning and Evaluation, US Department of Health and Human Services. December. 2021. https://aspe.hhs.gov/sites/default/files/documents/a1d5d810fe3433e18b192be42dbf2351/medicare-telehealth-report.pdf. Accessed 24 Nov 2021.
12. Czeisler ME, Marynak K, Clarke KEN, Salah Z, Shakya I, Thierry JM, et al. Delay or avoidance of medical care because of COVID-19-related concerns—United States, June 2020. MMWR Morb Mortal Wkly Rep. 2020;69(36):1250–7.
13. Koonin LM, Hoots B, Tsang CA, Leroy Z, Farris K, Jolly T, et al. Trends in the use of telehealth during the emergence of the COVID-19 pandemic—United States, January–March 2020. MMWR Morb Mortal Wkly Rep. 2020;69(43):1595–9.
14. Vosburg RW, Robinson KA. Telemedicine in primary care during the COVID-19 pandemic: provider and patient satisfaction examined. Telemed J E Health. 2021. https://doi.org/10.1089/tmj.2021.0174.
15. Pala P, Bergler-Czop BS, Gwizdz JM. Teledermatology: idea, benefits and risks of modern age—a systematic review based on melanoma. Postepy Dermatol Alergol. 2020;37(2):159–67. https://doi.org/10.5114/ada.2020.94834.
16. Pasquali P, Sonthalia S, Moreno-Ramirez D, Sharma P, Agrawal M, Gupta S, et al. Teledermatology and its current perspective. Indian Dermatol Online J. 2020;11(1):12–20. https://doi.org/10.4103/idoj.IDOJ_241_19.
17. Warshaw EM, Hillman YJ, Greer NL, Hagel EM, MacDonald R, Rutks IR, et al. Teledermatology for diagnosis and management of skin conditions: a systematic review. J Am Acad Dermatol. 2011;64(4):759–72. https://doi.org/10.1016/j.jaad.2010.08.026.
18. Finnane A, Dallest K, Janda M, Soyer HP. Teledermatology for the diagnosis and management of skin cancer: a systematic review. JAMA Dermatol. 2017;153(3):319–27. https://doi.org/10.1001/jamadermatol.2016.4361.

19. Hadeler E, Gitlow H, Nouri K. Definitions, survey methods, and findings of patient satisfaction studies in teledermatology: a systematic review. Arch Dermatol Res. 2021;313(4):205–15. https://doi.org/10.1007/s00403-020-02110-0.
20. Du-Harpur X, Watt FM, Luscombe NM, Lynch MD. What is AI? Applications of artificial intelligence to dermatology. Br J Dermatol. 2020;183(3):423–30. https://doi.org/10.1111/bjd.18880.
21. Pai VV, Pai RB. Artificial intelligence in dermatology and healthcare: an overview. Indian J Dermatol Venereol Leprol. 2021;87(4):457–67. https://doi.org/10.25259/IJDVL_518_19.
22. Rubegni P, Burroni M, Cevenini G, Perotti R, Dell'Eva G, Barbini P, et al. Digital dermoscopy analysis and artificial neural network for the differentiation of clinically atypical pigmented skin lesions: a retrospective study. J Invest Dermatol. 2002;119(2):471–4. https://doi.org/10.1046/j.1523-1747.2002.01835.x.
23. Brinker TJ, Hekler A, Enk AH, Klode J, Hauschild A, Berking C, et al. A convolutional neural network trained with dermoscopic images performed on par with 145 dermatologists in a clinical melanoma image classification task. Eur J Cancer. 2019;111:148–54. https://doi.org/10.1016/j.ejca.2019.02.005.
24. Haenssle HA, Fink C, Schneiderbauer R, Toberer F, Buhl T, Blum A, et al. Man against machine: diagnostic performance of a deep learning convolutional neural network for dermoscopic melanoma recognition in comparison to 58 dermatologists. Ann Oncol. 2018;29(8):1836–42. https://doi.org/10.1093/annonc/mdy166.
25. Tschandl P, Rosendahl C, Akay BN, Argenziano G, Blum A, Braun RP, et al. Expert-level diagnosis of nonpigmented skin cancer by combined convolutional neural networks. JAMA Dermatol. 2019;155(1):58–65. https://doi.org/10.1001/jamadermatol.2018.4378.
26. Rajpurkar P, Irvin J, Ball RL, Zhu K, Yang B, Mehta H, et al. Deep learning for chest radiograph diagnosis: a retrospective comparison of the CheXNeXt algorithm to practicing radiologists. PLoS Med. 2018;15(11):e1002686. https://doi.org/10.1371/journal.pmed.1002686.
27. Han SS, Park I, Eun Chang S, Lim W, Kim MS, Park GH, et al. Augmented intelligence dermatology: deep neural networks empower medical professionals in diagnosing skin cancer and predicting treatment options for 134 skin disorders. J Invest Dermatol. 2020;140(9):1753–61. https://doi.org/10.1016/j.jid.2020.01.019.
28. De A, Sarda A, Gupta S, Das S. Use of artificial intelligence in dermatology. Indian J Dermatol. 2020;65(5):352–7. https://doi.org/10.4103/ijd.IJD_418_20.
29. Chan S, Reddy V, Myers B, Thibodeaux Q, Brownstone N, Liao W. Machine learning in dermatology: current applications, opportunities, and limitations. Dermatol Ther (Heidelb). 2020;10(3):365–86. https://doi.org/10.1007/s13555-020-00372-0.
30. Chuchu N, Dinnes J, Takwoingi Y, Matin RN, Bayliss SE, Davenport C, et al. Teledermatology for diagnosing skin cancer in adults. Cochrane Database Syst Rev. 2018;12:CD013193. https://doi.org/10.1002/14651858.CD013193.
31. Deleuran M, Vestergaard C. Clinical heterogeneity and differential diagnosis of atopic dermatitis. Br J Dermatol. 2014;170(Suppl1):2–6. https://doi.org/10.1111/bjd.12933.
32. Malhi IS, Yiu ZZN. Algorithm-based smartphone apps to assess risk of skin cancer in adults: critical appraisal of a systematic review. Br J Dermatol. 2021;184(4):638–9. https://doi.org/10.1111/bjd.19502.
33. Raji D. How our data encodes systematic racism. Technol Rev. 2020. https://www.technologyreview.com/2020/12/10/1013617/racism-data-science-artificial-intelligence-ai-opinion/. Accessed 7 Dec 2021.
34. Hogarty DT, Su JC, Phan K, Attia M, Hossny M, Nahavandi S, et al. Artificial intelligence in dermatology—where we are and the way to the future: a review. Am J Clin Dermatol. 2020;21(1):41–7. https://doi.org/10.1007/s40257-019-00462-6.
35. Kaplan B. The influence of medical values and practices on medical computer applications. In: Anderson JG, Jay SJ, editors. Use and impact of computers in clinical medicine. New York, Berlin, Heidelberg, London, Paris, Tokyo: Springer-Verlag; 1987. p. 39–50.
36. Kaplan B. Revisiting health information technology ethical, legal, and social issues and evaluation: telehealth/telemedicine and COVID-19. Int J Med Inf. 2020;143(11):104239. https://doi.org/10.1016/j.ijmedinf.2020.104239.

37. Kaplan B. Ethical, legal, and social issues pertaining to virtual and digital representations of patients. In: Hsueh P-YS, Wetter T, Zhu X, editors. Personal health informatics: patient participation in precision health. Cham: Springer; 2022. p. 519–42.
38. Harrison MI, Koppel R, Bar-Lev S. Unintended consequences of information technologies in health care—an interactive sociotechnical analysis. J Am Med Inf Assoc. 2007;14(5):542–9. https://doi.org/10.1197/jamia.M2384.
39. Botrugno C. From divine healing powers to the tyranny of the virtual gaze: medical practice and the technological imperative in healthcare. In: Leone M, Mohr R, Branco P, Mohsen N, editors. Tools of meaning representation, objects, and agency in the technologies of law and religion. Rome: Aracne; 2018. p. 163–76.
40. Botrugno C. Information technologies in healthcare: enhancing or dehumanising doctor-patient interaction? Health (London). 2021;25(4):475–93. https://doi.org/10.1177/1363459319891213.
41. Le CG. Normal et le pathologique. Paris: Presses Universitaires de France; 2013.
42. Foucault M. The birth of the clinic. Paris: Presses Universitaires de France; 1977.
43. Jewson ND. The disappearance of the sick-man from medical cosmology, 1770–1870. Int J Epidemiol. 2009;38(3):622–33. https://doi.org/10.1093/ije/dyp180.
44. McLean TR. Telemedicine and the commoditization of medical services. DePaul J Health Care Law. 2007;10(2):131–76.
45. Botrugno C. La nuova geografia del diritto alla salute. Innovazione tecnologica, relazioni spaziali e forme di sapere. Rome: IF Press; 2021.
46. Sinha A. An overview of telemedicine: the virtual gaze of health care in the next century. Med Anthropol Q. 2000;14(3):291–309. https://doi.org/10.1525/maq.2000.14.3.291.
47. Kaplan B. Objectification and negotiation in interpreting clinical images: implications for computer-based patient records. Artif Intell Med. 1995;280(October):439–54.
48. Botrugno C, Ghirotto L. Getting closer at a distance: a focused ethnography in a teleconsultation service in North of Italy. In: Bollon FM, Suman AB, editors. Legal, social and ethical perspectives on health and technology. Presses Universitaires Savoie Mont Blanc; 2020. p. 169–87.
49. Koller L. The evolution of medical imaging technologies: electric meat and the physician's shifting gaze. EA-J. 2011;2(3):1–22.
50. Hatherley JJ. Limits of trust in medical AI. J Med Ethics. 2020;46(7):478–81. https://doi.org/10.1136/medethics-2019-105935.
51. Mattessich S, Tassavor M, Swetter SM, Grant-Kels JM. How I learned to stop worrying and love machine learning. Clin Dermatol. 2018;36(6):777–8. https://doi.org/10.1016/j.clinderma tol.2018.06.003.
52. Truong A. Are you ready to be diagnosed without a human doctor? A discussion about artificial intelligence, technology, and humanism in dermatology. Int J Womens Dermatol. 2019;5(4):267–8. https://doi.org/10.1016/j.ijwd.2019.05.001.
53. Elston DM. Availability bias and artificial intelligence. J Am Acad Dermatol. 2023;89(1):29–30. https://doi.org/10.1016/j.jaad.2019.07.051.
54. Reiser SJ. Medicine and the reign of technology. New York: Cambridge University Press; 1978.
55. Evans RG, Stoddart GL. Producing health, consuming health care. Soc Sci Med. 1990;31(12):1347–63. https://doi.org/10.1016/0277-9536(90)90074-3.
56. Pellegrino ED. The commodification of medical and health care: the moral consequences of a paradigm shift from a professional to a market ethic. J Med Philos. 1999;24(3):243–66. https://doi.org/10.1076/jmep.24.3.243.2523.
57. Le DP. Trasformazioni del rapporto comunicativo nella relazione interpersonale medico-paziente. Rassegna Italiana di Sociologia. 1984;25(4):547–71.
58. Da Gama AD. La crise de la medicine contemporaine ou la second mort d'hyppocrate. J Mal Vasc. 2001;26(5):287–9.
59. Garattini L, Zanetti M, Freemantle N. The Italian NHS: what lessons to draw from COVID-19? Appl Health Econ Health Policy. 2020;18(4):463–6. https://doi.org/10.1007/s40258-020-00594-5.

60. Botrugno C. The spread of telemedicine in daily practice: weighing risks and benefits. In: Ienca M, Pollicino O, Liguori L, Stefanini E, Andorno R, editors. Emerging technologies, emerging rights? The Cambridge Handbook of Information Technology, Life Sciences and Human Rights. Cambridge: Cambridge University Press; 2022. p. 102–12.
61. Smith AC, Thomas E, Snoswell CL, Haydon H, Mehrotra A, Clemensen J, et al. Telehealth for global emergencies: implications for coronavirus disease 2019 (COVID-19). J Telemed Telecare. 2020;26(5):309–13. https://doi.org/10.1177/1357633X20916567.
62. Ohannessian R, Duong TA, Odone A. Global telemedicine implementation and integration within health systems to fight the COVID-19 pandemic: a call to action. JMIR Public Health Surveill. 2020;6(2):e18810. https://doi.org/10.2196/18810.
63. van Deursen AJ. Digital inequality during a pandemic: quantitative study of differences in COVID-19-related internet uses and outcomes among the general population. J Med Internet Res. 2020;22(8):e20073.
64. Amnesty International. Preoccupazione di amnesty international italia per la situazione esplosiva nelle carceri italiane. 2021. https://www.amnesty.it/situazione-esplosiva-carceri/. Accessed 5 Dec 2021.
65. Sanfelici M. The impact of the COVID-19 crisis on marginal migrant populations in Italy. Am Behav Sci. 2021;65(10):1323–41.
66. Botrugno C. El papel de la tecnología en la gestión de la pandemia de CoViD-19. RedBioetica Unesco. 2020;21:13–20. https://redbioetica.com.ar/revista-redbioetica-unesco-no-21/. Accessed 7 Dec 2021.
67. McAuley A. Digital health interventions: widening access or widening inequalities? Public Health. 2014;128(12):1118–20. https://doi.org/10.1016/j.puhe.2014.10.008.
68. Latulippe K, Hamel C, Giroux D. Social health inequalities and ehealth: a literature review with qualitative synthesis of theoretical and empirical studies. J Med Internet Res. 2017;19(4):e136. https://doi.org/10.2196/jmir.6731.
69. Moor I, Spallek J, Richter M. Explaining socioeconomic inequalities in self-rated health: a systematic review of the relative contribution of material, psychosocial and behavioural factors. J Epidemiol Commun Health. 2017;71(6):565–75. https://doi.org/10.1136/jech-2016-207589.
70. Kontos E, Blake KD, Chou WY, Prestin A. Predictors of health usage: insights on the digital divide from the health information national trends survey 2012. J Med Internet Res. 2014;16(7):e172. https://doi.org/10.2196/jmir.3117.
71. Beaunoyer E, Dupere S, Guitton MJ. COVID-19 and digital inequalities: reciprocal impacts and mitigation strategies. Comput Human Behav. 2020;111:106424. https://doi.org/10.1016/j.chb.2020.106424.
72. Kaplan B. Ethics, guidelines, standards, and policy: telemedicine, COVID-19, and broadening the ethical scope. Camb Q Healthc Eth. 2022. https://doi.org/10.1017/S0963180121000852.
73. Subbian V, Solomonides A, Clarkson M, Rahimzadeh VN, Petersen C, Schreiber R, et al. Ethics and informatics in the age of COVID-19: challenges and recommendations for public health organization and public policy. J Am Med Inf Assoc. 2020;28(1):184–9. https://doi.org/10.1093/jamia/ocaa188.
74. Butt S, Butt H, Gnanappiragasam D. Unintentional consequences of artificial intelligence in dermatology for patients with skin of colour. Clin Exp Dermatol. 2021;46(7):1333–4. https://doi.org/10.1111/ced.14726.
75. Huckvale K, Venkatesh S, Christensen H. Toward clinical digital phenotyping: a timely opportunity to consider purpose, quality, and safety. NPJ Digit Med. 2019;2:88. https://doi.org/10.1038/s41746-019-0166-1.
76. Scott IA. Hope, hype and harms of big data. Intern Med J. 2019;49:126–9. https://doi.org/10.1111/imj.14172.
77. Challen R, Denny J, Pitt M, Gompels L, Edwards T, Tsaneva-Atanasova K. Artificial intelligence, bias and clinical safety. BMJ Qual Saf. 2019;28:231–7. https://doi.org/10.1136/bmjqs-2018-008370.

78. Mohr D, Zhang M, Schueller SM. Personal sensing: understanding mental health using ubiquitous sensors and machine learning. Annu Rev Clin Psychol. 2017;13:23–47. https://doi.org/10.1146/annurev-clinpsy-032816-044949.
79. Intersoft Consulting. General data protection regulation: rights of the data subject. https://gdpr-info.eu/chapter-3/. Accessed 6 Dec 2021.
80. Vogl R, Farhangi A, Casey B. Rethinking explainable machines: the next chapter in the GDPR's 'right to explanation' debate. 2018. https://www.law.ox.ac.uk/business-law-blog/blog/2018/05/rethinking-explainable-machines-next-chapter-gdprs-right-explanation. Accessed 6 Dec 2021.
81. Cohen IG, Evgeniou T, Gerke S, Minssen T. The European artificial intelligence strategy: implications and challenges for digital health. Lancet Digit Health. 2020;2(7):e376–9. https://doi.org/10.1016/S2589-7500(20)30112-6.
82. Cheshire WP. Loopthink: a limitation of medical artificial intelligence. Eth Med. 2017;33(1):7–12. https://doi.org/10.1016/j.jns.2019.06.024.
83. Ward-Peterson M, Acuña JM, Alkhalifah MK, Nasiri AM, Al-Akeel ES, Alkhaldi TM, et al. Association between race/ethnicity and survival of melanoma patients in the united states over 3 decades: a secondary analysis of SEER data. Medicine (Baltimore). 2016;95(17):e3315. https://doi.org/10.1097/MD.0000000000003315.
84. Cormier JN, Xing Y, Ding M, Lee JE, Mansfield PF, Gershenwald JE, et al. Ethnic differences among patients with cutaneous melanoma. Arch Intern Med. 2006;166(17):1907–14. https://doi.org/10.1001/archinte.166.17.1907.
85. Koppel R. Uses of the legal system that attenuate patient safety. DePaul L Rev. 2019;68(2):273–90.
86. Food and Drug Administration. Proposed regulatory framework for modifications to artificial intelligence/machine learning (AI/ML)-based software as a medical device (SaMD)—discussion paper and request for feedback. 2019. https://www.fda.gov/media/122535/download. Accessed 7 Dec 2021.
87. Food and Drug Administration. Artificial intelligence and machine learning (AI/ML) software as a medical device action plan. 2021. https://www.fda.gov/media/145022/download. Accessed 7 Dec 2021.
88. International Medical Device Regulators Forum. Software as a "medical device": possible framework for risk categorization and corresponding considerations. 2014. http://www.imdrf.org/docs/imdrf/final/technical/imdrf-tech-140918-samd-framework-risk-categorization-141013.pdf. Accessed 7 Dec 2021.
89. Kaplan B. Regulation of software as a medical device: opportunity for bioethics. Hastings Center Forum; 2021 [updated March 1, 2021]. https://www.thehastingscenter.org/regulation-of-software-as-a-medical-device-opportunity-for-bioethics. Accessed 1 Mar 2021.
90. Kaplan B. Seeing through health information technology: the need for transparency in software, algorithms, data privacy, and regulation. J Law Biosci. 2020;7:lsaa062. https://doi.org/10.1093/jlb/lsaa062.
91. Ross C. As the FDA clears a flood of AI tools, missing data raise troubling questions on safety and fairness. Stat. 2021. https://www.statnews.com/2021/02/03/fda-clearances-artificial-intelligence-data/. Accessed Dec 7 2021.
92. Botrugno C. Telemedicine in daily practice: addressing legal challenges while waiting for an EU regulatory framework. Health Policy Technol. 2018;7(2):131–6. https://doi.org/10.1016/j.hlpt.2018.04.003.
93. European Commission of the European Union. Proposal for a regulation laying down harmonised rules for artificial intelligence. 2021. https://eur-lex.europa.eu/resource.html?uri=cellar:e0649735-a372-11eb-9585-01aa75ed71a1.0001.02/DOC_1&format=PDF. Accessed 6 Dec 2021.
94. European Commission of the European Union. Fostering a European approach to artificial intelligence. Communication nr. 2021/205. 2021. https://digital-strategy.ec.europa.eu/en/library/communication-fostering-european-approach-artificial-intelligence. Accessed 6 Dec 2021.

95. European Commission of the European Union. Artificial intelligence for Europe. Communication nr. 2018/137. 2018. https://eur-lex.europa.eu/legal-content/EN/TXT/?uri=COM%3A2018%3A237%3AFIN. Accessed 6 Dec 2021.
96. European Commission of the European Union, High Level Expert Group on Artificial Intelligence. Ethics guidelines for trustworthy AI. 2019. https://ec.europa.eu/futurium/en/ai-alliance-consultation.1.html. Accessed 7 Dec 2021.
97. World Health Organization. Ethics and governance of artificial intelligence for health: WHO guidance. 2021 [updated June 28, 2021]. https://www.who.int/publications/i/item/9789240029200. Accessed 6 Dec 2021.
98. World Medical Association 2019. WMA statement on augmented intelligence in care. https://www.wma.net/policies-post/wma-statement-on-augmented-intelligence-in-medical-care/. Accessed 6 Dec 2021.
99. World Medical Association. WMA statement on the ethics of telemedicine. 2018 https://www.wma.net/policies-post/wma-statement-on-the-ethics-of-telemedicine/AA. Accessed 6 Dec 2021.
100. World Health Organization. Mhealth: new horizons for health through mobile technologies. 2011. www.who.int/goe/publications/goe_mhealth_web.pdf. Accessed 6 Dec 2021.
101. American Medical Association. AMA passes first policy recommendation on augmented intelligence. 2018. https://www.ama-assn.org/press-center/press-releases/ama-passes-first-policy-recommendations-augmented-intelligence. Accessed 6 Dec 2021.
102. Chaet D, Clearfield R, Sabin JE, Skimming K. Ethical practice in telehealth and telemedicine. J Gen Intern Med. 2017;32(10):1136–40. https://doi.org/10.1007/s11606-017-4082-2.
103. American Medical Association. Telehealth implementation playbook. 2020. https://www.ama-assn.org/system/files/2020-04/ama-telehealth-playbook.pdf. Accessed 6 Dec 2021.
104. American Medical Association. Augmented intelligence in health care. 2018. https://www.ama-assn.org/system/files/2019-08/ai-2018-board-report.pdf. Accessed 6 Dec 2021.
105. American Medical Association. Augmented intelligence in health care. Payment and regulation. 2019. https://www.ama-assn.org/system/files/2019-08/ai-2019-board-report.pdf. Accessed 6 Dec 2021.
106. American Medical Association. AMA adopts new guidance for ethical practice in telemedicine. AMA; 2016 [updated June 16, 2016]. https://www.ama-assn.org/press-center/press-releases/ama-adopts-new-guidance-ethical-practice-telemedicine. Accessed Oct 2016 and Apr 2018, 2020.
107. American Medical Association Council on Medical Service. Established patient relationships and telemedicine: CMS report 1-i-19. 2019. https://www.ama-assn.org/system/files/2019-12/i19-cms-report1-patient-relations-telemedicine.pdf. Accessed 6 Dec 2021.
108. American Medical Association. Augmented intelligence in health care. Medical education, professional development and credentialing. https://www.ama-assn.org/system/files/2019-08/ai-2019-cme-report.pdf. Accessed 6 Dec 2021.
109. American Academy of Dermatology Association. Position statement on augmented intelligence. 2019. https://server.aad.org/Forms/Policies/Uploads/PS/PS-Augmented%20Intelligence.pdf. Accessed 6 Dec 2021.
110. American Academy of Dermatology Association. Telemedicine: overview. https://www.aad.org/public/fad/telemedicine. Accessed 6 Dec 2021.
111. Shortliffe EH, Sepúlveda MJ. Clinical decision support in the era of artificial intelligence. JAMA. 2018;320(21):2199–200. https://doi.org/10.1001/jama.2018.17163.
112. Kuziemsky CE, Hunter I, Gogia SB, lyenger S, Kulatunga G, Rajput V, et al. Ethics in telehealth: comparison between guidelines and practice-based experience—the case for learning health systems. Yearb Med Inform. 2020;29(01):044–50. https://doi.org/10.1055/s-0040-1701976.

Technological Advancements in Lasers

Betty Nguyen, Fabio S. Frech, and Michael Abrouk

Abstract Since the first use of lasers in dermatology in 1963, laser technology has become widely utilized for medical and cosmetic treatments. Selecting the proper laser, wavelength, pulse, and fluence depends on factors including patients' Fitzpatrick skin type and clinical diagnoses. This chapter explores the fundamentals of lasers, including an overview of types of lasers used in dermatology, components of lasers, and key principles of Q-switching, population inversion, and selective photothermolysis. Common clinical applications of lasers in dermatology include treatment of acne, scars, and vascular lesions. Neodymium:yttrium aluminum garnet (Nd:YAG) lasers are best used for acne treatment. Hypertrophic scars, acne scars, and burn scars may be targeted with 585 and 595-nm pulsed dye lasers (PDL). PDL selectively targets hemoglobin and therefore is also the laser of choice for vascular lesions. Cosmetic uses of lasers include hair removal, tattoo removal, and skin resurfacing. Diode lasers (810 nm) are preferred over Nd:YAG for hair removal due to their high efficacy and low rates of adverse effects, especially in skin of color. Erbium:yttrium aluminum garnet (Er:YAG) (2940 nm) and fractional carbon dioxide (CO_2) (10,600 nm) lasers are commonly used for skin resurfacing. The type of laser used for tattoo removal varies depending on the color(s) of tattoo pigment involved. The development of fractional lasers and other technological advancements have improved the safety profile of lasers and decreased the healing time for patients. Further research on novel applications of lasers holds promise in treating alopecia, cellulite, onychomycosis, and hyperhidrosis.

Keywords Laser · Alexandrite · CO_2 · Diode · Er:YAG · Nd:YAG · Potassium titanyl phosphate · Pulsed dye · Ruby

B. Nguyen (✉) · F. S. Frech
Dr. Phillip Frost Department of Dermatology and Cutaneous Surgery, Miller School of Medicine, University of Miami, Miami, FL, USA
e-mail: bettynguyenmed@gmail.com

B. Nguyen
University of California, Riverside School of Medicine, Riverside, CA, USA

M. Abrouk
Laser and Cosmetic Center, Massachusetts General Hospital Dermatology, Boston, MA, USA

K. Nouri (ed.), *Telemedicine and Technological Advances in Dermatology*,
https://doi.org/10.1007/978-3-031-69091-4_23

Learning Objectives

1. Understand the fundamental principles behind laser technology
2. Determine which lasers are appropriate treatment modalities for certain dermatologic conditions.

1 Introduction

In 1963, Leon Goldman was the first to use lasers on the skin, issuing an era of laser treatment for dermatologic disease [1]. Over the past 50 years, advancements in laser technology have enabled dermatologists worldwide to expand the scope of treatment to include removal, repair, and resurfacing. Lasers are routinely used to treat hyperpigmentation, scars, telangiectasias, wounds, and congenital birthmarks, as well as to remove tattoos. New studies continue to prove laser efficacy in treating conditions such as alopecia, cellulite, fungal infections, and hyperhidrosis.

1.1 Fundamentals of Lasers

Lasers (Light Amplification by Stimulated Emission of Radiation) are devices that emit light of a certain wavelength and energy.

There are four main components of lasers [2]:

1. The laser medium
2. Resonator/optical cavity
3. Energy source
4. Delivery system.

The laser medium can be *solid*, *liquid*, or *gas*. *Solids* include ruby, alexandrite, neodymium:yttrium aluminum garnet (Nd:YAG), and erbium:yttrium aluminum garnet (Er:YAG). *Liquids* include pulsed dye. *Gases* include argon, carbon dioxide (CO_2), copper vapor, helium neon, and krypton. The name of each laser is derived from its medium component (e.g., Nd:YAG laser). The resonator contains two mirrors placed in parallel: one mirror that is opaque, and one with partial transparency to allow the photons to eventually exit as a laser beam. Light rays that are parallel to the axis are amplified, whereas light at an angle will exit the cylinder.

Lasers are based on the fundamental principle of quantum mechanics. When electrons absorb energy, they move to a higher quantum state ("excited state"). As these electrons relax and return to their ground state, they release light in packets of energy known as photons. The ability to produce a laser beam is dependent on how many atoms are in the excited state. The process of stimulated emission occurs when a photon hits an atom in the excited state, causing it to drop to a lower energy level and generate two photons of the same wavelength and direction of travel. Conversely, if a photon hits an atom in the ground state, no photon is generated. Hence, the creation of a laser beam is dependent on stimulated emission. When more atoms are in the excited state than the ground state, this is known as population inversion. Energy can be "pumped" into the system to excite atoms and achieve population inversion, leading to net optical amplification allowing intensification of light rays into a laser beam.

1.2 Q-Switching

Q-switching (QS) is a technique to discharge the laser beam in short outputs, in the range of nanoseconds, with high intensity. QS relies on an attenuator inside the resonator that enables population inversion to occur but prevents light from feedbacking to the medium, and therefore preventing lasing. Energy accumulates in the gain medium. When enough energy is pumped into the system to reach a maximum stored energy, known as gain saturation, the Q-switch can be turned from low to high, allowing light to feedback and amplify. Atoms in the excited state fall at the same time, emitting a short pulse of light. This method enables energy to be built up to high levels and then released quickly to produce a powerful and short output.

1.3 Selective Photothermolysis

Targeting precise tissue components is possible due to the concept of selective photothermolysis. Selective substances in tissues, such as ink pigment, melanin, or oxyhemoglobin, absorb a specific wavelength better than others. Lasers can utilize these specific wavelengths to selectively target tissue components, known as chromophores, without destroying the surrounding tissue. Destruction occurs when tissue components are heated more quickly than their thermal relaxation time, or the time it takes to cool by 50% of the initial maximum temperature.

1.4 Types of Lasers

Lasers can be broken down into three categories: *continuous wave*, *pulsed*, and *ultrafast*. *Continuous wave* lasers use CO_2 or argon to emit a constant beam of light over a long period of time. *Pulsed* lasers emit light in a non-continuous manner, typically with repetition. Pulsed lasers can have durations ranging from milliseconds to nanoseconds, as seen in QS lasers. *Ultrafast* lasers emit short pulses of light typically in the range of 5 fs to 100 ps.

Lasers can be *ablative* or *non-ablative*. *Ablative* lasers damage the superficial layer of the skin and promote re-epithelialization, whereas *non-ablative* lasers do not damage the epidermis but rather induce thermal injury in the dermis to stimulate collagen production. Ablative lasers may deliver results in fewer treatments but may also have more side effects.

Fractionating can be done to minimize recovery time and side effects. Lasers may target either an entire field or fractions of the skin. Fractional lasers target columns in the treatment area by delivering a beam divided into thousands of microscopic columns, creating tissue coagulation in the treatment area that stimulates growth of healthy tissue. The intervening areas of skin are unaffected. This allows for rapid migration of intervening healthy cells into treatment areas, reducing recovery time and side effects. Fractional lasers penetrate both the epidermis and dermis, making them popular resurfacing tools often used for wrinkles, pigmentation, photoaging, and acne scars.

Although not a laser, intense pulsed light (IPL) is another technique that uses the same principles as lasers. IPL is a non-ablative tool that delivers light of multiple wavelengths instead of only one wavelength. IPL delivers focused, high-intensity light across the 515–1200-nm spectrum at a fluence of up to 40 J/cm^2. IPL may be a more affordable alternative to PDL and fractional CO_2 lasers. Specific ranges of wavelengths can be selectively filtered for, such as 755 nm to stimulate collagen production, 695 nm to treat superficial leg veins, and 515 nm to treat rosacea [3].

1.5 Approach to Treatment

Patients should be evaluated for their dermatologic condition, and expectations should be set prior to treatment initiation. Improvements tend to be mild to moderate. Healing time after laser treatment varies by laser. The traditional CO_2 laser may be followed by several weeks to months of erythema. Postoperative erythema resolves more quickly for fractional lasers.

Selection of laser type and wavelength depends on a patient's dermatologic condition and Fitzpatrick skin type. Longer wavelengths of light can penetrate deeper into the skin than shorter wavelengths. Melanin preferentially absorbs light of shorter wavelengths and therefore may be excessively targeted and destroyed at these wavelengths. Epidermal cooling techniques, such as chilling skin with ice cubes, cryogen spurts prior to treatment or using continuous flowing air throughout treatment, can protect the epidermis and reduce risk of adverse effects [4].

2 Clinical Applications

Acne. Nd:YAG lasers hold the most promise in treating acne [5]. Other lasers such as CO_2, potassium titanyl phosphate, and 1565-nm non-ablative fractional lasers have limited evidence on efficacy [5]. Like other scars, PDL of 585-nm has been shown to significantly improve erythematous and hypertrophic acne scars [6].

Birthmarks. Birthmarks may be seen as a part of a person's identity, and removal may be a personal choice. Port wine stains (PWS), infantile hemangiomas, and various nevi can be treated with QS lasers. Lasers are the gold standard for treatment of PWS, and PDL are commonly used. Treatment of PWS at an early age may reduce the number of required treatments [7, 8]. Infantile hemangiomas are often managed conservatively or with propranolol, though lesions that are small, superficial, or ulcerated may be treated with PDL. Nevus of Ota, nevus of Ito, and nevus of Hori are commonly removed using QS alexandrite or Nd-YAG lasers [9, 10]. Nevus spilus may also be treated with QS lasers after ruling out malignancy [11]. Other birthmarks commonly treated with QS lasers include congenital dermal melanocytosis (1064 nm QS laser) and congenital nevomelanocytic nevi (QS and LP) [11].

Hair removal. Hair removal relies on a high-intensity laser to permanently reduce hair growth by destroying the hair follicle. Lasers with wavelengths ranging from 600 to 1100 nm can be used to target melanin in the hair shaft and bulb [12, 13]. Pulse durations should be less than or equal to the thermal relaxation time of the hair shaft [14]. Light is absorbed by melanin, which then generates heat energy that destroys the follicle [15]. Follicular stem cells nearby are also destroyed by diffusion of thermal energy, preventing future hair regrowth [16]. However, pigmented skin is more susceptible to adverse effects due to a higher concentration of melanin.

The diode and the long-pulsed Nd:YAG are the most common and reliable lasers for hair removal [14], though other types of lasers used include the *ruby laser*, *alexandrite laser*, and *IPL*. *Ruby laser* (694 nm) has been shown to be more effective for individuals with Fitzpatrick skin types I-III and dark hair [17], but has become less popular due to limitations in skin types and its high electricity usage [18]. *Alexandrite laser* (755 nm) penetrates deeper than the ruby laser but has less melanin absorption, and therefore may not be as effective. Alexandrite laser is most effective in individuals with Fitzpatrick skin types I–III and lighter hair. IPL (475–1200 nm) may be used on darker skin and was found to reduce hair count by 37–87% 6 months following treatment [19, 20], with mild burning and itching sensation as common adverse effects [20]. *IPL* has been successfully used to destroy hair follicles in patients with mild-to-moderate hidradenitis suppurativa and may be a future treatment for this condition [21]. IPL may also be an affordable option for home-based hair removal.

Diode lasers (810 nm) may be more efficacious than Nd:YAG in darker skin types (III V) [14] and have become the dominant mode of laser hair removal globally [18]. Long pulsed Nd:YAG (1064 nm) lasers were previously the preferred modality due to their safety profile for patients with Fitzpatrick skin types IV to VI [14, 22–24]. However, Nd:YAG may be more painful than diode lasers or IPL [14]. Recent studies with 810 nm diode lasers have shown high efficacy, high patient satisfaction, and low rates of adverse effects in Fitzpatrick types III–V [25, 26].

Pigmentation. In treating pigmentation, lasers should have an optimal wavelength that is highly absorbed by targeted pigments, such as melanin, and poorly absorbed by water or hemoglobin [11]. Pulse durations should be no more than 1/10th of the cooling (thermal relaxation) time of the target [11]. Lasers including the 755 nm Q-switched alexandrite, 1064 and 532 nm Q-switched Nd:YAG, 694 Q-switched ruby, and 595 nm PDL lasers are often used [11].

Conditions commonly treated by lasers include actinic lentigines (532 nm; 694 nm; 755 nm QS lasers or IPL), café au lait macules (1064 nm QS Nd:YAG; 694 nm QS ruby; QS and long pulsed 755 nm alexandrite), ephelides (532 nm QS lasers), hypermelanosis (532 nm and 755 nm QS lasers), lentigos simplex (532 nm; 694 nm; 755 nm QS lasers or IPL), and melasma (PDL, IPL, 1064 Nd:YAG [27]) [11]. However, café au lait spots have high recurrence from treatment with lasers and treatment results vary [11].

Resurfacing. Laser resurfacing is a mainstay treatment of photoaging, rhytides, skin laxity, and wrinkles. Commonly used lasers include Er:YAG (2940 nm) and fractional CO_2 (10,600 nm). Er:YAG has been shown to reduce superficial and mild-depth rhytides due to its ability to ablate up to the papillary dermis after multiple passes [28], and these effects remain notable several months after treatment [29]. The CO_2 laser's wavelength of 10,600 nm is primarily absorbed by intracellular water [30], leading to ablation of the superficial epidermis [31] and heat transfer to the dermis that promotes collagen remodeling [32]. Re-epithelialization occurs earlier from Er:YAG treatment (8–10 days) compared to CO_2 (10–12 days) [33], but CO_2 lasers generate greater histological improvements including collagen and elastin formation [34].

Tattoo removal. A tattoo is the presence of pigment granules in the dermis. This can be done intentionally through tattooing pigmented ink (e.g., cosmetic tattoos, medical tattoos, decorative tattoos) or may be due to trauma from particles such as gravel, metal, or graphite from pencils becoming embedded in the dermis. From the moment tattoo ink is deposited into the dermis, leukocytes begin actively removing the ink through the lymphatic system. Large ink pigments are unable to be absorbed by the lymphatic system. Laser removal techniques utilize the lasers to heat up the targeted ink particles to break them into smaller particles, enabling the lymphatic system to absorb the particles.

A variety of ingredients may be found in colored tattoo ink, including carbon and iron oxide (black), cobaltic aluminate (blue), chrome oxide (green), mercury sulfide or cadmium selenide (red), cadmium sulfide or ochre (yellow), and titanium dioxide or zinc oxide (white). Prior studies found that picosecond lasers are the most effective when treating blue, green, and yellow tattoo pigment [35]. Q-switched 532 nm Nd:YAG lasers are also an effective alternative for red, orange, and yellow pigment [36, 37], whereas the 1064 nm Nd:YAG is used for black and blue pigment [38]. Ruby (693 nm) [39] and alexandrite (755 nm) [40] lasers can be used for black, blue, or green ink. White, tan, or brown pigment tattoos, or tattoos that may have undergone "color correction" may darken from laser treatment due to reduction of titanium dioxide or ferric oxide, and spot testing should be done prior to treatment [37]. These pigments may require ablation with a CO_2 or Er:YAG laser [37].

Keloids and scars. Hypertrophic scars form due to excessive collagen formation during wound healing after trauma or burn injuries [41]. PDL of 585 and 595-nm are the most commonly used lasers for scar remodeling [42], though Nd:YAG may also be used. A randomized study with 20 patients in Egypt found that both Nd:YAG and PDL significantly improved keloids and hypertrophic scars, with no significant difference between the modalities [43].

Burn scars also benefit from PDL treatment, including on sensitive areas such as the face [44]. Fractional CO_2 lasers have been successfully used on burn scars to improve pigmentation, scar height, vascularity, and pliability [45, 46], with mild and tolerable side effects. Traditional or nonfractional CO_2 and argon lasers are no longer used due to concerns about postoperative pain, prolonged erythema, and high rates of recurrence and infection [42].

Vascular lesions. In vascular lesions, oxyhemoglobin is the major chromophore targeted and is absorbed maximally in the range of yellow to green light (500–600 nm) [47]. Lasers can be used to treat a variety of vascular lesions, such as telangiectasias, hemangiomas, Kaposi sarcoma, pyogenic granulomas, and superficial vascular malformations. Treatment is most effective when started early, as superficial blood vessels are more responsive to treatment than deeper, larger vessels. PDL selectively targets hemoglobin and therefore is the laser of choice for vascular lesions. PDL (585–600 nm) has a low-risk profile and superior clinical efficacy compared to other lasers. Vbeam® (Syneron *Candela*, Wayland, MA) is a type of PDL with long pulse duration commonly used to treat vascular lesions. Due to the longer duration of energy, Vbeam is able to target pathologies with wider capillary diameters, including hemangiomas and pyogenic granulomas [48]. In addition, Vbeam has fewer side effects than PDL [49], such as formation of purpura, hypopigmentation, and hyperpigmentation. Other types of lasers used to treat vascular lesions include Nd:YAG, argon, argon pumped tunable dye (APTD), krypton, frequency-doubled Nd:YAG (also known as the potassium titanyl phosphate (KTP) laser), copper vapor, and copper bromide.

3 Novel Applications

Alopecia. Absorption of red to near-infrared light is known to enhance growth factor synthesis, cell signaling, and ATP production in mitochondria via photobiomodulation [50]. Low-level laser therapy (LLLT) at 655 nm has been shown to significantly improve hair regrowth in a double-blinded randomized controlled trial (RCT) of male patients with androgenetic alopecia through photobiomodulation [51]. A total of 17 patients with pediatric alopecia areata have been treated with 308 nm excimer laser with a 58.8% response rate [52]. Side effects include mild erythema and desquamation.

Cellulite. In Brazil, 52 patients with cellulite were treated with 1064-nm Nd:YAG lipolysis with fat transplantation, yielding significant clinical improvements [53]. The authors concluded that lipolysis with Nd:YAG has many benefits including neocollagenesis and stimulated skin tightening, likely due to Nd:YAG's penetration of all affected layers of cellulite including the dermis, connective tissue, and fat.

Fungal infections. CO_2 lasers combined with topical agents have been shown to significantly increase efficacy of treating onychomycosis by 5.38 times compared to topical agents alone ($p < 0.00001$) [54].

Hyperhidrosis. Nd:YAG and diode lasers have been used to treat axillary hyperhidrosis (AH). Four studies have reported use of subdermal 1064 nm [55], long-pulsed 1064 nm [55, 56], 1320 nm [57], and 1440 nm [58] Nd:YAG in treating AH in 39 total patients and found clinical improvements in 82.3–100% of patients [59]. However, another study by Aydin et al. found that treatment with Nd:YAG 1064 nm increased sweating, potentially through stimulation of the eccrine sweat glands [60]. The diode laser has been studied in two RCTs with a total of 131 patients [59]. The 800 nm pulsed laser found no statistically significant difference between the treatment and control axilla despite independent statistical significance, suggesting that effects may be due to placebo [61]. Another RCT including 100 patients found that the 924/975 nm diode laser followed by curettage yielded better outcomes than the 975 nm diode laser, curettage, and the 924/975 diode monotherapies [62].

4 Conclusion

Laser technology has enabled the advancement of non-cosmetic and cosmetic treatments. Technological advancements, including the development of fractional lasers, have decreased healing time and adverse effects of laser treatments. Today, lasers are a safe and mainstay treatment for acne, birthmarks, hyperpigmentation, scars, tattoo removal, and skin resurfacing. Ongoing research has enabled increased patient satisfaction and reduced adverse effects of laser treatments, especially in patients of diverse skin tones. Further research for novel applications of lasers holds promise in treating alopecia, cellulite, onychomycosis, and hyperhidrosis.

References

1. Goldman L, et al. Effect of the laser beam on the skin. Preliminary report. J Invest Dermatol. 1963;40:121–2.
2. Kurniadi I, et al. Laser tattoo removal: fundamental principles and practical approach. Dermatol Ther. 2021;34(1):e14418.
3. Hultman CS, et al. Shine on: review of laser- and light-based therapies for the treatment of burn scars. Dermatol Res Pract. 2012;2012:243651.
4. Kelly KM, et al. Description and analysis of treatments for port-wine stain birthmarks. Arch Facial Plast Surg. 2005;7(5):287–94.
5. Li MK, Liu C, Hsu JTS. The use of lasers and light devices in acne management: an update. Am J Clin Dermatol; 2021.

6. Alster TS, McMeekin TO. Improvement of facial acne scars by the 585 nm flashlamp-pumped pulsed dye laser. J Am Acad Dermatol. 1996;35(1):79–81.
7. Reyes BA, Geronemus R. Treatment of port-wine stains during childhood with the flashlamp-pumped pulsed dye laser. J Am Acad Dermatol. 1990;23(6 Pt 1):1142–8.
8. Tan OT, Sherwood K, Gilchrest BA. Treatment of children with port-wine stains using the flashlamp-pulsed tunable dye laser. N Engl J Med. 1989;320(7):416–21.
9. Badawi A, Osman MA, Kassab AN. Treatment of nevus of Ota and Ito and epidermal nevus syndrome. Hautarzt. 2020;71(12):926–31.
10. Yu P, et al. Comparison of clinical efficacy and complications between Q-switched alexandrite laser and Q-switched Nd:YAG laser on nevus of Ota: a systematic review and meta-analysis. Lasers Med Sci. 2016;31(3):581–91.
11. Passeron T, et al. Laser treatment of hyperpigmented lesions: position statement of the European Society of Laser in Dermatology. J Eur Acad Dermatol Venereol. 2019;33(6):987–1005.
12. McDaniel DH, et al. Laser hair removal: a review and report on the use of the long-pulsed alexandrite laser for hair reduction of the upper lip, leg, back, and bikini region. Dermatol Surg. 1999;25(6):425–30.
13. Gan SD, Graber EM. Laser hair removal: a review. Dermatol Surg. 2013;39(6):823–38.
14. Puri N. Comparative study of diode laser versus neodymium-yttrium aluminum: garnet laser versus intense pulsed light for the treatment of hirsutism. J Cutan Aesthet Surg. 2015;8(2):97–101.
15. Altshuler GB, et al. Extended theory of selective photothermolysis. Lasers Surg Med. 2001;29(5):416–32.
16. Fayne RA, et al. Laser and light treatments for hair reduction in Fitzpatrick skin types IV–VI: a comprehensive review of the literature. Am J Clin Dermatol. 2018;19(2):237–52.
17. Dierickx CC, et al. Permanent hair removal by normal-mode ruby laser. Arch Dermatol. 1998;134(7):837–42.
18. Thomas MM, Houreld NN. The "in's and outs" of laser hair removal: a mini review. J Cosmet Laser Ther. 2019;21(6):316–22.
19. Alster TS, Tanzi EL. Effect of a novel low-energy pulsed-light device for home-use hair removal. Dermatol Surg. 2009;35(3):483–9.
20. Trelles MA, Ash C, Town G. Clinical and microscopic evaluation of long-term (6 months) epilation effects of the iPulse personal home-use intense pulsed light (IPL) device. J Eur Acad Dermatol Venereol. 2014;28(2):160–8.
21. Andersen PL, et al. Intense pulsed light treatment for hidradenitis suppurativa: a within-person randomized controlled trial. Eur J Dermatol. 2020;30(6):723–9.
22. Lanigan SW. Incidence of side effects after laser hair removal. J Am Acad Dermatol. 2003;49(5):882–6.
23. Ismail SA. Long-pulsed Nd:YAG laser vs. intense pulsed light for hair removal in dark skin: a randomized controlled trial. Br J Dermatol. 2012;166(2):317–21.
24. Dorgham NA, Dorgham DA. Lasers for reduction of unwanted hair in skin of colour: a systematic review and meta-analysis. J Eur Acad Dermatol Venereol. 2020;34(5):948–55.
25. Agarwal M, Velaskar S, Gold MH. Efficacy of a low fluence, high repetition rate 810 nm diode laser for permanent hair reduction in Indian patients with skin types IV–VI. J Clin Aesthet Dermatol. 2016;9(11):29–33.
26. Royo J, et al. Six-month follow-up multicenter prospective study of 368 patients, phototypes III to V, on epilation efficacy using an 810-nm diode laser at low fluence. Lasers Med Sci. 2011;26(2):247–55.
27. Micek I, et al. Treatment of melasma with a low-fluence 1064 nm Q-switched Nd:YAG laser: laser toning in Caucasian women. Lasers in Surgery and Medicine. 2021.
28. Perez MI, Bank DE, Silvers D. Skin resurfacing of the face with the Erbium:YAG laser. Dermatol Surg. 1998;24(6): 653–8; discussion 658–9.
29. Kopelman J. Erbium:YAG laser–an improved periorbital resurfacing device. Semin Ophthalmol. 1998;13(3):136–41.

30. Reilly MJ, et al. Molecular effects of fractional carbon dioxide laser resurfacing on photodamaged human skin. Arch Facial Plast Surg. 2010;12(5):321–5.
31. Orringer JS, et al. Connective tissue remodeling induced by carbon dioxide laser resurfacing of photodamaged human skin. Arch Dermatol. 2004;140(11):1326–32.
32. Fitzpatrick RE, Rostan EF, Marchell N. Collagen tightening induced by carbon dioxide laser versus erbium:YAG laser. Lasers Surg Med. 2000;27(5):395–403.
33. Adrian RM. Pulsed carbon dioxide and erbium-YAG laser resurfacing: a comparative clinical and histologic study. J Cutan Laser Ther. 1999;1(1):29–35.
34. Alster TS, Lupton JR. Erbium:YAG cutaneous laser resurfacing. Dermatol Clin. 2001;19(3):453–66.
35. Gurnani P, et al. Comparing the efficacy and safety of laser treatments in tattoo removal: a systematic review. J Am Acad Dermatol. 2020.
36. Ferguson JE, August PJ. Evaluation of the Nd/YAG laser for treatment of amateur and professional tattoos. Br J Dermatol. 1996;135(4):586–91.
37. Naga LI, Alster TS. Laser tattoo removal: an update. Am J Clin Dermatol. 2017;18(1):59–65.
38. Kilmer SL, et al. The Q-switched Nd:YAG laser effectively treats tattoos. A controlled, dose-response study. Arch Dermatol. 1993;129(8):971–8.
39. Taylor CR, et al. Treatment of tattoos by Q-switched ruby laser. A dose-response study. Arch Dermatol. 1990;126(7):893–9.
40. Alster TS. Q-switched alexandrite laser treatment (755 nm) of professional and amateur tattoos. J Am Acad Dermatol. 1995;33(1):69–73.
41. Magee DJ, et al. Pathology and intervention in musculoskeletal rehabilitation, 2nd ed. ed. Musculoskeletal rehabilitation series. Maryland Heights, Missouri: Elsevier; 2016. p. xv, 1219 pages.
42. Chowdhury B, et al. Laser in surgical scar clearance: an update review. J Cosmet Dermatol. 2021.
43. Al-Mohamady Ael S, Ibrahim SM, Muhammad MM. Pulsed dye laser versus long-pulsed Nd:YAG laser in the treatment of hypertrophic scars and keloid: a comparative randomized split-scar trial. J Cosmet Laser Ther. 2016;18(4):208–12.
44. Donelan MB, Parrett BM, Sheridan RL. Pulsed dye laser therapy and z-plasty for facial burn scars: the alternative to excision. Ann Plast Surg. 2008;60(5):480–6.
45. Choi KJ, et al. Fractional CO_2 laser treatment for burn scar improvement: a systematic review and meta-analysis. Burns. 2021;47(2):259–69.
46. Peng W, et al. The efficacy and safety of fractional CO_2 laser therapy in the treatment of burn scars: a meta-analysis. Burns. 2021.
47. Iwasaka M, Miyakoshi J, Ueno S. Optical absorbance of hemoglobin and red blood cell suspensions under magnetic fields. IEEE Trans Magn. 2001;37(4):2906–8.
48. Kishi Y, et al. Dye laser treatment for hemorrhagic vascular lesions. Laser Ther. 2018;27(1):61–4.
49. Kono T, et al. Comparison study of a traditional pulsed dye laser versus a long-pulsed dye laser in the treatment of early childhood hemangiomas. Lasers Surg Med. 2006;38(2):112–5.
50. Glass GE. Photobiomodulation: the clinical applications of low-level light therapy. Aesthet Surg J. 2021;41(6):723–38.
51. Leavitt M, et al. HairMax LaserComb laser phototherapy device in the treatment of male androgenetic alopecia: a randomized, double-blind, sham device-controlled, multicentre trial. Clin Drug Investig. 2009;29(5):283–92.
52. Barton VR, et al. Treatment of pediatric alopecia areata: a systematic review. J Am Acad Dermatol. 2021.
53. Goldman A, et al. Cellulite: a new treatment approach combining subdermal Nd:YAG laser lipolysis and autologous fat transplantation. Aesthet Surg J. 2008;28(6):656–62.
54. Han Y, et al. The effects of CO_2 laser and topical agent combination therapy for onychomycosis: a meta-analysis. Dermatol Ther. 2021; e15136.
55. Goldman A, Wollina U. Subdermal Nd-YAG laser for axillary hyperhidrosis. Dermatol Surg. 2008;34(6):756–62.

56. Letada PR, et al. Treatment of focal axillary hyperhidrosis using a long-pulsed Nd:YAG 1064 nm laser at hair reduction settings. J Drugs Dermatol. 2012;11(1):59–63.
57. Kotlus BS. Treatment of refractory axillary hyperhidrosis with a 1320-nm Nd:YAG laser. J Cosmet Laser Ther. 2011;13(4):193–5.
58. Caplin D, Austin J. Clinical evaluation and quantitative analysis of axillary hyperhidrosis treated with a unique targeted laser energy delivery method with 1-year follow up. J Drugs Dermatol. 2014;13(4):449–56.
59. Cervantes J, et al. Laser treatment of primary axillary hyperhidrosis: a review of the literature. Lasers Med Sci. 2018;33(3):675–81.
60. Aydin F, et al. Axillary hair removal with 1064-nm Nd:YAG laser increases sweat production. Clin Exp Dermatol. 2010;35(6):588–92.
61. Bechara FG, et al. Effects of a long-pulsed 800-nm diode laser on axillary hyperhidrosis: a randomized controlled half-side comparison study. Dermatol Surg. 2012;38(5):736–40.
62. Leclere FM, et al. Efficacy and safety of laser therapy on axillary hyperhidrosis after one year follow-up: a randomized blinded controlled trial. Lasers Surg Med. 2015;47(2):173–9.

Advances in Aesthetic Dermatology

Loren Elizabeth de la Caridad Hernandez, Francelia J. Eckembrecher, Daphne G. Eckembrecher, Noreen Mohsin, Shelley Uppal, Marwa Hakimi, Ashley Vander Does, and Keyvan Nouri

Abstract Aesthetic dermatology is a growing division of dermatology that aims to improve personal appearance and promote aesthetic rejuvenation. According to the American Society for Dermatologic Surgery (ASDS), over 10.3 million cosmetic treatments were performed by dermatologists in 2019. It is critical that practitioners remain updated on advancements in aesthetic dermatology given the high demand for cosmetic procedures. From the implementation of biotechnology in skincare to advancements in minimally invasive procedures, aesthetic treatments have rapidly diversified, expanding the spectrum of treatments available for patients. This chapter will present these innovations and provide practitioners with an updated review of aesthetic treatments.

Keywords Aesthetic dermatology · Biotechnology · Enzymes · Non-invasive body contouring

1 Introduction

Aesthetic dermatology, also known as cosmetic dermatology, is a rapidly growing division of dermatology that aims to ameliorate the aging process and improve personal appearance. Aging is an inevitable process that can be subdivided into intrinsic and extrinsic components. Intrinsic aging, a form of irreversible tissue degeneration, is characterized histologically by flattening of the epidermal-dermal interface, loss of dermal papillae, and dermal atrophy [1]. In addition, elastic tissue is lost, and type I and III collagen production are markedly decreased. Intrinsic aging is

L. E. de la Caridad Hernandez (✉) · F. J. Eckembrecher · D. G. Eckembrecher · N. Mohsin · A. Vander Does · K. Nouri
Dr Phillip Frost Department of Dermatology and Cutaneous Surgery, Miller School of Medicine, University of Miami, 1600 NW 10th Ave, Miami, FL 33136, USA
e-mail: loren.hernandez@med.miami.edu

S. Uppal · M. Hakimi
The Kimberly and Eric J. Waldman Department of Dermatology, Mount Sinai, New York, NY, USA

K. Nouri (ed.), *Telemedicine and Technological Advances in Dermatology*,
https://doi.org/10.1007/978-3-031-69091-4_24

also distinguished by a lower epidermal turnover rate and less melanocyte activity [2, 3]. Extrinsic aging is influenced by environmental factors, including photoaging from UV radiation exposure, but can also be affected by other factors such as cigarette smoking and gravity. It is characterized by the presence of elastosis secondary to degeneration of dermal tissue, resulting in an increased production and deposition of elastin [1, 3, 4]. As a result, the skin becomes more lax and there is a redistribution of subcutaneous fat as well as soft-tissue volume loss [3]. Recent advancements aim to target both intrinsic and extrinsic causes of the aging process to promote aesthetic rejuvenation.

2 Biotechnology

Biotechnology involves creating products through genetic engineering, such as recombinant DNA technology, and/or fermentation processes with a wide array of microorganisms including bacteria, yeast, and fungi. Some of the products include ingredients such as kojic acid, hyaluronic acid, resveratrol, human epidermal growth factor, stem cells, enzymes, and peptides. This section will discuss the applications of these ingredients in cosmetic dermatology.

2.1 Kojic Acid

Kojic acid (5-hydroxy-2-hydroxymethyl-4-pyranone) is produced from the microbial fermentation of fungal species, such as *A. fumigatus*, *A. flavus* and *A. candidus* [5]. Kojic acid is naturally produced by the species of Acetobacter, Penicillium, and a variety of acetic acid bacilli [6]. It is commonly used for hyperpigmentation as a skin lightener in cosmeceuticals [7]. There are many causes of hyperpigmentation such as endocrine, nutritional, and metabolic abnormalities, medications (i.e. oral contraceptive pills, chlorpromazine and hydroxychloroquine), genetic factors, skin cancer, and injury [8]. Nonetheless, the root cause of hyperpigmentation is abnormal melanin production. Ultraviolet (UV) radiation stimulates the production of proopiomelanocortin (POMC) a precursor of both alpha-melanocyte stimulating hormone (α-MSH) and adrenocorticotropic hormone (ACTH) [9]. ACTH and α-MSH are agonists of the melanocortin 1 receptor (MC1R), a G-protein coupled receptor located on melanocytes [10]. It is also thought that fibroblasts may contribute to hyperpigmentation through a variety of extracellular signaling pathways involved in the synthesis of melanin. Melanin is derived from L-tyrosine via the enzyme tyrosinase, which converts L-tyrosine to L-3,4-dihydroxyphenylalanine (L-DOPA) and L-DOPA into dopaquinone [6]. There are two primary types of melanin pigment that contribute to skin pigmentation—pheomelanin and eumelanin—and both are produced from L-tyrosine [9, 11]. Tyrosinase contains a copper ion in its active site, which is captured by kojic acid, inhibiting tyrosinase activity and decreasing melanin production [6].

Kojic acid can be used in the treatment of hyperpigmentation disorders such as melasma, solar lentigos, post-inflammatory hyperpigmentation, and hyperestrogenic states, such as pregnancy, that are known to affect skin pigmentation [6]. Melasma, also referred to as the "mask of pregnancy" affects between 15 and 50% of pregnant patients and presents as gray-brown macules predominantly on the face [12]. In a split-face study, the efficacy of kojic acid was assessed in four patients in the treatment of facial melasma. In this study, a topical gel containing 2% kojic acid, 10% glycolic acid, and 2% hydroquinone was applied to one half of a subject's face and another topical gel containing 10% glycolic acid and 2% hydroquinone was applied to the other half. The topical gels were applied for a total of 12 weeks and results were assessed through clinical evaluation, self-assessment questionnaires, and photographs every 4 weeks. Topical kojic acid was found to clear more than half of lesions in 60% of subjects treated with the topical gel containing kojic acid cleared [13]. Kojic acid has the potential to benefit patients with melasma, particularly those who have a poor response or intolerance of topical hydroquinone. However, studies comparing topical kojic acid and hydroquinone have mixed results. In another study, topical creams containing hydroquinone and kojic acid were compared in patients with facial melasma. Approximately 60 patients with facial melasma were randomized to receive either 4% hydroquinone cream or 0.75% kojic acid cream with 2.5% vitamin C. Subjects were instructed to apply creams daily in the evening, and were evaluated for clinical response at 4-week intervals for a total of 12 weeks using the Melasma Area and Severity Index (MASI) score. Interestingly, subjects receiving 4% hydroquinone cream experienced statistically significant changes in MASI scores that were greater than those in patients receiving 0.75% kojic acid cream [14]. Nonetheless, topical kojic acid has the potential to treat other disorders of localized hyperpigmentation, such as post-inflammatory hyperpigmentation secondary to atopic dermatitis, lichen planus and acne. Kojic acid can be used in conjunction with other topical agents, such as hydroquinone and glycolic acid, for a synergistic effect [15, 16]. An important adverse effect associated with topical kojic acid is contact dermatitis, characterized by erythema, pruritus, irritation, and inflammation of the skin [17–19]. The Cosmetic Ingredient Review (CIR) Expert Panel, however, has concluded that kojic acid preparations are safe for use up to a concentration of 1% [20]. The effects of hyperpigmentation of the skin can be undesirable to patients and produce negative perception of one's self-image, resulting in depression and anxiety, thus treatment is often critical [21].

Kojic acid can also be helpful in treating wrinkles through its ability to scavenge reactive oxygen species (ROS), which can be deleterious to the skin [22]. In addition to hyperpigmentation, kojic acid has been shown to be fungistatic against the pathogenic yeast, Cryptococcus neoformans, due to its ability to inhibit melanin, a necessary component in Cryptococcal infections [19].

2.2 *Hyaluronic Acid*

Hyaluronic acid (HA) is a non-sulfated glycosaminoglycan (GAG) present in the extracellular matrix of the skin dermis, vitreous fluid of the eye, umbilical cord, joint synovial fluid, smooth connective tissue, and intervertebral discs [23]. As a GAG, HA contains repeating disaccharide units of N-acetyl-D-glucosamine and D-glucuronic acid, which contributes to its structural stability and ability to hold 1000 times its weight of water [24, 25]. HA is versatile and highly biocompatible, biodegradable, viscous, viscoelastic, and mucoadhesive [26]. Because of these properties, HA is able to hydrate the skin and improve skin elasticity and appearance, which is why it is commonly found in a variety of cosmetic formulations, such as emulsions, gels, and serums [25]. Multiple human clinical studies have evaluated the efficacy of HA in the treatment of facial wrinkles.

HA is also a component of the most common dermal fillers [27, 28]. Dermal fillers are used for facial contouring and the correction of facial volume loss and facial wrinkles [29]. HA dermal fillers are also commonly used to treat atrophic acne scars, although studies assessing their efficacy in this setting are limited [30, 31]. HA dermal fillers are safe and effective, and the effects of HA fillers can be easily reversed by the enzyme hyaluronidase. Hyaluronidase is often utilized in cases where filler has been injected too superficially causing blue discoloration [32]. There are a variety of HA fillers that are differentiated by degree of molecular cross-linking, size of HA molecules, and HA concentration, and optimized for certain anatomopathological regions based on these properties [27, 28].

HA originates from microbial fermentation of the Streptococcus species [33]. However, given the pathogenic potential of this organism, HA purification remains of utmost importance. As a result, microorganisms have been genetically modified to produce endotoxin-free HA without the potential for pathogenesis [26].

Injectable HA fillers are contraindicated in patients with a history of bleeding disorders, hypersensitivity or severe allergic reactions to HA (including anaphylaxis), hypersensitivity reactions to gram-positive bacterial proteins from bacterial sources, and hypersensitivity reactions to lidocaine. HA injections into "off-label" sites is also a contraindication. Because the safety of HA fillers in pregnant or breastfeeding patients has not been established, administration of fillers in this special population is not recommended [32]. Topical HA, however, is considered to be safe in both pregnant and breastfeeding patients.

Adverse reactions to HA fillers can be divided into immediate effects, which occur about 1–2 weeks after the injection, and long-term effects, which occur several weeks to months after the injection. Local injection site reactions, such as pain, swelling, tenderness, and bruising are common immediate reactions that occur with injectable HA derivatives [34]. Application of firm pressure and ice-packs before and/or after the procedure can help minimize post-injection swelling or bruising. Post-injection reactions are typically mild and resolve in less than one week [35]. Patients taking anticoagulant and anti-platelet medications (i.e. aspirin, clopidogrel, warfarin, dabigatran, enoxaparin, ticlopidine, and dipyridamole) in the prevention of embolic and thrombotic phenomenon, such as patients with coagulopathies and atrial fibrillation, should not discontinue their medications prior to receiving fillers and counseled on the increased risk of bruising and bleeding post-injection. Physicians should consider assessing and monitoring the INR in patients taking warfarin and receiving regular HA injections. An INR greater than 3 is considered supratherapeutic in most cases and may warrant postponing or delaying injections [36, 37]. It is recommended that patients discontinue NSAIDs 5 days prior to the injection of dermal fillers and 7 days for aspirin, if it is not medically necessary [38]. Infections are also a possible but rare adverse effect with dermal fillers.

The CDC recently reported that swelling at or near the site of dermal filler injections may occur following administration of the COVID-19 mRNA vaccine [39]. As this effect is often temporary, HA fillers are not a contraindication to receiving the COVID-19 vaccination. It is advised that patients receiving injectable dermal fillers contact their physician if they develop swelling at or near sites of filler injection after receiving the COVID-19 vaccination [39].

Unless patients develop severe adverse reactions, patient monitoring is not required after using products with HA derivatives and receiving HA dermal fillers. Patients should be advised that the effects of HA treatments are temporary, as results may last for at least 8–16 weeks depending on the exact filler used [30, 32].

2.3 *Resveratrol*

Resveratrol is a polyphenolic phytoalexin naturally found in variety of plants such as the skin of red grapes, berries, and cocoa [40]. It is also a prominent component of traditional Chinese and Japanese medicine and is available in topical formulations and oral herbal supplements [41].

In plants, resveratrol serves as a defense mechanism against stressors, such as bacterial and fungal infections and UV radiation [42]. It has also been shown to have anti-angiogenic, anti-inflammatory, anti-microbial and antioxidant properties [43]. While resveratrol exists in both trans- and cis-isomers, the trans-isomer, 3,5,4′-trihydroxy-trans-stilbene, is the biologically active isomer [44]. Upon exposure to UV radiation, oxygen, and fluctuations in pH, the trans-isomer converts to the cis-isomer, decreasing its activity and bioavailability [45]. Given that resveratrol can isomerize into an inactive form depending on environmental conditions, it is vital to produce a stable formulation of the trans-isomer for maximal efficacy. In cosmetics, resveratrol serves as an antioxidant and is effective in neutralizing ROS by decreasing the expression of NF-kB and AP-1 transcription factors. Through this mechanism, resveratrol reduces oxidative damage and photoaging of the skin [43]. Resveratrol is also an anti-inflammatory agent that can bind to estrogen receptors (ER-α and ER-β), downregulating IL-6—a pro-inflammatory cytokine—and stimulating type I and II collagen production [43].

One study sought to evaluate the efficacy of a 1% resveratrol, 0.5% baicalin, and 1% vitamin E proprietary blend in the treatment of mild to moderately photodamaged skin. Patients were assessed with clinical assessments and ultrasound measurements of the periorbital area. The study found a statistically significant improvement in skin firmness, fine lines and wrinkles, skin elasticity, skin laxity, radiance, skin roughness, and hyperpigmentation after 12 weeks of cream use compared to baseline. Ultrasound measurements found an 18.9% improvement in dermal thickness [46]. Given that the resveratrol in a mixture of three different ingredients, it is difficult to attribute the study results solely to resveratrol.

Clinical and in vivo studies have also shown that resveratrol and its analogs are effective as skin-lightening agents [47]. Trans-resveratrol is produced via biotechnology using the yeasts *Pichia pastoris* and *Saccharomyces cerevisiae*, which are efficacious in the production of resveratrol due to their ability to produce large quantities of resveratrol rapidly [43, 48]. Resveratrol is currently incorporated into a variety of topical serums, creams, and gels. Patients can incorporate topical resveratrol into their skincare regimen to improve the appearance of fine lines, skin texture, hyperpigmentation, and overall radiance. Patients are recommended to apply resveratrol serum or moisturizer after cleansing the skin or applying toner at least once a day. Table 1 lists commercially available serums and creams containing resveratrol.

Side effects of topical resveratrol have not been studied extensively. Documented effects of resveratrol have been attributed to its oral formulation, and include nephrotoxicity and gastrointestinal effects [49, 50]. Ingestion of resveratrol has also been documented to enhance the anticoagulant effects of warfarin and increase circulating levels of sex hormone binding globulin, similar to estrogen [51–54].

Growth factors are secreted molecules that induce cellular responses by activating signaling cascades responsible for cellular growth, division, and/or differentiation [55]. Growth factors can bind to receptors at the cell surface or intracellularly

Table 1 Currently available serums and creams containing resveratrol

The Ordinary Resveratrol 3% + Ferulic Acid 3%
Typology 3% Ferulic Acid + 3% Resveratrol Antioxidant Serum
Caudalie Resveratrol-Lift Instant Firming Serum
Caudalie Resveratrol-Lift Firming Cashmere Cream
SkinCeuticals Resveratrol B E
Resvera-F Antioxidant Serum S12 with 5% Resveratrol and 3% Ferulic Acid
Versed on The Rise Firming Serum—peptide blend and resveratrol
Tracie Martyn Firming Serum
HydroPeptide LumaPro-C Skin Brightening Pigment Corrector
iS Clinical Hydra-Intensive Cooling Masque
Allies of Skin Mandelic Pigmentation Corrector Night Serum
Estee Lauder Advanced Night Repair Intense Rest Concentrate
Philosophy Anti-Wrinkle Miracle Worker + Line-Correcting Moisturizer

depending on their specific molecular properties. Important growth factors secreted include transforming growth factor-beta (TGF-β), granulocyte–macrophage colony-stimulating factor (GM-CSF), vascular endothelial growth factor (VEGF), epidermal growth factor (EGF), and platelet-derived growth factor (PDGF) [56]. Growth factors have been studied extensively in the context of wound healing, given their vital role all phases of wound healing [56]. In the first phases—the inflammatory phase—PDGF and TGF-β attract macrophages and neutrophils to the site of injury. During the proliferative phase, macrophages attract fibroblasts to the area of injury and the fibroblasts produce a collagen network [56]. Macrophages also secrete two enzymes at the wound site: TGF-β, which promotes fibrosis, and EGF, which stimulates fibroblasts to produce collagenase [57]. Collagenases are critical components of wound healing, and are involved in maintaining a clean and well-vascularized wound bed that can then successfully progress through the stages of wound healing [58]. Collagenases are also involved early in the proliferative phase with debridement of devitalized tissue from the wound bed, an essential component of wound bed preparation [58]. Given their ability to assist with wound healing, growth factors are being utilized in the cosmetics industry for the purpose of skin rejuvenation [57]. Topical and subcutaneous growth factors are formulations that are commercially available [59]. Topical application of growth factors has been shown to promote the proliferation of fibroblasts, keratinocytes, and the extracellular matrix, and reduce signs of skin photoaging [60]. However, penetration of topical growth factors is limited by its large molecular size (15,000 Da), which prevents it from effectively traversing the stratum corneum [61].

Commercial topical serums and creams have incorporated collagenases with their formulation, and often combined with other skincare ingredients, such as hyaluronic acid and retinol. Perricone MD®, a popular cosmeceutical producer, offers a facial serum (Perricone MD® High Potency Growth Factor Firming & Lifting Serum) and eye serum (Perricone MD® High Potency Growth Factor Firming & Lifting Eye Serum) with polyamine growth factors. In Perricone's clinical study with 38 female subjects, Perricone's facial serum improved skin redness, radiance, and brightness in 89% of patients, the appearance of skin tone in 78% of patients, and skin firmness in 76% of patients after 56 days. In another of Perricone's clinical studies, the efficacy of Perricone's growth factor eye serum was assessed in 33 female subjects. The eye serum improved skin hydration, and reduced the appearance of deep wrinkles, crow's feet, lines, and wrinkles in all patients after 4 weeks eye serum application. In addition, 88% of patients noticed a reduction of under-eye puffiness and improvement in skin elasticity.

The adverse effects of topically applied growth factors have been studied in the context of its use in wound healing. No adverse reactions or toxic effects have been recorded by the direct application of growth factors on skin wounds [62–65]. However, there are no studies that evaluate the adverse effects of topical growth factors for the purpose of anti-aging. Other possible adverse effects associated with topical application of any cream, serum, and ointment include erythema, edema, discomfort, and pruritus. Patients are advised to discontinue these products in the event that an adverse effect occurs.

3 Enzymes

Enzymes work by catalyzing the rate of biochemical reactions and are highly specific for their substrate. Without enzymes, most cellular reactions would not occur at a fast enough pace for organ function and sustaining life. Current enzymes used in aesthetics include superoxide dismutase, proteases, and DNA repair enzymes.

3.1 Superoxide Dismutase (SOD)

Superoxide dismutase (SOD), also referred to as mitochondrial superoxide dismutase 2 (SOD2 or MnSOD), is a metalloenzyme that acts as an antioxidant against ROS. SOD2 reduces oxidative stress by converting superoxide anions to hydrogen peroxide, which are then converted to water and oxygen by glutathione peroxidase and catalase [66, 67]. The free radical theory of aging postulates that aging is a result of the accumulation of damage due to ROS [68]. However, there have been multiple studies that contradict this, and many suggest that aging is secondary to cumulative damage from many types of stimuli [69–71]. UV-radiation [72, 73] and keratinocyte-mediated release of IL-1α, IL-1β, and TNF-α [74] are known upregulators of SOD2 in human fibroblasts. Because SOD is susceptible to physical and chemical instability, SOD mimetics and conjugates have been studied and shown to increase SOD stability and longevity in vivo [75, 76].

Currently, SOD is an ingredient in topical serums and mists, and has been marketed as an anti-aging treatment. In vitro studies have shown that SOD1 protects human keratinocytes from UVB radiation by reducing the ability of UVB to induce keratinocyte apoptosis [77]. SOD is also thought to help breakdown and soften scar tissue, accelerating wound healing [77]. Because safety studies of SOD in humans are limited, use of SOD is currently not recommended for women who are pregnant and/or breast-feeding.

3.2 Proteases

Proteases perform proteolysis by cleaving peptide bonds that hold together proteins. Proteins are broken down into polypeptides and amino acids via proteolysis. There is a great biodiversity of proteases that play key physiological roles and are found in all organisms. Most enzymes are subdivided into the following six groups based on the amino acid in the enzymes' active site: cysteine proteases, serine proteases, threonine proteases, aspartate proteases, glutamic acid proteases, and metalloproteinases [78]. Dermatologically, proteases have been utilized for the debridement of necrotic tissue, particularly in the setting of burns and pressure ulcers [79, 80]. Proteases are also used in cosmetics as they promote skin exfoliation through desquamation of the stratum corneum and enhanced the absorption of topical serums and ointments [81]. Proteases are also thought to ameliorate the effects of endogenous, pro-inflammatory proteins that interfere with adequate wound healing [82, 83]. Examples of proteases used commercially in cosmetics include papain, bromelain, and chymotrypsin. Bromelain, specifically, is a powerful sensitizing substance and sensitization that usually follows its inhalation so use should be cautioned in patients presenting with allergic reactions to foods that may cross-react with the enzyme [84, 85]. Proteases can be incorporated into facial cleaners and topical formulations, such as moisturizers and serums, and optimize moisturization and barrier repair effects more than standard skincare products [86]. A 3-protease blend of bromelain, ficin, and actinidin has been incorporated into a moisturizing lotion and a cleansing wash, and in vitro studies have shown that the blend can decrease the effects of pro-inflammatory cytokines, substance P, and metalloproteinases, thereby decreasing cutaneous inflammation [86]. By reducing inflammation, protease-containing formulations have the potential to become adjunctive therapy for patients with inflammatory dermatoses.

Clinicians must also take into consideration the non-protease ingredients in the vehicle formulation when advising patients about protease-containing products. Safety, efficacy, and cosmetic outcomes may vary between different products depending on the vehicle used. With newer products entering the market, further clinical studies will need to be conducted to measure clinical outcomes and elucidate changes in the skin microenvironment that may occur after treatment with these protease-containing products [86].

3.3 DNA Repair Enzymes

DNA repair enzymes, such as photolyase, T4 endonuclease, UV endonuclease, and DNA glycosylase, have also been studied for cosmetic purposes. Photolyases are enzymes that utilize blue light from visible light to eliminate pyrimidine dimers and reverse DNA mutations induced by UV radiation [87]. As flavoenzymes, photolyases require flavin cofactors to absorb UV-radiation and act as catalysts, transferring energy to DNA to break cyclobutene-type pyrimidine dimers (CPD). Flavin reactions, in the setting of DNA repair, have been demonstrated in both in vitro and in vivo studies [88]. Given that exposure to UV radiation contributes to the pathogenesis of skin cancers and skin photoaging, photolyases have the potential for therapeutic benefit in aesthetic rejuvenation and skin cancer management. In one study, photolyases were found to decrease the number of actinic keratoses (AK) in sun-exposed skin. Another study showed that sunscreen with and without photolyase reduced CPDs by 93% and 62%, respectively, after one week of UV exposure [89]. Other studies have shown that sunscreen containing photolyases—encapsulated in liposomes that transport the enzymes into keratinocytes—reduced both the number of existing AKs and the appearance of new lesions [90]. Application of DNA repair enzymes—photolyase, UV endonuclease, and OGG1 endonuclease encapsulated in liposomes—twice a day over the course of 4 weeks has also been shown to reduce

Table 2 Commercially sunscreens containing photolyases in the United States

Product	Company	SPF	DNA repair ingredients
Neova Everyday® Facial Fluid Broad Spectrum SPF 44	Pharma Cosmetics, Oradell, New Jersey, United States	44	Liposomal encapsulated photolyase
Neova Active® Optimal Defense Broad Spectrum SPF 43 Water Resistant [80 min] [166]		43	
Neova Silc Sheer 2.0® Photo Finish Tint Broad Spectrum SPF 40 Water Resistant [80 Minutes]		40	
Neova Smart Moisture® Daily Defense Broad Spectrum SPF 30		30	Encapsulated photolyase
Priori Tetra fx251® Sunscreen Lotion Broad Spectrum SPF 55	PRIORI Skincare, San Diego, California, United States	55	DNA enzyme complex

the appearance of crow's feet [91]. Currently, photolyases are incorporated into topical sunscreens and creams for their ability to reverse UV-induced skin damage and photoaging. Per the American Academy of Dermatology (AAD) guidelines, sunscreen should meet the following criteria to maximize these benefits: have broad spectrum coverage, offer a minimum of SPF 30 protection, and be water resistant [92]. Table 2 lists commercially available sunscreens containing photolyases in the United States.

4 Stem Cells

Stem cells are undifferentiated cells that carry the potential to become specialized cells in the human body and have the ability of self-renewal [93]. Stem cells have been implicated in the aging process, as UV-radiation has been shown to induce a decrease in epidermal stem cell function and shorten telomeres [94]. Human stem cells can be divided into either embryonic stem cells or adult stem cells, based on their degree of developmental potency. As a stem cell becomes more specialized, developmental potency is reduced, which means that a stem cell (i.e. unipotent stem cell) is not able to differentiate into as many types of cells as other types of stem cells (i.e. pluripotent stem cells) [93]. Totipotent cells carry the highest differentiation potential and are able to differentiate into both embryonic and extra-embryonic structures, such as the placenta. Pluripotent stem cells, in contrast, can differentiate into cells of all germ layers, but not extra-embryonic structures. Examples of pluripotent stem cells include embryonic stem cells and induced pluripotent stem cells [93]. Multipotent stem cells have a narrower spectrum of differentiation potential than both totipotent and pluripotent stem cells and can differentiate into discrete cells of specific cell lineages [93]. Similarly, oligopotent stem cells uphold the ability to differentiate into select cell types, and an example includes myeloid stem cells. Unipotent stem cells have the narrowest differentiation potential and can only become one cell type [93].

Similar to humans, plants are equipped with a robust mechanism for tissue regeneration and repair when injury has occurred. Plant stem cells, however, are unique in that they are entirely totipotent and have robust plasticity [95, 96]. Plant cells are able to initiate cell division for mostly any tissue, and have been shown to regenerate tissues, organs and entire plants though a process of cell dedifferentiation and subsequent differentiation [96]. Studies have shown that stem cells derived from plants are UV-protective, stimulate cellular DNA repair, regulate fibroblast growth and collagen synthesis, assist with repair of epidermal damage, and increase epidermal flexibility [96, 97]. Plant stem cells are currently being artificially produced via in vitro cell cultures through a micropropagation method for cosmetic purposes. Mibelle AG Biochemistry (Switzerland) has produced plant stem cell extracts from the plant species, *Argania spinosa* (PhytoCellTec™; Argan, Switzerland), *Saponaria pumila* (PhytoCellTec™ nunatak®; Buchs, Switzerland), *Vitis vinifera* (PhytoCellTec™; Solar Vitis, Switzerland), and *Uttwiler Spätlauber* (PhytoCellTec™; Thugaru, Switzerland), a rare subtype of the Swiss apple or *Malus domestica* [97]. Cultured apple stem cells from *Malus domestica* (PhytoCellTec™) have been shown to reduce the appearance of facial wrinkles in prior studies [98]. Other plant stem cells that have been investigated include: *Lycopersicon esculentum* from tomatoes, *Syringa vulgaris*, *Coffea bengalensis*, *Nicotiana sylvestris*, *Zingiber officinale* from ginger leaves, and Citrustem™ from oranges. *Lycopersicon esculentum* has been shown to have anti-inflammatory and antioxidant properties. *Syringa vulgaris* (lilac leaf) stem cell extract has been shown to have anti-inflammatory and antioxidant effects due its essential ingredient, verbascosides, which is a phenylpropanoid glycoside [99]. *Coffea bengalensis* and *Nicotiana sylvestris* are species that have been shown to stimulate fibroblasts to produce collagen, which in turn leads to skin regeneration [100, 101]. *Zingiber officinale* is a plant species that has been shown to improve skin texture by decreasing sebum production and reducing the appearance of skin pores [100]. Finally, Citrustem™, which contains *Citrus aurantium dulcis* derived from orange peels, has demonstrated the ability to renew overall skin appearance by enhancing skin elasticity, reducing the appearance of wrinkles, and increasing collagen synthesis [99, 102].

Mesenchymal stromal cells (MSCs), either fetal- or adult-associated cells, are the most frequently used form of stem cells for aesthetic purposes [103]. In an 8 week placebo-controlled clinical trial evaluating the effectiveness of topical amniotic membrane stem cell-condition media (AMSC-CM) and microneedling (for transdermal drug delivery) found that AMSC-CM was associated with improvement in photoaging parameters, including the pores, wrinkles, spot polarized, spot UV, and skin tone [104]. Another study evaluating the efficacy of topical human embryonic stem cells with microneedling demonstrated a greater improvement in size and appearance of wrinkles and pores after five treatments compared to placebo [104] In these studies, post-treatment safety monitoring was not necessary, and adverse events were mild and only reported by a small number of participants [103, 104].

Recent studies have also assessed the efficacy of stem cells therapy with laser treatment for skin rejuvenation and the treatment of acne scars [58, 104]. Defensins, which activate the body's dormant stem cells to generate new epidermal cells, are also being studied for skin rejuvenation [32, 58]. Studies on defensin-containing products and stem cell therapy combined with laser therapy have reported positive results. However, sample sizes in these trials were small, reducing the power of these studies and increasing the margin of error [105, 106].

While the effects of stem cell therapies in skin rejuvenation appears to be promising, more research is needed before this treatment can be clinically recommended. In July 2020, the U.S. Food and Drug Administration (FDA) issued a consumer alert to warn consumers about illegally marketed regenerative medicine products—stem cells, fat-derived cells, umbilical cord blood and/or cord blood stem cells, and amniotic fluids—that may pose risks to patients, given the lack of FDA-regulated trials and human safety data [107]. The FDA has received reports of blindness, tumor formation, and infections due to the use of these unapproved products [107]. Currently, hematopoietic progenitor cells are the only FDA-approved stem cell products, derived from the umbilical cord blood and used in patients with hematopoietic system disorders [32].

5 Peptides

Peptides are proteins that are involved in a wide array of physiological processes, such as growth, reproduction, homeostasis, and immunity [108]. Peptides can be categorized into the following subtypes: signal peptides, carrier peptides, enzyme-inhibiting peptides, and neurotransmitter-inhibiting peptides [109]. Signal peptides, such as matricins, act as cellular messengers to stimulate neocollagenesis, thereby giving the skin a firmer appearance [110, 111]. Commonly used signal peptides are Palmitoyl Tripeptide-1, Palmitoyl hexapeptide-12, and Palmitoyl tetrapeptide-7. Palmitoyl Tripeptide-1 stimulates neocollagenesis in human fibroblast cultures and prevents collagen degradation caused by exposure to UVA radiation [112]. Palmitoyl hexapeptide-12 has been shown to stimulate the production of extracellular matrix molecules, collagen, elastin, fibronectin, and glycosaminoglycans (GAGs). Palmitoyl Tetrapeptide-7, a fragment of immunoglobulin-G, has been shown to decrease IL-6 secretion and inflammation upon exposure to UVB radiation [113]. A combination of Palmitoyl Tetrapeptide-7 and Palmitoyl Tripeptide-1, Maytrixyl®-3000, can induce fibroblast activity and promote new collagen production [111]. Other signaling peptides include palmitoyl hexapeptide-12, palmitoyl pentapeptide-4, palmitoyl tripeptide-5, lipospondin, hexapeptide-11, tripeptide-10 citrulline, PKEK, GEKG, and SA1-III.

Carrier peptides, such as copper tripeptide, are a peptide subtype that function by stabilizing trace elements within enzymes, thereby promoting enzymatic activity and wound healing. Copper tripeptides are currently incorporated in topical moisturizers and serums for their anti-aging and skin renewal effect and their potential to stimulate hair growth [111]. Multiple studies have investigated the efficacy of copper peptide as an anti-aging ingredient. The application of a facial cream with glycyl-l-histidyl-l-lysine(GHK)-copper to the face of 71 women for 12 weeks was found to reduce the appearance of fine lines, the depth of wrinkles, and the extent of skin laxity while increasing skin density and thickness [114]. Another study found that the application of GHK-copper to skin located on the thigh for 12 weeks resulted in improved collagen production in 70% of subjects, in contrast to 40% and 50% of subjects treated with retinoic acid and vitamin C cream, respectively [115].

Pentapeptide-3, an antagonist of the acetylcholine receptor, is an example of a neurotransmitter-inhibiting peptide that acts to promote muscle relaxation by blocking binding of acetylcholine at the post-synaptic membrane [111]. Pentapeptide-3 has been reported to decrease wrinkle size and skin roughness in in vitro and in vivo studies [116]. Other neurotransmitter-inhibiting peptides include acetyl hexapeptide-3, pentapeptide-18, tripeptide-3, and acetyl octapeptide-1/-3.

Collagen peptides have also been marketed antiaging products, however, most studies have failed to show any clinically significant benefit with use of oral collagen peptides [117–120]. Clinicians should advise patients who are using or considering using these products that they are categorized as dietary supplements and are, therefore, FDA-regulated. Furthermore, patients using these products should ensure that they have been verified by third-party organizations, such as the USP or NSF, who will verify that supplements truly contain the ingredients on label [103].

Generally, no monitoring is required after using peptide-containing products. While no significant side effects have been reported in studies, it is important to note that the safety and efficacy of peptides is dependent on the vehicle formulation, which affect peptide stability and product delivery. Because vehicle formulations vary greatly between products, further research is required to assess the effect of vehicle formulation on peptide stability, absorption, and activity on biological targets [121]. In summary, although studies of peptides have reported favorable cosmetic outcomes, there is insufficient scientific data to support clinical use for antiaging purposes.

6 Sculptra® Aesthetic

Sculptra® Aesthetic, also known as Poly-L-lactic acid, was first approved by the FDA in 2004 for the treatment of facial lipoatrophy in patients with human immunodeficiency virus (HIV) [122]. As of 2009, Sculptra® Aesthetic was approved by the FDA for use in facial wrinkles and nasolabial folds. Specifically, Sculptra® is indicated for use in patients who are immunocompetent for the correction of nasolabial contour deficiencies and facial wrinkles through a cross-hatch injection technique. It is, however, used off-label for other anatomic areas, including the hands, cheeks, neck, thighs, buttocks, and chest wall [123]. Injection with Sculptra® has been shown assist with the restoration of facial fullness and volume over time, giving patients a more youthful appearance [124, 125] In contrast to other dermal fillers, Sculptra®

is considered a stimulatory filler in that it creates its effect through neocollagenesis—the production of novel collagen—when injected [126]. Upon initial injection of Sculptra®, there is a temporary augmentation at the site of injection, secondary to reconstitution of injected material and tissue edema. Soon thereafter, particles of poly-L-lactic acid are phagocytosed by macrophages, causing a local inflammatory response that leads to the conversion of poly-L-lactic acid into monomeric lactic acid. Monomeric lactic acid is subsequently broken down into water and carbon dioxide, inducing production of type I collagen [124]. On average, 3 treatments of Sculptra® over a few months are required to achieve optimal results. Patients should be counseled that changes are seen gradually and may last for at least two years.

Patients who have a history of keloid formation, hypertrophic scarring, or are allergic to any ingredient present in Sculptra® are unable to receive treatment. Because safety has not been established in patients under the age of 18 years old, pregnant patients, and lactating or breastfeeding patients, Sculptra® is contraindicated in these patient populations. Sculptra® should also be avoided in areas of the skin with active inflammation, such as skin affected by acne, cysts, rashes, or urticaria, or infection present.

Other side effects of Sculptra® include injection-side reactions that are associated with the injection of poly-L-lactic acid. Signs and symptoms indicative of injection-site reactions include erythema, edema, bruising, and pain at the injection site. Injection-site reactions are usually transient and resolve spontaneously [127–130]. If Sculptra® is inadvertently injected into a patient's vessel, vascular embolization can occur, which may lead to tissue ischemia, and/or infarction [131]. More serious but rare events include tissue necrosis, blindness, and cerebral ischemia or cerebral hemorrhage leading to a stroke. Infection at the injection site is another possible complication secondary to disruption of the epidermis/dermis, thus it vital to appropriately cleanse the injection site to prevent infection [132]. Other adverse effects include inflammatory reactions leading to the formation of papules, nodules, and granulomas. Papules and nodules can occur several weeks after injection of poly-L-lactic acid, and typically do not cause symptoms or progress in size. Furthermore, they remain the same size until they are treated, resorbed, or removed [122]. Papules may be surgically excised, however, patients should be counseled on the possibly of scar development secondary to the procedure [133, 134]. If patients wish to temporarily improve the appearance of papules or nodules, HA dermal filler can also be injected into the site [135].

Studies have shown that the incidence of papule and nodule formation after injection of Sculptra® ranges from 6 to 44% [128–130, 136–138]. Papules and nodules tend to occur more frequently around the periocular and perioral regions [139]. The location of papules and nodules may also suggest their etiology. If the Sculptra® is placed too superficially, visible, well-defined papules will be present. If Sculptra® is placed too deep, such as in or through musculature, nodules will arise from product containment within muscle fibers. The presence of diffuse papules and/or nodules may suggest improper reconstitution. As filler material is freeze dried, reconstitution with 4–5 mL of sterile water and 1 mL lidocaine with epinephrine is recommended to allow for efficient and uncomplicated injection of Sculptra®. The presence of crystals on the periphery of the vial that that do not disappear with adding water and shaking the product vial as well as poor product suspension of product suggest improper reconstitution [135]. The risk of developing papules and nodules can be minimized by ensuring adequate product reconstitution as well as utilization of proper injection technique and placement of product [122, 140]. It has been shown that increased product hydration time and reconstitution volume, greater duration of time between treatments, and clinical expertise about injection sites and injection depth for the desired effect can improve clinical outcomes [141].

True granulomas are a form of chronic inflammation and their incidence is less than 0.1% [142–144]. Unlike papules or nodules, granulomas arise months or years after injection of product. Granulomas have the potential to grow over time and persist, but are also able to regress and resolve spontaneously [122]. Because granulomas have poorly defined borders, surgical excision is not a recommended treatment option. In addition, surgical removal of granulomas has been shown to be associated with the formation of abscesses, fistulas, and scars [122]. Instead, steroid injections (intramuscular, intralesional, or systemic), with or without the addition of immune-modulating agents, may be used for treatment [122]. Other treatment options include intralesional injection of 5-fluorouracil with or without betamethasone or acetonide [134]. Intense pulsed light is an excellent option for vascular granulomas, defined by the presence of capillaries [122].

7 Platelet Rich Plasma (PRP)

Platelet rich plasma (PRP) is plasma highly concentrated with platelets derived from a patient's blood via centrifugation. The process of plasma centrifugation concentrates the growth factors and cytokines present in the alpha-granules of platelets [145]. The preparation of PRP varies slightly in published literature, but the fundamental steps of PRP preparation are as follows: blood is drawn into a tube often treated with an anticoagulant, blood is centrifuged and platelets are activated via a chemical agent (i.e. calcium chloride, bovine, or autologous thrombin), and platelets coagulate creating a gel-like substance from which PRP is extracted. Because there is no standardized harvest protocol in place for harvesting, platelet concentration can vary with different users and treatments. A minimum platelet concentration of 1 million/mL, however, has been found to be effective therapeutically [146].

PRP has been shown to have desirable cosmetic effects by stimulating the processes of neocollagenesis, angiogenesis, and adipogenesis [147]. Many small studies on the use of PRP for skin rejuvenation have shown promising cosmetic results, including increased skin firmness and smoothness and reduction in wrinkle count [103, 148]. PRP has also been associated with favorable cosmetic outcomes in patients with conditions including acne, androgenic alopecia, psoriasis, and chronic vitiligo [148]. It can improve the appearance of both acne and traumatic scars by activating the regenerative skin process [149, 150]. PRP can also be used in the treatment of androgenic alopecia, where it is thought induce the differentiation of stem cells in hair follicles, promote angiogenesis, increase fibroblast survival in the dermal papilla, and activate anti-apoptotic pathways [147, 151–153]. PRP has been shown to have synergistic effects when combined with lasers and microneedling, and it is thought that these effects are due to enhanced absorption of PRP through disturbances in the skin barrier [147]. Furthermore, application of PRP after treatment with CO_2 or erbium fractional resurfacing has also showed positive cosmetic results, including increased fibroblasts, improved skin elasticity, and thickened collagen bundles [154]. In contrast, areas only treated with laser resurfacing did not undergo these changes [154]. However, larger randomized, controlled trials are warranted before the benefits and limitations of PRP therapy can be definitively outlined.

Currently, there is no standardized protocol for the preparation and administration of PRP. PRP can be used for skin rejuvenation via dermal injections or can be applied topically during microneedling procedures [155]. One study comparing intradermal and topical application of PRP in thirty patients found no significant clinical differences between both applications of PRP [156]. Larger standardized trials, however, are necessary to assess efficacy of PRP applications and determine optimal preparation and administration methods.

Adverse effects of PRP reported have been observed in studies, and include swelling, burning sensation, erythema, or ecchymosis at the site of administration. These effects appear to be transient, resolving within two weeks, and generally do not require post-treatment monitoring [156]. PRP has been shown to be safe and associated with low risk of serious adverse effects in a multitude of studies. However, one case report documented an adverse event of irreversible blindness after administration of PRP into the glabella [157]. Injections of any type into the glabella are high-risk, in general, due to complex vascularity and anatomy of the face [158].

8 Radiofrequency (RF) Microneedling

Radiofrequency (RF) is a non-ionizing electromagnetic radiation in the frequency range of 3 kHz–300 GHz [159]. In contrast to most lasers, RF is chromophore-independent, meaning it does not require a skin component with a distinct and intrinsic color (i.e. melanin) to be the target of the laser [159]. Instead, RF depends on electrical properties of the target tissue, and thus is expected to have a better safety profile for all skin types. In 2008, the FDA approved fractional RF for skin rejuvenation, given the ability for depth control of RF thermal zones which allows it to spare the epidermis, contributing to rapid healing and decreasing the incidence adverse events such as post-inflammatory hyperpigmentation (PIH) associated with epidermal injury [159]. RF microneedling combines the aesthetic benefits of RF and microneedling and combines them into one treatment [54]. RF generates heat within the tissue of interest by generating an electrical current, inducing neocollagenesis and the contraction of collagen fibrils [54]. There are two types of radiofrequency delivery modalities: monopolar RF and bipolar RF. Monopolar RF involves energy flow in one direction from the electrode in the user's handpiece to a grounding pad on the patient [160]. Bipolar RF, in contrast, involves energy flow between 2 adjacent electrodes [160]. Microneedling involves use of a device with short, sterile needles that create microtraumas in the skin, which stimulates new collagen production through the release of growth factors [161]. RF microneedling generates thermal lesions that are fractionally generated within the reticular dermis, which induces a vigorous wound healing process leading to dermal remodeling and the generation of new collagen, elastin and hyaluronic acid [159].

In RF microneedling, there are different devices available that vary based on their mode of radiofrequency delivery and needle type. As for needle type, there are non-insulated and insulted microneedles. Non-insulated needles deliver electrical energy through the entirety of their length as opposed to insulated needles, which are more protective of the epidermis and only deliver energy to the tip of the needle [162]. The heat generated by RF allows the microneedles to penetrate deeper into the dermis and induce tissue remodeling and neocollagenesis. Furthermore, RF has been studied in a number of clinical trials in the setting of treating acne scars and wrinkles [92, 157]. RF microneedling is currently used for the treatment striae distensae or "stretch marksand experts consider RF microneedling to be the treatment of choice for this condition [163]. In the setting of aesthetic rejuvenation, RF microneedling has been shown to decrease the appearance of wrinkles and improve skin laxity [121, 164, 165].

Microneedling is often used in conjunction with PRP. Studies comparing combination treatment of microneedling and PRP with microneedling alone have shown mixed results. A split-face study from 2021 showed no advantage of combination therapy with microneedling and PRP over microneedling alone in the treatment of acne scars [62]. However, another study concluded that microneedling combined with PRP is more effective than microneedling in the treatment of atrophic acne scars [63]. Similarly, it was found that combination treatment of microneedling and PRP was more effective than microneedling alone in the treatment of stria distensae [64].

RF microneedling, specifically, is also performed with the addition of PRP by dermatologists and plastic surgeons, alike. However, there are not many studies that have reviewed the effects of these modalities used in conjunction. One study comparing RF microneedling and PRP in the treatment of mild and moderate skin laxity showed that both monotherapy and combination therapy were safe and effective, although the efficacy of both modalities were inconclusive in comparison [66]. Another study found that RF microneedling using fractional bipolar RF treatment is effective for the treatment of photoaged skin in Asian patients with darker skin types and poses little risk of PIH [159].

Commercially available fractional and penetrating microneedle devices include Fractora™, eMatrix™, Infini™, Intensif™, and Profound™. There are also exist radiofrequency devices marketed for at-home use. In general, RF microneedling is well tolerated but is considered to be an ablative therapy given the risk of edema and ecchymosis post-treatment. Other common side effects include pain, erythema, and bleeding at the treatment site, and are usually temporary, lasting several hours to days

[162, 166]. Of note, microneedling has a very low risk of causing cutaneous infection and inducing pigmentary alterations, even for individuals with highly pigmented skin [163, 167]. While transdermal passage of microorganisms after microneedling has been shown in in vitro studies, clinical studies have shown that there is no increased risk of infection with microneedling, if standard hygienic measures are implemented [168]. Several studies have reported using topical and/or oral antibiotic prophylaxis in patients undergoing microneedling, however, benefits were marginal as bacterial infections were rarely reported in patients undergoing microneedling [166, 168, 169].

Contraindications to RF microneedling include active acne, active herpes labialis or other localized infections, moderate-to-severe chronic skin conditions (i.e. eczema or psoriasis), pregnancy, and active immunosuppression (including chemotherapy) [162]. A history of extreme keloidal tendencies is also a relative contraindication to microneedling [162]. Clinicians should also be cautious of RF microneedling near sites treated with chemodenervation injections (i.e. botulinum toxin) in order to avoid toxin diffusion [162].

Treatment intervals between RF microneedling sessions should be at least 3 weeks [170]. Post-treatment, patients should rest 24 h before resuming regular activities [162]. Patients should be advised to wear sun-screen, avoid excessive sun exposure, and minimize contact with harsh chemical products for at least 7 days after treatment [162]. It is important to note that the effects of RF microneedling may not be apparent for between 3 and 6 months post-treatment, due to the gradual nature of neocollagenesis.

There are several advantages of RF microneedling including rapid recovery time, relatively low cost of treatment, and good safety profile [162]. Additionally, an advantage for clinicians is that the technique is not complicated and easily understandable. Nonetheless, despite encouraging data for efficacy in a number of dermatologic conditions, there is still a need for large randomized-controlled clinical trials to assess the efficacy of RF microneedling and compare it with standard of care treatment options.

9 Plasma Exeresis

Plasma exeresis is a minimally invasive procedure that relies on plasma to produce a variety of aesthetic effects [171]. Plasma exeresis works through an instrument (plasma exeresis device) that ionizes gases in the space between the instrument's tip (i.e., sprayer) and the tissue being treated. The plasma exeresis device is a hand-operated, cordless microsurgical device that transfers heat to the tissues of interest [171]. Electrical energy, in the form of a voltage difference, develops into a small electric arc from surrounding atmospheric gases present between the instrument tip and tissue, causing sublimation of fluids in the tissue of the epidermis and producing plasma. This reaction occurs without disrupting the basement membrane and underlying dermal structures [171, 172]. In order for the plasma exeresis device to function, it must remain in direct contact with the tissue being treated at all times. Plasma exeresis has been implemented in the treatment of active acne lesions [173]. It is also used as an alternative to blepharoplasties [174–176] and in combination with autologous threads, mesotherapy, and PRP for aesthetic rejuvenation and anti-aging [177]. One study with 20 subjects assessed the efficacy of plasma exeresis in treating epidermoid cysts. The study found that plasma exeresis effectively removed epidermoid cysts in subjects, without any side effects and minimal scarring (scars that developed were less than 3 mm). Furthermore, this research suggests that plasma exeresis could be a safe and effective treatment option for cyst removal [178]. While plasma exeresis has demonstrated promising effects on collagen remodeling in small studies, larger randomized, controlled clinical studies are needed to evaluate the safety and efficacy in large-scale populations.

10 Non-invasive Body Contouring

The goal of non-invasive body contouring is to improve the contours of the body through non-invasive removal of adipose tissue. Currently, there are five FDA-approved modalities: laser, high-intensity focused electromagnetic field (EF), high-intensity focused ultrasound, radiofrequency, and cryolipolysis. Non-invasive body contouring is ideal for patients with persistent fatty areas, despite optimal dietary intake and exercise regimens. However, it is not recommended for patients interesting in achieving weight loss. It is also important to note that while these modalities are unable to reproduce results seen with invasive procedures, such as liposuction, they are less expensive, effective treatments with a shorter recovery time.

10.1 Low-Level Laser Therapy (LLLT)

Low-Level Laser Therapy (LLLT) was approved by the FDA in 2010 for the reduction of adipose tissue. The mechanism by which LLLT reduces adipose tissue is currently unknown, but there are multiple hypotheses postulated. One purported hypothesis is that the application of LLLT disrupts the cell membranes of adipocytes, allowing lipids to become released from the cell [179]. Another proposed mechanism is that LLLT induces triglyceride mobilization from unaffected cells [180]. A more recent study proposes that LLLT reduces subcutaneous adipose tissue by modulating systemic lipid metabolism [181].

A commercially available, FDA-approved LLLT laser is the Erchonia® Zerona™ Laser (Erchonia Medical, Inc., McKinney, TX) with a light-emitting diode that emits light with a frequency of 532 nm. In one study, treatments with the Erchonia® Zerona™ Laser twice a week for 6 weeks decreased subjects' baseline weight by 3%

in 30% of subjects with a BMI of 25.0 to 29.9 kg/m^2 [182]. Another study investigated LLLT emitting light with a frequency of 635 nm for non-invasive contouring of the hips, waist, and thighs in 80 subjects treated every-other-day for 2 weeks. Circumferential measurements were taken of subjects' hips, waist, and bilateral thighs prior to treatment and one week after all treatments were completed. After 2 weeks of treatment, there was a statistically significant reduction in subjects' hips, waist, and thigh measurements by 0.769 cm, 1.12 cm, and 1.17 cm, respectively [183]. While studies support the use of LLLT for weight loss, larger randomized controlled trials are required to assess the safety and efficacy of these LLLT treatments [184–188].

No monitoring is necessary following LLLT treatments. Although most studies have reported no significant side effects, one study consisting of twenty-four patients documented skin ulcers in irradiated areas post-LLLT treatment in two patients [184–188]. However, most lasers operate several centimeters away from the skin unlike those utilized in the study [136]. It is important to note that patients should avoid exposing eyes and skin affected by infection or trauma to the laser in order to avoid vision damage and further cutaneous damage. In addition, LLLT is contraindicated in pregnant patients and in specific anatomic regions, including the face, neck, and breasts. Clinicians should advise patients that the results of post-LLLT treatment will not be immediately apparent and may take several sessions to achieve the desire effect.

LLLT was discovered in the late 1960s, but it has only recently been applied in dermatology as a potential modality to reduce the appearance of wrinkles, acne scars, and hypertrophic scars [189]. In addition to weight loss, LLLT may have other applications in dermatology. LLLT has been studied for its ability to assist with healing burns and has shown benefits for certain inflammatory diseases, such as psoriasis and acne [190].

10.2 Radiofrequency (RF)

Radiofrequency (RF) is form of electromagnetic energy that produces resistance in tissue layers, creating an electrical current which is then converted to thermal energy [191]. RF causes skin tightening by inducing thickening and contraction of collagen fibers in the extracellular matrix [191]. TF's tissue effects differ from that of other lasers in that chromophores, such as melanin, are not targeted in the skin, allowing RF to be safely used in patients with skin of color. As mentioned previously, RF is divided into monopolar and dipolar RF. Monopolar RF uses an electrode from the user's handpiece to deliver an electric current to the tissue via a second grounding electrode on the patient [192]. Bipolar RF, in contrast, utilizes symmetric and closely placed electrodes to pass current through a defined volume of tissue [193].

Monopolar radiofrequency devices currently approved by the FDA include Thermage®, TruSculpt™, Exilis™, Exilis Protege™, ThermiTight™, ThermiRase™, ThermiVa™, and ThermiSmooth™. Most studies evaluating the efficacy of monopolar

RF as an anti-aging treatment have found both objective and subjective improvements in brow height, skin laxity, and the appearance of wrinkles and acne lesions and scarring. The most recent iteration of Thermage® is Thermage® FLX, which has been shown to have reduce treatment time and work more effectively than its predecessor, Thermage® CPT. Thermage® FLX treatments are subdivided into two categories: radiofrequency current alone or radiofrequency current in combination with skin vibrational energy. Most patients treated with Thermage® FLX experience measurable results between 2 and 6 months after each treatment session. The results produced can last for 1–2 years, varying between patients. During the procedure, patients may feel heat, which is counteracted with the device's cooling system. Side effects of Thermage® FLX including erythema or swelling at the treatment site typically resolve within 24 h.

TruSculpt™ iD applies an electric field perpendicular to skin-fat and fat-muscle interfaces to reduce the subcutaneous fat layer between skin and muscle layers. TruSculpt 3D™ is another monopolar radiofrequency device targets subcutaneous fat. TruSculpt™ iD and TruSculpt 3D™ differ in their handpieces, as truSculpt™ iD includes six individuals handpieces whereas truSculpt 3D™ has one gliding hand-held handpiece. In addition, each truSculpt™ iD treatment lasts approximately 15 min, with no down-time or post-treatment monitoring required, whereas each truSculpt™ 3D session lasts approximately 60 min.

Another monopolar RF device with bipolar capabilities (i.e. through a bipolar handpiece) is the Accent™ RF system. Other bipolar radiofrequency devices include Aurora™, Polaris WR™, VelaSmooth™, VelaShapeIII™, Reaction™, Apollo™, Forma™, and BodyFx™. VelaSmooth™ is a device that combines radiofrequency and infrared light for the purpose of reducing cellulite.

FDA guidelines state that the delivery of radiofrequency energy is indicated for electrocoagulation and hemostasis and for the treatment of periorbital and facial wrinkles. Combination treatment with radiofrequency and skin vibration is indicated for the above indications, temporary improvement of cellulite and local circulation, and the symptomatic improvement of minor muscle aches and spasms. RF can also be used for selective lipolysis, using the following devices: Vanquish ME™ and BodyFX™. In general, RF is well tolerated by patients and has a low risk of significant side effects. After treatment, patients can resume their normal activities and no post-treatment monitoring is required.

Isotretinoin use within 6 months of RF treatment is a contraindication to RF, due to concerns for impaired wound healing with concomitant isotretinoin therapy [194]. Additionally, having pacemakers, defibrillators, and implants in the treatment area is a contraindication to RF treatment [195]. Radiofrequency should be avoided during pregnancy because the effects of RF on the fetus are currently unknown.

10.3 Microfocused Ultrasound

Microfocused ultrasound generates heat over 55 °C and produces thermal coagulation points (TCPs) in tissue. The development of TCPs results in tissue healing, during which neocollagenesis and neoelastogenesis occur [196]. Ultherapy® is a commercially available, FDA approved microultrasound device for the treatment of wrinkles and décolletage lines [197], and the non-invasive lifting of the neck, brow [198, 199], and chin [199].

Patients in their 30–40 s with mild to moderate skin laxity are the ideal candidates for microfocused ultrasound skin tightening [200]. With each patient, goals of treatment should be discussed, as treatment with microfocused ultrasound is not a replacement for surgical facelift.

Microfocused ultrasound treatments typically last between 30 and 90 min, but times also vary depending on the area being treated. During the procedure, patients may report feeling either a warm or tingling sensation. However, this sensation only occurs briefly—initially when the ultrasound energy is being delivered—and is dependent patient tolerance, as level of comfort differs from patient to patient. After the procedure, patients experience no downtime and are able to resume normal activity without post-treatment monitoring. Typically, most patients require only 1 treatment to see noticeable results. However, other patients may benefit from additional treatment sessions. Degree of response to microultrasound therapy is dependent on patient skin characteristics, including degree of skin laxity and response to their first microultrasound treatment. Nonetheless, as microfocused ultrasound stimulates neocollagenesis, results appear over 2–3 months post-procedure and may last, at a minimum, for 1 year.

After treatment with microfocused ultrasound, patients may experience mild tenderness, edema, and erythema at the treatment site but symptoms are transient in nature [201]. Rare adverse events that have been reported include welting, bruising, and nerve-related symptoms, such as paresthesia and paresis. In rare cases, where improper technique was implemented, surface thermal injuries were observed [201]. In patients with Fitzpatrick skin types IV–VI or when depths of 1.5 mm are used, post-inflammatory dyspigmentation is a rare, but potential adverse effect that is observed [202]. Other more serious adverse events reported in literature include cutaneous necrosis, cutaneous and subcutaneous tissue atrophy, blistering, erosion, and ulceration [202]. Although the aforementioned effects are rare, these may be underreported and more significant than reported.

10.4 High-Intensity Focused Ultrasound (HIFU)

High-intensity focused ultrasound (HIFU) allows for noninvasive body contouring by inducing coagulative necrosis and cell death of targeted adipose tissue [203]. HIFU can result in cavitation by promoting lysis of adipocytes without damaging surrounding areas of tissue. Although the initial indication for HIFU was for brow lifting, HIFU is currently being used for body contouring as well as facial tightening, rejuvenation, and lifting [204, 205]. Currently available HIFU devices include Ultra 4D, LIPOcel™, Liposonix, Artec EVA®, and many others [198]. Although HIFU has gained popularity, there is sparse large-scale research trials on its safety, efficacy, and frequency for optimal use.

One study found that after two sessions of HIFU, 150 J/cm applied in the first session and 135 J/cm applied in the second session, adults with a body mass index $\leq$ 30 kg/m and abdominal subcutaneous fat tissue thickness $\geq$ 2.5 cm experienced an average reduction of 3.43 cm in waist circumference after 8 weeks. Another study found that a single HIFU treatment produced a statistically significant decrease in infraumbilical circumference (by 0.6%) in males with BMI $\leq$ 30 kg/cm^2 and $\geq$ 2.0 cm of abdominal fat [206]. While many studies have shown improvements in body contouring with HIFU, few studies have assessed the durability of these changes [203, 207–210]. One study showed that results of HIFU used for wrinkles and skin laxity were apparent three months after the final treatment and were maintained at the six-month post-treatment follow-up visit [211]. Another study found that the effects of lipolysis with HIFU were maintained for up to 1 year after treatment [209].

The most common side effects with HIFU reported from clinical studies are pain and erythema at treatment site [212]. Patients have also reported ecchymosis and edema after treatment, but these effects are temporary and rare [198, 213]. Furthermore, no monitoring is necessary after HIFU treatment.

Because HIFU has mainly been studied in patients with a BMI < 30, further studies are required to study the safety and efficacy of HIFU as a body contouring option for individuals with a BMI $\geq$ 30 [214]. HIFU should be avoided in patients with a history of heart conditions, thrombosis, cancer, diabetes, epilepsy, autoimmune conditions, transplant surgery, liver or kidney disease, and patients with alcohol use disorder [215]. HIFU should also be avoided in patients who are pregnant or breastfeeding, and in patients with metal prosthesis located in targeted treatment areas [215].

10.5 High-Intensity Focused Electromagnetic (HIFEM) Treatments

For decades, HIFEM has been used in medicine in the fields of neurology, psychiatry, urology, and physical therapy. Only recently has HIFEM been used in the fields of dermatology and plastic surgery for body contouring [216]. HIFEM treatments utilize very low frequency magnetic waves, 3–5 kHz, to induce muscle contraction and subcutaneous adipose tissue loss [217]. A circular coil passes an electric current over the treated area, and fluctuating electric currents induce magnetic waves, generating additional electric currents [217]. The electrical currents cause depolarization of motor neurons, producing muscle contractions. HIFEM, specifically, causes sustained stimulation of muscles without relaxation, producing supramaximal muscular contractions and causing micro-damage to muscular tissue and muscular hypertrophy [217]. As the energy expenditure of supramaximal muscle contraction is too great to be met by glycogenolysis alone, lipolysis occurs to meet the high energy demand, causing fat loss from subcutaneous adipose tissue [217].

One study reported an 18.6% reduction in adipose tissue and an 15.4% increase in rectus abdominus thickness 2 months after HIFEM treatment [218]. Another study consisting of 33 patients showed that, on average, patients had a 23.3% reduction in adipose tissue 3 months after treatment [219]. Several other studies have, similarly, found positive results, however large, randomized controlled studies are lacking [216, 220]. Additional research is needed to definitively determine the optimal treatment intervals and maintenance treatment for patients interested in achieving fat loss and toning.

In 2017, Emsculpt, a HIFEM treatment, was FDA-approved for the treatment of muscle spasms. However, it has been recently approved for non-invasive lipolysis and reduction of abdominal circumference [219]. CoolTone is another device that uses electromagnetic fields to stimulate muscular contraction. CoolTone was FDA-approved in 2019 for strengthening, toning, and firming abdominal, buttock, and thigh muscles [221]. In general, patients receive four 30 min treatments that are administered several days apart and over a 2 week period [218, 221]. It is common for subjects to report muscle soreness 24 h after the procedure [218, 221]. Based on the available data from smaller studies, HIFEM has not been associated with any significant side effects, and monitoring is not required after treatment [218, 220]. Women who are pregnant or attempting to become pregnant should not receive HIFEM treatment because the safety of these treatments during pregnancy has not been established. Additionally, patients with implantable cardioverter defibrillators and pacemakers should avoid receiving HIFEM treatment.

10.6 Cryotherapy

Cryolipolysis refers to the targeted application of cool air to tissue for localized reduction of subcutaneous fat. Cryolipolysis functions based off the principle that adipocytes are very sensitive to the effects of extreme temperatures, both heat and cold, and undergo cell-death when exposed to extreme temperatures. CoolSculpting® and CoolSculpting® Elite are two modalities that take advantage of this principle and utilize cryolipolysis for non-invasive body contouring. CoolSculpting® was cleared by the FDA in 2010 for the treatment of unwanted fat in areas that are resistant to fat loss despite adequate dieting and exercise. Areas that are targeted during treatments include the submental and submandibular areas, thighs, flanks, abdomen, buttocks, upper arms, chest, and back. CoolSculpting® Elite was FDA approved in 2021 and offers multiple changes to its predecessor, CoolSculpting®, including inclusion of a C-shaped applicator that optimizes contact between the applicator and skin surface. Inclusion of a C-shaped applicator has been shown to enhance treatment effects, allowing 20–25% fat loss per treatment with CoolSculpting® Elite as compared to

18–20% with CoolSculpting®. Furthermore, results are seeing more rapidly and in fewer treatments with CoolSculpting® Elite compared to CoolSculpting®. It is important to note that that CoolSculpting® and CoolSculpting® Elite are not intended to produce drastic weight-loss, and have not been tested in men and pregnant females or lactating females. Not every patient is a candidate for the CoolSculpting® or CoolSculpting® Elite procedures, and it should be noted that patients with cryoglobulinemia, paroxysmal cold hemoglobinuria, or cold agglutinin disease should not be treated with CoolSculpting® or CoolSculpting® Elite. Table 3 lists relative contraindications to CoolSculpting® or CoolSculpting® Elite.

After cryolipolysis, adipocytes are metabolized and removed by the body's lymphatic system. Post-treatment changes are typically visualized 1–3 months after the procedure while final results can take at least 6 months to appear. Patients can receive multiple treatments per treatment site and this is dependent on the treatment area. A minimum interval of 8 weeks between treatments should be allowed between treatments for resolution of treatment-induced inflammation [222]. A recent prospective study sought to evaluate the effects of an intensive regimen of CoolSculpting® in 28 patients. During an initial treatment session, patients underwent $\leq$ 4 cycles of treatment per body area and if needed, $\leq$ 4 cycles of treatment 4 weeks thereafter. Patients were followed for $\geq$ 12 weeks and over 58 body areas were treated. 27 of the 28 patients were considered treatment "responders" with an average skinfold thickness of 35.4 $\pm$ 9.9 mm prior to treatment and 22.2 $\pm$ 7.6 mm 12 weeks after treatment [223].

During CoolSculpting® and CoolSculpting® Elite, it is normal for patients to experience sensations of tugging, pulling, cold, pinching, aching, tingling, stinging, and cramping at the treatment site. These sensations tend to subside as the area becomes numb during treatment. Adverse events are often minimal and may include persistent numbness and/or paresthesia, and bruising, edema, and erythema at the treatment site. Other symptoms, such as blanching, cramping, aching, or itching of the skin, may

Table 3 List of relative contraindications to CoolSculpting® and CoolSculpting® Elite

Cold sensitivity	Cold urticaria, Raynaud's disease, pernio, chilblains
Allergies and/or sensitivity	Isopropyl alcohol, propylene glycol, fructose, glycerin
Neuropathic	Nerve pain (post-herpetic neuralgia, diabetic neuropathy), impaired skin sensation, chronic pain
Infection	Open or infected wounds
Hematologic	Bleeding disorders, patients on blood thinners
Anatomical	Recent surgery or scar at the treatment area; hernia in or adjacent to the treatment area
Cardiovascular	Impaired peripheral circulation, active implanted device such as defibrillators or pacemakers
Psychololgical	Anxiety disorder
Dermatological	Active skin conditions such as eczema, rashes, or dermatitis at the treatment area

also occur immediately after treatment. Symptoms—erythema, bruising, swelling, cramping, and tenderness—occur, most often, 1–2 weeks after treatment. Numbness, however, may persist for up to several weeks after treatment. After cryolipolysis of submental and/or submandibular, patients often report experiencing a sensation of fullness at the back of their throat. Other adverse effects include tongue deviation, lower lip weakness, and decreased saliva production, due to cold exposure to the hypoglossal nerve, marginal mandibular nerve, and submandibular gland, respectively. However, more serious adverse events include paradoxical adipose hyperplasia, skin hyperpigmentation, severe and/or persistent pain, dysesthesia, and motor neuropathy [224]. Paradoxical adipose hyperplasia typically occurs 2–5 months after cryolipolysis and requires surgical intervention to treat. Hyperpigmentation may occur at the treatment site but typically resolves spontaneously. Other adverse events include burns (first and second degree), subcutaneous induration characterized by discrete nodules and/or generalized hardness, worsening of pre-existing hernias or formation of new hernias, treatment area demarcation, and cold panniculitis. Of note, cold panniculitis may be mild, where patients may experience erythema, swelling, warmth, tenderness, skin nodules, and possible low-grade fever, or severe and life-threatening. If severe, fat necrosis can occur, which requires immediate medical or surgical intervention.

11 Laser Therapy

Lasers are pivotal in the field of dermatology and their history in this specialty is both broad and complex. The mechanisms by which lasers work is discussed in-depth in the chapter titled "Telecosmetics and Lasers." This section will provide a brief overview of laser therapy in aesthetic dermatology and will discuss ablative, non-ablative, and fractional resurfacing. In ablative skin resurfacing, the epidermal and dermal layers of the skin are destroyed by the laser. Ablative laser therapy is indicated for the treatment of wrinkles, photoaging, acne scars, scar revisions, and seborrheic keratoses [225]. The two most common lasers used in ablative skin resurfacing are the CO_2 (10,600 nm) and erbium:yttrium aluminum garnet (Er:YAG; 2940 nm) lasers. Ablative skin resurfacing is thought to produce its anti-aging effects by denaturing collagen and stimulating neocollagenesis. Non-ablative skin resurfacing, in contrast to ablative skin resurfacing, does not damage the epidermal layer. Lasers commonly used in non-ablative skin resurfacing include the following: Nd:YAG laser (1064 nm and 1320 nm), intense pulsed light (IPL; 500–1200 nm), diode (980 nm and 1450 nm), and erbium:glass (Er:glass; 1540 nm) lasers. Non-ablative skin resurfacing produces desirable effects by stimulating neocollagenesis, like ablative skin resurfacing, with a more rapid post-operative recovery due to less epidermal damage. In fractional resurfacing, the laser targets only a portion of the tissue and thermally ablates columns of epidermal and dermal tissue, and the microtraumas produced enhance skin tone and texture [226].

12 Conclusion

Advancements in aesthetic dermatology includes implementation of biotechnology in skincare, such as kojic acid, enzymes, peptides, and hyaluronic acid in topical formulations, plasma exeresis, RF microneedling, minimally invasive body contouring, and laser therapy. It is important for dermatologists to be familiar with advancements in aesthetic treatments to be able to choose appropriate treatments for their patients based on their aesthetic goals and desires. This chapter described recent advances in the field of aesthetic dermatology and provides an overview of treatments currently available on the market.

Key Points

- Aesthetic dermatology is a growing field that is becoming diversified in treatment options available for patients.
- Aesthetic dermatology continues to evolve, providing patients with more minimally invasive options for skin rejuvenation and anti-aging.

Conflicts of Interest The authors have no conflicts of interest to declare.

References

1. El-Domyati M, Attia S, Saleh F, et al. Intrinsic aging vs. photoaging: a comparative histopathological, immunohistochemical, and ultrastructural study of skin. Exp Dermatol. 2002;11(5):398–405.
2. Shah AR, Kennedy PM. The aging face. Med Clin North Am. 2018;102(6):1041–54.
3. Zhang S, Duan E. Fighting against skin aging: the way from bench to bedside. Cell Transplant. 2018;27(5):729–38.
4. Montagna W, Kirchner S, Carlisle K. Histology of sun-damaged human skin. J Am Acad Dermatol. 1989;21(5 Pt 1):907–18.
5. El-Kady IA, Zohri AN, Hamed SR. Kojic acid production from agro-industrial by-products using fungi. Biotechnol Res Int. 2014;2014: 642385.
6. Saeedi M, Eslamifar M, Khezri K. Kojic acid applications in cosmetic and pharmaceutical preparations. Biomed Pharmacother. 2019;110:582–93.
7. Beelik A. Kojic acid. Adv Carbohydr Chem. 1956;48(11):145–83.
8. Nicolaidou E, Katsambas AD. Pigmentation disorders: hyperpigmentation and hypopigmentation. Clin Dermatol. 2014;32(1):66–72.
9. Maranduca MA, Branisteanu D, Serban DN, et al. Synthesis and physiological implications of melanic pigments. Oncol Lett. 2019;17(5):4183–7.
10. Serre C, Busuttil V, Botto JM. Intrinsic and extrinsic regulation of human skin melanogenesis and pigmentation. Int J Cosmet Sci. 2018;40(4):328–47.
11. Ashari SE, Mohamad R, Ariff A, Basri M, Salleh AB. Optimization of enzymatic synthesis of palm-based kojic acid ester using response surface methodology. J Oleo Sci. 2009;58(10):503–10.
12. Basit H, Godse KV, Al Aboud AM. Melasma. In: StatPearls. Treasure Island; FL; 2021.
13. Lim JT. Treatment of melasma using kojic acid in a gel containing hydroquinone and glycolic acid. Dermatol Surg. 1999;25(4):282–4.

14. Monteiro RC, Kishore BN, Bhat RM, Sukumar D, Martis J, Ganesh HK. A comparative study of the efficacy of 4% hydroquinone vs 0.75% kojic acid cream in the treatment of facial melasma. Indian J Dermatol. 2013;58(2):157.
15. Deo KS, Dash KN, Sharma YK, Virmani NC, Oberai C. Kojic acid vis-a-vis its combinations with hydroquinone and betamethasone valerate in melasma: a randomized, single blind, comparative study of efficacy and safety. Indian J Dermatol. 2013;58(4):281–5.
16. Garcia A, Fulton JE Jr. The combination of glycolic acid and hydroquinone or kojic acid for the treatment of melasma and related conditions. Dermatol Surg. 1996;22(5):443–7.
17. Tejera-Vaquerizo A, Garcia-Gavin J. Allergic contact dermatitis to kojic acid. Actas Dermosifiliogr (Engl Ed). 2019;110(3):243–4.
18. Serra-Baldrich E, Tribo MJ, Camarasa JG. Allergic contact dermatitis from kojic acid. Contact Dermatitis. 1998;39(2):86–7.
19. Mata TL, Sanchez JP, De La Cuadra Oyanguren J. Allergic contact dermatitis due to kojic acid. Dermatitis. 2005;16(2):89; quiz 55–86.
20. Burnett CL, Bergfeld WF, Belsito DV, et al. Final report of the safety assessment of kojic acid as used in cosmetics. Int J Toxicol. 2010;29(6 Suppl):244S – 273.
21. Franca K, Keri J. Psychosocial impact of acne and postinflammatory hyperpigmentation. An Bras Dermatol. 2017;92(4):505–9.
22. Niwa Y, Akamatsu H. Kojic acid scavenges free radicals while potentiating leukocyte functions including free radical generation. Inflammation. 1991;15(4):303–15.
23. Papakonstantinou E, Roth M, Karakiulakis G. Hyaluronic acid: a key molecule in skin aging. Dermatoendocrinol. 2012;4(3):253–8.
24. Fallacara A, Baldini E, Manfredini S, Vertuani S. Hyaluronic acid in the third millennium. Polymers (Basel). 2018;10(7).
25. Bukhari SNA, Roswandi NL, Waqas M, et al. Hyaluronic acid, a promising skin rejuvenating biomedicine: a review of recent updates and pre-clinical and clinical investigations on cosmetic and nutricosmetic effects. Int J Biol Macromol. 2018;120(Pt B):1682–95.
26. de Oliveira JD, Carvalho LS, Gomes AM, Queiroz LR, Magalhaes BS, Parachin NS. Genetic basis for hyper production of hyaluronic acid in natural and engineered microorganisms. Microb Cell Fact. 2016;15(1):119.
27. Pierre S, Liew S, Bernardin A. Basics of dermal filler rheology. Dermatol Surg. 2015;41(Suppl 1):S120-126.
28. Choi MS. Basic rheology of dermal filler. Arch Plast Surg. 2020;47(4):301–4.
29. Kontis TC. Contemporary review of injectable facial fillers. JAMA Facial Plast Surg. 2013;15(1):58–64.
30. Boen M, Jacob C. A review and update of treatment options using the acne scar classification system. Dermatol Surg. 2019;45(3):411–22.
31. Price RD, Berry MG, Navsaria HA. Hyaluronic acid: the scientific and clinical evidence. J Plast Reconstr Aesthet Surg. 2007;60(10):1110–9.
32. Walker K BB, Goyal A, et al. Hyaluronic Acid. [Updated 7 July 2021]. In: StatPearls [Internet]. StatPearls Publishing; Treasure Island, FL; 2021. Available from: https://www.ncbi.nlm.nih.gov/books/NBK482440/.
33. Liu L, Liu Y, Li J, Du G, Chen J. Microbial production of hyaluronic acid: current state, challenges, and perspectives. Microb Cell Fact. 2011;10:99.
34. Narins RS, Brandt F, Leyden J, Lorenc ZP, Rubin M, Smith S. A randomized, double-blind, multicenter comparison of the efficacy and tolerability of Restylane versus Zyplast for the correction of nasolabial folds. Dermatol Surg. 2003;29(6):588–95.
35. Mohammed H, Abduljabbar MAB. Complications of hyaluronic acid fillers and their managements. J Dermatol Dermatol Surg. 2016;20(2):100–6.
36. Kirkorian AY, Moore BL, Siskind J, Marmur ES. Perioperative management of anticoagulant therapy during cutaneous surgery: 2005 survey of Mohs surgeons. Dermatol Surg. 2007;33(10):1189–97.
37. Callahan S, Goldsberry A, Kim G, Yoo S. The management of antithrombotic medication in skin surgery. Dermatol Surg. 2012;38(9):1417–26.

38. Hamman MS, Goldman MP. Minimizing bruising following fillers and other cosmetic injectables. J Clin Aesthet Dermatol. 2013;6(8):16–8.
39. https://www.cdc.gov/vaccines/covid-19/info-by-product/clinical-considerations.html.
40. Galiniak S, Aebisher D, Bartusik-Aebisher D. Health benefits of resveratrol administration. Acta Biochim Pol. 2019;66(1):13–21.
41. Zhang H, Li C, Kwok ST, Zhang QW, Chan SW. A review of the pharmacological effects of the dried root of *Polygonum cuspidatum* (Hu Zhang) and its constituents. Evid Based Complement Alternat Med. 2013;2013: 208349.
42. Park EJ, Pezzuto JM. The pharmacology of resveratrol in animals and humans. Biochim Biophys Acta. 2015;1852(6):1071–113.
43. Anna Ratz-Łyko JA. Resveratrol as an active ingredient for cosmetic and dermatological applications: a review. J Cosmet Laser Ther. 2019;21(2):84–90.
44. Orallo F. Comparative studies of the antioxidant effects of cis- and trans-resveratrol. Curr Med Chem. 2006;13(1):87–98.
45. Salehi B, Mishra AP, Nigam M, et al. Resveratrol: a double-edged sword in health benefits. Biomedicines. 2018;6(3).
46. Farris P, Yatskayer M, Chen N, Krol Y, Oresajo C. Evaluation of efficacy and tolerance of a nighttime topical antioxidant containing resveratrol, baicalin, and vitamin E for treatment of mild to moderately photodamaged skin. J Drugs Dermatol. 2014;13(12):1467–72.
47. Boo YC. Human skin lightening efficacy of resveratrol and its analogs: from in vitro studies to cosmetic applications. Antioxidants (Basel). 2019;8(9).
48. Ibrahim GG, Yan J, Xu L, Yang M, Yan Y. Resveratrol production in yeast hosts: current status and perspectives. Biomolecules. 2021;11(6).
49. Howells LM, Berry DP, Elliott PJ, et al. Phase I randomized, double-blind pilot study of micronized resveratrol (SRT501) in patients with hepatic metastases–safety, pharmacokinetics, and pharmacodynamics. Cancer Prev Res (Phila). 2011;4(9):1419–25.
50. Poulsen MM, Vestergaard PF, Clasen BF, et al. High-dose resveratrol supplementation in obese men: an investigator-initiated, randomized, placebo-controlled clinical trial of substrate metabolism, insulin sensitivity, and body composition. Diabetes. 2013;62(4):1186–95.
51. Huang TY, Yu CP, Hsieh YW, Lin SP, Hou YC. Resveratrol stereoselectively affected (+/-)warfarin pharmacokinetics and enhanced the anticoagulation effect. Sci Rep. 2020;10(1):15910.
52. Chiba T, Kimura Y, Suzuki S, Tatefuji T, Umegaki K. Trans-resveratrol enhances the anticoagulant activity of warfarin in a mouse model. J Atheroscler Thromb. 2016;23(9):1099–110.
53. Qasem RJ. The estrogenic activity of resveratrol: a comprehensive review of in vitro and in vivo evidence and the potential for endocrine disruption. Crit Rev Toxicol. 2020;50(5):439–62.
54. Gehm BD, McAndrews JM, Chien PY, Jameson JL. Resveratrol, a polyphenolic compound found in grapes and wine, is an agonist for the estrogen receptor. Proc Natl Acad Sci U S A. 1997;94(25):14138–43.
55. Stone WL, Leavitt L, Varacallo M. Physiology, growth factor. In: StatPearls. Treasure Island, FL; 2021.
56. Agarwal A, Gupta S, Sikka S. The role of free radicals and antioxidants in reproduction. Curr Opin Obstet Gynecol. 2006;18(3):325–32.
57. Fabi S, Sundaram H. The potential of topical and injectable growth factors and cytokines for skin rejuvenation. Facial Plast Surg. 2014;30(2):157–71.
58. Das A, Datta S, Roche E, et al. Novel mechanisms of Collagenase Santyl Ointment (CSO) in wound macrophage polarization and resolution of wound inflammation. Sci Rep. 2018;8(1):1696–1696.
59. Sundaram H, Mehta RC, Norine JA, et al. Topically applied physiologically balanced growth factors: a new paradigm of skin rejuvenation. J Drugs Dermatol. 2009;8(5 Suppl Skin Rejuenation):4–13.
60. Pamela RD. Topical growth factors for the treatment of facial photoaging: a clinical experience of eight cases. J Clin Aesthet Dermatol. 2018;11(12):28–9.

61. Mehta RC, Fitzpatrick RE. Endogenous growth factors as cosmeceuticals. Dermatol Ther. 2007;20(5):350–9.
62. Wang SCX, Fu X, Zhou L, Ma J, Yan S. Recombinant human basic fibroblast growth factor in treating burns and other skin injuries. Chin J Traumatol. 1999;15:196–9.
63. Ma BCD, Xia ZF, Ben DF, Lu W, Cao ZF, Wang Q, He J, Chai JK, Shen CA, Sun YH, Zhang GA, Hu XH. Randomized, multicenter, double-blind, and placebo-controlled trial using topical recombinant human acidic fibroblast growth factor for deep partial-thickness burns and skin graft donor site. Wound Repair Regen. 2007;15(6):795–9.
64. Chai J, Sun Y, Xia Z, et al. A randomized, multi-center and parallel control clinical trial for acidic fibroblast growth factor in the treatment of deep second degree burn. China Pharmacist. 2015;4:589–91.
65. Wang S. Experimental observation on ADRs of recombinant human epidermal growth factor (rhEGF) in healthy and burned volunteers. Chin New Drugs J. 2000;9:34–6.
66. Chung WH. Unraveling new functions of superoxide dismutase using yeast model system: beyond its conventional role in superoxide radical scavenging. J Microbiol. 2017;55(6):409–16.
67. Lobo V, Patil A, Phatak A, Chandra N. Free radicals, antioxidants and functional foods: impact on human health. Pharmacogn Rev. 2010;4(8):118–26.
68. Wickens AP. Ageing and the free radical theory. Respir Physiol. 2001;128(3):379–91.
69. Ziada AS, Smith MR, Cote HCF. Updating the free radical theory of aging. Front Cell Dev Biol. 2020;8: 575645.
70. Vina J. The free radical theory of frailty: mechanisms and opportunities for interventions to promote successful aging. Free Radic Biol Med. 2019;134:690–4.
71. Gladyshev VN. The free radical theory of aging is dead. Long live the damage theory! Antioxid Redox Signal. 2014;20(4):727–31.
72. Meewes C, Brenneisen P, Wenk J, et al. Adaptive antioxidant response protects dermal fibroblasts from UVA-induced phototoxicity. Free Radic Biol Med. 2001;30(3):238–47.
73. Poswig A, Wenk J, Brenneisen P, et al. Adaptive antioxidant response of manganese-superoxide dismutase following repetitive UVA irradiation. J Invest Dermatol. 1999;112(1):13–8.
74. Naderi-Hachtroudi L, Peters T, Brenneisen P, et al. Induction of manganese superoxide dismutase in human dermal fibroblasts: a UV-B-mediated paracrine mechanism with the release of epidermal interleukin 1 alpha, interleukin 1 beta, and tumor necrosis factor alpha. Arch Dermatol. 2002;138(11):1473–9.
75. Mansuroglu B, Derman S, Yaba A, Kizilbey K. Protective effect of chemically modified SOD on lipid peroxidation and antioxidant status in diabetic rats. Int J Biol Macromol. 2015;72:79–87.
76. Kakimoto K, Kojima Y, Ishii K, Onoue K, Maeda H. The suppressive effect of gelatin-conjugated superoxide dismutase on disease development and severity of collagen-induced arthritis in mice. Clin Exp Immunol. 1993;94(2):241–6.
77. Rosa AC, Corsi D, Cavi N, Bruni N, Dosio F. Superoxide dismutase administration: a review of proposed human uses. Molecules. 2021;26(7):1844.
78. Lopez-Otin C, Bond JS. Proteases: multifunctional enzymes in life and disease. J Biol Chem. 2008;283(45):30433–7.
79. Rosenberg L, Krieger Y, Bogdanov-Berezovski A, Silberstein E, Shoham Y, Singer AJ. A novel rapid and selective enzymatic debridement agent for burn wound management: a multi-center RCT. Burns. 2014;40(3):466–74.
80. Ramundo J, Gray M. Enzymatic wound debridement. J Wound Ostomy Continence Nurs. 2008;35(3):273–80.
81. Suzuki Y, Nomura J, Koyama J, Horii I. The role of proteases in stratum corneum: involvement in stratum corneum desquamation. Arch Dermatol Res. 1994;286(5):249–53.
82. Baskovich B, Sampson EM, Schultz GS, Parnell LK. Wound dressing components degrade proteins detrimental to wound healing. Int Wound J. 2008;5(4):543–51.

83. Parnell LK. Protein degradation and protection observed in the presence of novel wound dressing components. J Funct Biomater. 2011;2(4):338–54.
84. van Kampen V, Merget R, Bruning T. Occupational allergies to bromelain. Pneumologie. 2007;61(3):159–61.
85. Nettis E, Napoli G, Ferrannini A, Tursi A. IgE-mediated allergy to bromelain. Allergy. 2001;56(3):257–8.
86. Del Rosso JQ. Application of protease technology in dermatology: rationale for incorporation into skin care with initial observations on formulations designed for skin cleansing, maintenance of hydration, and restoration of the epidermal permeability barrier. J Clin Aesthet Dermatol. 2013;6(6):14–22.
87. Sancar A. Mechanisms of DNA repair by photolyase and excision nuclease (nobel lecture). Angew Chem Int Ed Engl. 2016;55(30):8502–27.
88. Banas AK, Zglobicki P, Kowalska E, Bazant A, Dziga D, Strzalka W. All you need is light. Photorepair of UV-induced pyrimidine dimers. Genes (Basel). 2020;11(11):1304.
89. Berardesca E, Bertona M, Altabas K, Altabas V, Emanuele E. Reduced ultraviolet-induced DNA damage and apoptosis in human skin with topical application of a photolyase-containing DNA repair enzyme cream: clues to skin cancer prevention. Mol Med Rep. 2012;5(2):570–4.
90. Puig S, Granger C, Garre A, Trullas C, Sanmartin O, Argenziano G. Review of clinical evidence over 10 years on prevention and treatment of a film-forming medical device containing photolyase in the management of field cancerization in actinic keratosis. Dermatol Ther (Heidelb). 2019;9(2):259–70.
91. Walfield AM, Yarosh DB. It's never too late: DNA repair and photo-aging. Cosm Toil. 2007;122:7.
92. Sunscreen FAQs. Published 2021. Accessed 14 Nov 2021.
93. Zakrzewski W, Dobrzynski M, Szymonowicz M, Rybak Z. Stem cells: past, present, and future. Stem Cell Res Ther. 2019;10(1):68.
94. Shen Q, Jin H, Wang X. Epidermal stem cells and their epigenetic regulation. Int J Mol Sci. 2013;14(9):17861–80.
95. Trehan S, Michniak-Kohn B, Beri K. Plant stem cells in cosmetics: current trends and future directions. Future Sci OA. 2017;3(4):FSO226.
96. Barbulova A, Apone F, Colluci G. Plant cell cultures as source of cosmetic active ingredients. Cosmetics. 2014;1:94–104.
97. Georgiev V, Slavov A, Vasileva I, Pavlov A. Plant cell culture as emerging technology for production of active cosmetic ingredients. Eng Life Sci. 2018;18:1–20.
98. Schmid D, Schurch C, Blum P, Belser E, Zull F. Plant stem cell extract for longevity of skin and hair. SOFW J. 2008;134(5):30–5.
99. Miastkowska M, Elzbieta S. Anti-aging properties of plant stem cells extracts. Cosmetics. 2018;5:55.
100. Tito A, Carola A, Bimonte M, et al. A tomato stem cell extract, containing antioxidant compounds and metal chelating factors, protects skin cells from heavy metal-induced damages. Int J Cosmet Sci. 2011;33(6):543–52.
101. Apone F, Tito A, Carola A, et al. A mixture of peptides and sugars derived from plant cell walls increases plant defense responses to stress and attenuates ageing-associated molecular changes in cultured skin cells. J Biotechnol. 2010;145(4):367–76.
102. CitrustemTM. https://www.centerchem.com/Products/citrustem/. Accessed 4 Oct 2021.
103. Wang JV, Schoenberg E, Saedi N, Ibrahim O. Platelet-rich plasma, collagen peptides, and stem cells for cutaneous rejuvenation. J Clin Aesthet Dermatol. 2020;13(1):44–9.
104. Prakoeswa CRS, Pratiwi FD, Herwanto N, et al. The effects of amniotic membrane stem cell-conditioned medium on photoaging. J Dermatolog Treat. 2019;30(5):478–82.
105. Taub A, Bucay V, Keller G, Williams J, Mehregan D. Multi-center, double-blind, vehicle-controlled clinical trial of an alpha and beta defensin-containing anti-aging skin care regimen with clinical, histopathologic, immunohistochemical, photographic, and ultrasound evaluation. J Drugs Dermatol. 2018;17(4):426–41.

106. Zhou BR, Zhang T, Bin Jameel AA, et al. The efficacy of conditioned media of adipose-derived stem cells combined with ablative carbon dioxide fractional resurfacing for atrophic acne scars and skin rejuvenation. J Cosmet Laser Ther. 2016;18(3):138–48.
107. Center for Biologics Evaluation and Research; 2021. From https://www.fda.gov/vaccines-blood-biologics/consumers-biologics/important-patient-and-consumer-information-about-regenerative-medicine-therapies. Accessed.
108. Pai VV, Bhandari P, Shukla P. Topical peptides as cosmeceuticals. Indian J Dermatol Venereol Leprol. 2017;83(1):9–18.
109. Ferreira MS, Magalhaes MC, Sousa-Lobo JM, Almeida IF. Trending anti-aging peptides. Cosmetics. 2020;7(4):91.
110. Husein El Hadmed H, Castillo RF. Cosmeceuticals: peptides, proteins, and growth factors. J Cosmet Dermatol. 2016;15(4):514–9.
111. Schagen SK. Topical peptide treatments with effective anti-aging results. Cosmetics. 2017;4:16.
112. Lintner K, Peschard O. Biologically active peptides: from a laboratory bench curiosity to a functional skin care product. Int J Cosmet Sci. 2000;22(3):207–18.
113. Mondon P, Hillion M, Peschard O, et al. Evaluation of dermal extracellular matrix and epidermal-dermal junction modifications using matrix-assisted laser desorption/ionization mass spectrometric imaging, in vivo reflectance confocal microscopy, echography, and histology: effect of age and peptide applications. J Cosmet Dermatol. 2015;14(2):152–60.
114. Leyden J, Stephens T, Finkey M, Appa Y, Barkovic S. Skin care benefits of copper peptide containing facial cream. Paper presented at: Proceedings of the American Academy of Dermatology 60th Annual Meeting; New Orleans, LA, USA; 2002.
115. Abdulghani ASA, Shirin S, Solodkina G, Tapia E, Wolf B, Gottlieb AB. Effects of topical creams containing vitamin C, a copper-binding peptide cream and melatonin compared with tretinoin on the ultrastructure of normal skin—a pilot clinical, histologic, and ultrastructural study. Dis Manag Clin Outcomes. 1998;1:136–41.
116. Errante F, Ledwon P, Latajka R, Rovero P, Papini AM. Cosmeceutical peptides in the framework of sustainable wellness economy. Front Chem. 2020;8: 572923.
117. Asserin J, Lati E, Shioya T, Prawitt J. The effect of oral collagen peptide supplementation on skin moisture and the dermal collagen network: evidence from an ex vivo model and randomized, placebo-controlled clinical trials. J Cosmet Dermatol. 2015;14(4):291–301.
118. Genovese L, Corbo A, Sibilla S. An insight into the changes in skin texture and properties following dietary intervention with a nutricosmeceutical containing a blend of collagen bioactive peptides and antioxidants. Skin Pharmacol Physiol. 2017;30(3):146–58.
119. Kim DU, Chung HC, Choi J, Sakai Y, Lee BY. Oral intake of low-molecular-weight collagen peptide improves hydration, elasticity, and wrinkling in human skin: a randomized, double-blind, placebo-controlled study. Nutrients. 2018;10(7).
120. Proksch E, Segger D, Degwert J, Schunck M, Zague V, Oesser S. Oral supplementation of specific collagen peptides has beneficial effects on human skin physiology: a double-blind, placebo-controlled study. Skin Pharmacol Physiol. 2014;27(1):47–55.
121. Alexiades M, Berube D. Randomized, blinded, 3-arm clinical trial assessing optimal temperature and duration for treatment with minimally invasive fractional radiofrequency. Dermatol Surg. 2015;41(5):623–32.
122. Lam SM, Azizzadeh B, Graivier M. Injectable poly-L-lactic acid (Sculptra): technical considerations in soft-tissue contouring. Plast Reconstr Surg. 2006;118(3 Suppl):55S-63S.
123. Sickles CK, Nassereddin A, Gross GP. Poly-L-lactic Acid. In: StatPearls. Treasure Island, FL; 2021.
124. Stein P, Vitavska O, Kind P, Hoppe W, Wieczorek H, Schurer NY. The biological basis for poly-L-lactic acid-induced augmentation. J Dermatol Sci. 2015;78(1):26–33.
125. Goldberg D, Guana A, Volk A, Daro-Kaftan E. Single-arm study for the characterization of human tissue response to injectable poly-L-lactic acid. Dermatol Surg. 2013;39(6):915–22.
126. Lacombe V. Sculptra: a stimulatory filler. Facial Plast Surg. 2009;25(2):95–9.

127. Andre P, Lowe NJ, Parc A, Clerici TH, Zimmermann U. Adverse reactions to dermal fillers: a review of European experiences. J Cosmet Laser Ther. 2005;7(3–4):171–6.
128. Engelhard P, Humble G, Mest D. Safety of Sculptra: a review of clinical trial data. J Cosmet Laser Ther. 2005;7(3–4):201–5.
129. Moyle GJ, Lysakova L, Brown S, et al. A randomized open-label study of immediate versus delayed polylactic acid injections for the cosmetic management of facial lipoatrophy in persons with HIV infection. HIV Med. 2004;5(2):82–7.
130. Valantin MA, Aubron-Olivier C, Ghosn J, et al. Polylactic acid implants (New-Fill) to correct facial lipoatrophy in HIV-infected patients: results of the open-label study VEGA. AIDS. 2003;17(17):2471–7.
131. Sanchez-Carpintero I, Candelas D, Ruiz-Rodriguez R. Dermal fillers: types, indications, and complications. Actas Dermosifiliogr. 2010;101(5):381–93.
132. Fiore R 2nd, Miller R, Coffman SM. Mycobacterium mucogenicum infection following a cosmetic procedure with poly-L-lactic acid. J Drugs Dermatol. 2013;12(3):353–7.
133. Goldman MP. Cosmetic use of poly-L-lactic acid: my technique for success and minimizing complications. Dermatol Surg. 2011;37(5):688–93.
134. Lemperle G, Gauthier-Hazan N. Foreign body granulomas after all injectable dermal fillers: part 2 treatment options. Plast Reconstr Surg. 2009;123(6):1864–73.
135. Vleggaar D, Fitzgerald R, Lorenc ZP. Understanding, avoiding, and treating potential adverse events following the use of injectable poly-L-lactic acid for facial and nonfacial volumization. J Drugs Dermatol. 2014;13(4 Suppl):s35-39.
136. Mest DR, Humble G. Safety and efficacy of poly-L-lactic acid injections in persons with HIV-associated lipoatrophy: the US experience. Dermatol Surg. 2006;32(11):1336–45.
137. Lafaurie M, Dolivo M, Porcher R, Rudant J, Madelaine I, Molina JM. Treatment of facial lipoatrophy with intradermal injections of polylactic acid in HIV-infected patients. J Acquir Immune Defic Syndr. 2005;38(4):393–8.
138. Moyle GJ, Brown S, Lysakova L, Barton SE. Long-term safety and efficacy of poly-L-lactic acid in the treatment of HIV-related facial lipoatrophy. HIV Med. 2006;7(3):181–5.
139. Levy RM, Redbord KP, Hanke CW. Treatment of HIV lipoatrophy and lipoatrophy of aging with poly-L-lactic acid: a prospective 3-year follow-up study. J Am Acad Dermatol. 2008;59(6):923–33.
140. Fitzgerald R, Vleggaar D. Facial volume restoration of the aging face with poly-l-lactic acid. Dermatol Ther. 2011;24(1):2–27.
141. Vleggaar D, Fitzgerald R, Lorenc ZP. The history behind the use of injectable poly-L-lactic acid for facial and nonfacial volumization: the positive impact of evolving methodology. J Drugs Dermatol. 2014;13(4 Suppl):s32-34.
142. Lowe NJ, Maxwell CA, Patnaik R. Adverse reactions to dermal fillers: review. Dermatol Surg. 2005;31(11 Pt 2):1616–25.
143. Vleggaar D. Soft-tissue augmentation and the role of poly-L-lactic acid. Plast Reconstr Surg. 2006;118(3 Suppl):46S-54S.
144. Jham BC, Nikitakis NG, Scheper MA, Papadimitriou JC, Levy BA, Rivera H. Granulomatous foreign-body reaction involving oral and perioral tissues after injection of biomaterials: a series of 7 cases and review of the literature. J Oral Maxillofac Surg. 2009;67(2):280–5.
145. Andersen C, Wragg NM, Shariatzadeh M, Wilson SL. The use of platelet-rich plasma (PRP) for the management of non-union fractures. Curr Osteoporos Rep. 2021;19(1):1–14.
146. Dhurat R, Sukesh M. Principles and methods of preparation of platelet-rich plasma: a review and author's perspective. J Cutan Aesthet Surg. 2014;7(4):189–97.
147. Sand JP, Nabili V, Kochhar A, Rawnsley J, Keller G. Platelet-rich plasma for the aesthetic surgeon. Facial Plast Surg. 2017;33(4):437–43.
148. Lin M-Y, Lin C-S, Hu S, Chung W-H. Progress in the use of platelet-rich plasma in aesthetic and medical dermatology. J Clin Aesthet Dermatol. 2020;13(8):28–35.
149. Zhu JT, Xuan M, Zhang YN, et al. The efficacy of autologous platelet-rich plasma combined with erbium fractional laser therapy for facial acne scars or acne. Mol Med Rep. 2013;8(1):233–7.

150. Lee JW, Kim BJ, Kim MN, Mun SK. The efficacy of autologous platelet rich plasma combined with ablative carbon dioxide fractional resurfacing for acne scars: a simultaneous split-face trial. Dermatol Surg. 2011;37(7):931–8.
151. Gupta AK, Carviel J. A mechanistic model of platelet-rich plasma treatment for androgenetic alopecia. Dermatol Surg. 2016;42(12):1335–9.
152. Cervelli V, Garcovich S, Bielli A, et al. The effect of autologous activated platelet rich plasma (AA-PRP) injection on pattern hair loss: clinical and histomorphometric evaluation. Biomed Res Int. 2014;2014: 760709.
153. Gkini MA, Kouskoukis AE, Tripsianis G, Rigopoulos D, Kouskoukis K. Study of platelet-rich plasma injections in the treatment of androgenetic alopecia through an one-year period. J Cutan Aesthet Surg. 2014;7(4):213–9.
154. Na JI, Choi JW, Choi HR, et al. Rapid healing and reduced erythema after ablative fractional carbon dioxide laser resurfacing combined with the application of autologous platelet-rich plasma. Dermatol Surg. 2011;37(4):463–8.
155. Peng GL. Platelet-rich plasma for skin rejuvenation: facts, fiction, and pearls for practice. Facial Plast Surg Clin North Am. 2019;27(3):405–11.
156. Gawdat HI, Hegazy RA, Fawzy MM, Fathy M. Autologous platelet rich plasma: topical versus intradermal after fractional ablative carbon dioxide laser treatment of atrophic acne scars. Dermatol Surg. 2014;40(2):152–61.
157. Kalyam K, Kavoussi SC, Ehrlich M, et al. Irreversible blindness following periocular autologous platelet-rich plasma skin rejuvenation treatment. Ophthalmic Plast Reconstr Surg. 2017;33(3S Suppl 1):S12–S16.
158. Walker L, King M. This month's guideline: visual loss secondary to cosmetic filler injection. J Clin Aesthet Dermatol. 2018;11(5):E53–5.
159. Seo KY, Yoon MS, Kim DH, Lee HJ. Skin rejuvenation by microneedle fractional radiofrequency treatment in Asian skin; clinical and histological analysis. Lasers Surg Med. 2012;44(8):631–6.
160. Weiner SF. Radiofrequency microneedling: overview of technology, advantages, differences in devices, studies, and indications. Facial Plast Surg Clin North Am. 2019;27(3):291–303.
161. Rodrigues M, Kosaric N, Bonham CA, Gurtner GC. Wound healing: a cellular perspective. Physiol Rev. 2019;99(1):665–706.
162. Singh A, Yadav S. Microneedling: advances and widening horizons. Indian Dermatol Online J. 2016;7(4):244–54.
163. Ryu HW, Kim SA, Jung HR, Ryoo YW, Lee KS, Cho JW. Clinical improvement of striae distensae in Korean patients using a combination of fractionated microneedle radiofrequency and fractional carbon dioxide laser. Dermatol Surg. 2013;39(10):1452–8.
164. Alexiades-Armenakas M, Newman J, Willey A, et al. Prospective multicenter clinical trial of a minimally invasive temperature-controlled bipolar fractional radiofrequency system for rhytid and laxity treatment. Dermatol Surg. 2013;39(2):263 73.
165. Alexiades-Armenakas M, Rosenberg D, Renton B, Dover J, Arndt K. Blinded, randomized, quantitative grading comparison of minimally invasive, fractional radiofrequency and surgical face-lift to treat skin laxity. Arch Dermatol. 2010;146(4):396–405.
166. Gowda A, Healey B, Ezaldein H, Merati M. A systematic review examining the potential adverse effects of microneedling. J Clin Aesthet Dermatol. 2021;14(1):45–54.
167. Alster TS, Li MK. Microneedling treatment of striae distensae in light and dark skin with long-term follow-up. Dermatol Surg. 2020;46(4):459–64.
168. Majid I. Microneedling therapy in atrophic facial scars: an objective assessment. J Cutan Aesthet Surg. 2009;2(1):26–30.
169. Sharad J. Combination of microneedling and glycolic acid peels for the treatment of acne scars in dark skin. J Cosmet Dermatol. 2011;10(4):317–23.
170. Rossi E, Paganelli A, Mandel VD, Pellacani G. Plasma exeresis treatment for epidermoid cysts: a minimal scarring technique. Dermatol Surg. 2018;44(12):1509–15.
171. Sotiris TG, Nittari G, Sagaro GG, Amenta F. A descriptive study on the applications of plasma exeresis in dermatology. J Clin Aesthet Dermatol. 2021;14(3):E58–62.

172. Gloustianou G, Sifaki M, Tsioumas SG, Scarano A. Presentation of old and new histological results after plasma exeresis (plexr) application (regeneration of the skin tissue with collagen III). Pinnacle Med Med Sci. 2016;3(3):983–90.
173. Stamatina G, Sotiris T, Aglaia V. Plexr in acne treatment. Pinnacle Med Med Sci. 2015;2(1):1–5.
174. Rossi E, Farnetani F, Trakatelli M, Ciardo S, Pellacani G. Clinical and confocal microscopy study of plasma exeresis for nonsurgical blepharoplasty of the upper eyelid: a pilot study. Dermatol Surg. 2018;44(2):283–90.
175. Ferreira FC, Sathler C, Hida IY, et al. Upper eyelid blepharoplasty using plasma exeresis: evaluation of outcomes, satisfaction, and symptoms after procedure. J Cosmet Dermatol. 2021;20(9):2758–64.
176. Hassan AM, Rady AAE, Shalaby OE, Shafik HM, Shaker ESE. Evaluation of plasma exeresis as a new technique for non surgical treatment of dermatochalasis. J Dermatolog Treat. 2020:1–6.
177. Sotiris TG. Combination of autologous treatments for non-invasive blepharoplasty and non-surgical full face lift. J Clin Exp Dermatol Res. 2017;8(5):1–5.
178. Avci P, Gupta A, Sadasivam M, et al. Low-level laser (light) therapy (LLLT) in skin: stimulating, healing, restoring. Semin Cutan Med Surg. 2013;32(1):41–52.
179. Neira R, Arroyave J, Ramirez H, et al. Fat liquefaction: effect of low-level laser energy on adipose tissue. Plast Reconstr Surg. 2002;110(3):912–22; discussion 923–915.
180. Caruso-Davis MK, Guillot TS, Podichetty VK, et al. Efficacy of low-level laser therapy for body contouring and spot fat reduction. Obes Surg. 2011;21(6):722–9.
181. Jankowski M, Gawrych M, Adamska U, Ciescinski J, Serafin Z, Czajkowski R. Low-level laser therapy (LLLT) does not reduce subcutaneous adipose tissue by local adipocyte injury but rather by modulation of systemic lipid metabolism. Lasers Med Sci. 2017;32(2):475–9.
182. Croghan IT, Hurt RT, Schroeder DR, et al. Low-level laser therapy for weight reduction: a randomized pilot study. Lasers Med Sci. 2020;35(3):663–75.
183. McRae E, Boris J. Independent evaluation of low-level laser therapy at 635 nm for non-invasive body contouring of the waist, hips, and thighs. Lasers Surg Med. 2013;45(1):1–7.
184. Nestor MS, Zarraga MB, Park H. Effect of 635 nm low-level laser therapy on upper arm circumference reduction: a double-blind, randomized, sham-controlled trial. J Clin Aesthet Dermatol. 2012;5(2):42–8.
185. Montazeri K, Mokmeli S, Barat M. The effect of combination of red, infrared and blue wavelengths of low-level laser on reduction of abdominal girth: a before-after case series. J Lasers Med Sci. 2017;8(Suppl 1):S22-s26.
186. Rubenstein R, Roenigk HH Jr, Stegman SJ, Hanke CW. Atypical keloids after dermabrasion of patients taking isotretinoin. J Am Acad Dermatol. 1986;15(2 Pt 1):280–5.
187. Thornfeldt CR, Thaxton PM, Hornfeldt CS. A six-week low-level laser therapy protocol is effective for reducing waist, hip, thigh, and upper abdomen circumference. J Clin Aesthet Dermatol. 2016;9(6):31–5.
188. Jackson RF, Stern FA, Neira R, Ortiz-Neira CL, Maloney J. Application of low-level laser therapy for noninvasive body contouring. Lasers Surg Med. 2012;44(3):211–7.
189. Seaton ED, Mouser PE, Charakida A, Alam S, Seldon PM, Chu AC. Investigation of the mechanism of action of nonablative pulsed-dye laser therapy in photorejuvenation and inflammatory acne vulgaris. Br J Dermatol. 2006;155(4):748–55.
190. Jackson RF, Dedo DD, Roche GC, Turok DI, Maloney RJ. Low-level laser therapy as a non-invasive approach for body contouring: a randomized, controlled study. Lasers Surg Med. 2009;41(10):799–809.
191. Greene RM, Green JB. Skin tightening technologies. Facial Plast Surg. 2014;30(1):62–7.
192. Burns JA. Thermage: monopolar radiofrequency. Aesthet Surg J. 2005;25(6):638–42.
193. Eckhouse S, Onder M, Fritz K. Bipolar radiofrequency.
194. Paasch U, Bodendorf MO, Grunewald S, Simon JC. Skin rejuvenation by radiofrequency therapy: methods, effects and risks. J Dtsch Dermatol Ges. 2009;7(3):196–203.

195. Atiyeh BS, Chahine F. Evidence-based efficacy of high-intensity focused ultrasound (HIFU) in aesthetic body contouring. Aesthetic Plast Surg. 2021;45(2):570–8.
196. Casabona G, Kaye K. Facial skin tightening with microfocused ultrasound and dermal fillers: considerations for patient selection and outcomes. J Drugs Dermatol. 2019;18(11):1075–82.
197. Fabi SG, Goldman MP, Dayan SH, Gold MH, Kilmer SL, Hornfeldt CS. A prospective multicenter pilot study of the safety and efficacy of microfocused ultrasound with visualization for improving lines and wrinkles of the decollete. Dermatol Surg. 2015;41(3):327–35.
198. Alam M, White LE, Martin N, Witherspoon J, Yoo S, West DP. Ultrasound tightening of facial and neck skin: a rater-blinded prospective cohort study. J Am Acad Dermatol. 2010;62(2):262–9.
199. Brobst RW, Ferguson M, Perkins SW. Ulthera: initial and six month results. Facial Plast Surg Clin North Am. 2012;20(2):163–76, vi.
200. Fabi SG, Joseph J, Sevi J, Green JB, Peterson JD. Optimizing patient outcomes by customizing treatment with microfocused ultrasound with visualization: gold standard consensus guidelines from an expert panel. J Drugs Dermatol. 2019;18(5):426–32.
201. Hitchcock TM, Dobke MK. Review of the safety profile for microfocused ultrasound with visualization. J Cosmet Dermatol. 2014;13(4):329–35.
202. Friedmann DP, Bourgeois GP, Chan HHL, Zedlitz AC, Butterwick KJ. Complications from microfocused transcutaneous ultrasound: case series and review of the literature. Lasers Surg Med. 2018;50(1):13–9.
203. Fatemi A, Kane MA. High-intensity focused ultrasound effectively reduces waist circumference by ablating adipose tissue from the abdomen and flanks: a retrospective case series. Aesthetic Plast Surg. 2010;34(5):577–82.
204. Fonseca VM, Campos PS, Certo TF, et al. Efficacy and safety of noninvasive focused ultrasound for treatment of subcutaneous adiposity in healthy women. J Cosmet Laser Ther. 2018;20(6):341–50.
205. Suh DH, Shin MK, Lee SJ, et al. Intense focused ultrasound tightening in Asian skin: clinical and pathologic results. Dermatol Surg. 2011;37(11):1595–602.
206. Guth F, Bitencourt S, Bedinot C, Sinigaglia G, Tassinary JAF. Immediate effect and safety of HIFU single treatment for male subcutaneous fat reduction. J Cosmet Dermatol. 2018;17(3):385–9.
207. Hong JY, Ko EJ, Choi SY, et al. Efficacy and safety of high-intensity focused ultrasound for noninvasive abdominal subcutaneous fat reduction. Dermatol Surg. 2020;46(2):213–9.
208. Lim Y, Park JH, Kang SH, Lee JH. Highly-focused ultrasound in non-invasive body contouring: long-term follow-up in Korean patients. Dermatol Ther. 2018;31(5): e12664.
209. Robinson DM, Kaminer MS, Baumann L, et al. High-intensity focused ultrasound for the reduction of subcutaneous adipose tissue using multiple treatment techniques. Dermatol Surg. 2014;40(6):641–51.
210. Shek SY, Yeung CK, Chan JC, Chan HH. Efficacy of high-intensity focused ultrasonography for noninvasive body sculpting in Chinese patients. Lasers Surg Med. 2014;46(4):263–9.
211. Karkhi A, Kisyova R. High intensity focused ultrasound (HIFU) technology for body contouring. J Aesthetic Nurs. 2019;8(Sup1):34–7.
212. Aşiran Serdar Z, Aktaş Karabay E, Tatlıparmak A, Aksoy B. Efficacy of high-intensity focused ultrasound in facial and neck rejuvenation. J Cosmet Dermatol. 2020;19(2):353–8.
213. Saket P, Shobeihi S, Mehrdadi S. Study of efficacy of esthetic high-intensity focused ultrasound system on Iranian skin for reducing the laxity and wrinkles of aging. J Cosmet Dermatol. 2017;16(3):336–41.
214. Park H, Kim E, Kim J, Ro Y, Ko J. High-intensity focused ultrasound for the treatment of wrinkles and skin laxity in seven different facial areas. Ann Dermatol. 2015;27(6):688–93.
215. Kilmer SL, Cox SE, Zelickson BD, et al. Feasibility study of electromagnetic muscle stimulation and cryolipolysis for abdominal contouring. Dermatologic surgery : official publication for American Society for Dermatologic Surgery [et al]. 2020;46(Suppl 1(1)):S14–S21.
216. Giesse S. A German prospective study of the safety and efficacy of a non-invasive, high-intensity, electromagnetic abdomen and buttock contouring device. J Clin Aesthet Dermatol. 2021;14(1):30–3.

217. Jacob CI, Paskova K. Safety and efficacy of a novel high-intensity focused electromagnetic technology device for noninvasive abdominal body shaping. J Cosmet Dermatol. 2018;17(5):783–7.
218. U.S. Food and Drug Administration. (2019). K192224. Retrieved November 2, from https://www.accessdata.fda.gov/cdrh_docs/pdf19/K192224.pdf.
219. Katz B, Bard R, Goldfarb R, Shiloh A, Kenolova D. Ultrasound assessment of subcutaneous abdominal fat thickness after treatments with a high-intensity focused electromagnetic field device: a multicenter study. Dermatol Surg. 2019;45(12):1542–8.
220. Kinney BM, Lozanova P. High intensity focused electromagnetic therapy evaluated by magnetic resonance imaging: Safety and efficacy study of a dual tissue effect based non-invasive abdominal body shaping. Lasers Surg Med. 2019;51(1):40–6.
221. U.S. Food and Drug Administration. (2019). K192940. Retrieved November 2, from https://www.accessdata.fda.gov/cdrh_docs/pdf19/K192940.pdf.
222. Avram MM, Harry RS. Cryolipolysis for subcutaneous fat layer reduction. Lasers Surg Med. 2009;41(10):703–8.
223. McKeown DJ, Payne J. Significant improvement in body contour with multiple cycles of CoolSculpting: results of a prospective study. Dermatol Ther. 2021;34(2): e14850.
224. Hedayati B, Juhasz M, Chu S, Mesinkovska NA. Adverse events associated with cryolipolysis: a systematic review of the literature. Dermatol Surg. 2020;46(Suppl 1):S8–13.
225. Krupa Shankar D, Chakravarthi M, Shilpakar R. Carbon dioxide laser guidelines. J Cutan Aesthet Surg. 2009;2(2):72–80.
226. Update on fractional laser technology. J Clin Aesthet Dermatol. 2010;3(1):42–50.

Three-Dimensional Printing in Dermatology

Isabella Dreyfuss, Daphne G. Eckembrecher, Francelia J. Eckembrecher, Amanda Ramnot, and Keyvan Nouri

Abstract This chapter will discuss skin tissue engineering using 3D printing and its implications for the future of dermatology, particularly for wound care. The use of three-dimensional (3D) printing comes from the modernization of moulages, a nineteenth century hot wax used for the representation of life-like dermatologic and venerologic conditions. The technological design of this topic consists of skin tissue engineering, which is accomplished using computer- controlled cell deposition into precise 3D geometrical pattern (Tarassoli et al. in J Plast Reconstr Aesthet Surg 71:615–623, 2018 [1]). The principles of 3D printing have shown favorable in delivery of cells for the replication of skin anisotropy. Additionally, this chapter will discuss the current modalities of use and the case studies that pertain to 3D printing. Other aspects that will also be discussed are the benefits and the current limitations in 3D printing and its future directions. Overall, continued research on 3D printing in dermatology is vital as it has the potential to greatly impact skin reconstruction and wound healing, thus enhancing patient health outcome and the quality of life.

Keywords 3-dimensional printing · Wound care · Skin tissue engineering · Human hair keratinic extract · Skin substitute · Electrospinning

Key Concepts

1. Three-Dimensional printing comes from the modernization of moulages
2. Three-Dimensional printing in dermatology improves treatments of wounds, severe burns, and autografts.
3. The limitations of three-dimensional include the positioning of the cells, thermal temperatures, and amount of titrated material.

I. Dreyfuss (✉) · D. G. Eckembrecher · F. J. Eckembrecher · A. Ramnot · K. Nouri
Dr. Phillip Frost Department of Dermatology and Cutaneous Surgery, Miller School of Medicine, University of Miami, Miami, USA
e-mail: id233@mynsu.nova.edu

K. Nouri
e-mail: knouri@med.miami.edu

K. Nouri (ed.), *Telemedicine and Technological Advances in Dermatology*,
https://doi.org/10.1007/978-3-031-69091-4_25

Learning Objectives

1. To understand the technological design and current usage of three-dimensional printing.
2. Evaluate what the benefits of three-dimensional printing are and how these benefits impact patients.
3. Learn about the overall limitations of three-dimensional printing.

1 Overview

1.1 Introduction

The use of three-dimensional (3D) printing comes from the modernization of moulages [2]. The creation of 3D models known as moulages in dermatology can be traced back to the nineteenth century [2]. These moulages were used to represent the life-like dermatologic and venerologic conditions and they were used as clinical teaching models through the utilization of hot wax until the mid-1900s [2]. 3D bioprinting is a modern regenerative medicine approach in which cells and cell-based materials are utilized in order to mimic native tissue [3]. Four main components of the functional replacement of tissue includes a moist environment for the skin to adhere to, an ability to enhance the natural wound-healing response, sufficient oxygen exchange for the environment, and limited harm and infiltration for infection from bacteria, viruses, and pathogens [3]. This chapter will discuss skin tissue engineering using 3D printing and its implications for the future of dermatology, particularly for wound care.

1.2 Technological Design

Skin tissue engineering is accomplished using computer controlled cell deposition into precise 3D geometrical pattern [1]. The principles of 3D printing have shown favorable in delivery of cells for the replication of skin anisotropy [1]. The major reason why there is success in functional skin depends on the material and cells used, as well as the biomaterial aspects that should be considered such as biocompatibility, biodegradability, bioinertness, strength, durability, and ductility [1]. Additionally, the biomaterial that it utilized should be printable, this encompasses two attributes. According to Tarassoli et al., these attributes consist of rheology, which include shear thinning and viscosity, and the cross-linking abilities, through physical, chemical, stereocomplex or ionic mechanisms [1]. Lastly, cell selection is the second key component for 3D bioprinting of skin, thus far research has focused on the use of keratinocytes, due to their easy propagation in culture and fibroblasts since they have multilineage potential [1].

1.3 Current Modalities

Tissue engineered substitutes include epidermal, dermal, and dermo-epidermal and substitutes. Epidermal substitutes can be cultured from autografts, yet most of these substitutes have a risk of infection and downside of cost. Ingetra bases their scaffolding off a crosslink of bovine and collagen, which has been found to have successful aesthetic but poor adhesion. AlloDerm provides vascularization via a human acellular dermis in lyophilized form. Dermagraft is a synthetic bioabsorabable polyglactin with neonatal human foreskin fibrolasts used in chronic wounds, yet cellulitis has been reported. Dermo-epidermografts include PermaDerm and DenovoSkin that are working towards clinical trials [3, 4]. Current modalities use these epidermal substitutes with ECM and major growth factors, such as epidermal growth factor (EGF), basic fibroblast growth factor (bFGF), transforming growth factor-beta (TGF-beta), platelet derived growth factor (PDGF), vascular endothelial growth factor (VEGF), interleukin (IL)-1, IL-6, and tumor necrosis factor-alpha (TNF-alpha), to re-epithelialize and provide the moist wound environment needed.

Bioprinting assembles biomaterials to 3D print patient-tailored skin replacements. The components used to create this material includes ECM components, growth factors, and cell types. The type of printer and bioink formulation are imperative. The bioink formulation is comprised of synthetic polymers to support cell proliferation. The inkjet printer is dispensed in droplets onto a collector plate from a piezoelectric actuator or heater. Inks are heated to over 200 degrees Celsius for short bursts so that the ink can purposefully recover from temperature change.

Limitations in bioprinting include the positioning of the cells, thermal temperatures, and amount of titrated material. The temperature of must remain consistent in order for the viscosity range to remain 3.5–12 mPa/s range, yet specifically 1–300 mPa/s range with the LIFT schematic. Clogging of the released gelatine polymers can also occur and the vapor bubble of the machine is not monitored. This requires diligent monitoring of the ink nozzle dispense amount.

Mechanical or robotic extrusion printers is another bioprinting methodology used, instead of the droplet method. Here, the viscosity ranges, from 30 to 6×10^7 mPa/s, are higher and can more easily achieve physiologic cell density levels.

Skin printing is another is the layer-by-layer construction of adult human dermal fibroblasts and primary adult human epidermal keratinocytes, nebulized by $NahCO_3$ vapor. Spatial cell organization where 2 upper layers of keratinocytes are organized with 3 lower layers are distributed throughout has also been tested by Lee et al. [5].

2 Examples

Various synthetic and bioengineered skin substitutes have failed to provide results that are equivalent to autologous skin graft, however, 3D printing can be a potential solution to major skin defects due to trauma, burns, or tumors excisions [6].

According to Bauermeister et al., ideal skin alternatives must be durable, prevent loss of water, lack antigenicity, resist infection, and be able to conform to irregular wound surfaces [6]. The use of 3D printers has allowed for the reproduction of the histologic architecture of skin through the inclusion of layer/depth specific cellular deposition [6].

3 Case Studies (3)

In a recent August 2021 study, multi-layered skin substitutes mimicked the genuine skin anatomy of multiple layers. This specific skin substitute combined human-derived keratinic extract-loaded nano- and micro-fiber using electrospinning and structure using 3D printing. The polycaprolactone PCL/keratin electrospun scaffold showed better cell adhesion and proliferation than the keratin-free PCL. Co-cultured with keratinocytes and fibroblasts better promoted regeneration of the epidermal and dermal layers in deep skin defects, producing artificial skin using multiple cells [7].

3D printing models in order to use Mohs Micrographic Surgery have also proved to be an alternative that clinical trials are using. Under ClinicalTrials.gov Identifier NCT03461965, 82 patients in a randomized, parallel assignment at the Cleveland Medical Center at the Chagrin Highlands and Westlake locations used 3D printing. The models were used to measure the skin flaps used to successfully proceed with the Mohs Micrographic Surgeries.

In 2016, 100 cm^2 standard P100 tissue cultured plates were printed in 35 min, as well as 30 min for fibrin gelatin. This was successfully transplanted in immunodeficient mice long-term [8].

4 Benefits

The benefits of 3D printing in dermatology include improved treatments of wounds, severe burns, and autografts. Current wound treatments include bandages and gauze that can adhere to the wound. This can result in damage to the fluid extrusions and an incorrect healing process. Hydrocolloids have made progress in the wound environment and bioactive molecules [9]. Severe burns can be treated with skin grafts from a donor or from the patient. Advances in spray-on autologous cells have been applied to partial thickness burns. Autographs provide adhesion and a decreased chance of graft-versus-host disease [3, 9].

Other benefits with the use of 3D printing are that it is economically feasible due to its increasing availability [6]. Additionally, 3D printing does not need large-scale production to reduce its costs due to the first custom 3D implant being as inexpensive as the previous one [6].

5 Limitations

Tissue-engineered skin can be enhanced by the addition of growth factors and other biomolecules, regulating several wound-healing-related processes, as the ECM has been an important factor in growth factor regulation and delivery. Major growth factors and cytokines that can be added to modulate wound healing are epidermal growth factor (EGF), basic fibroblast growth factor (bFGF), transforming growth factor-beta (TGF-beta), platelet-derived growth factor (PDGF), vascular endothelial growth factor (VEGF), interleukin (IL)-1, IL-6, and tumor necrosis factor-alpha (TNF-alpha). These influence re-epithelialization, granulation tissue formation, matrix formation and remodeling, and inflammation levels. When added unaided, proteases at the wound site have shown to interfere with efficacy. Therefore, combining growth factors with wound dressings and/or tissue-engineered skin grafts improves healing by creating an appropriate wound environment. To improve the therapeutic efficacy of growth factors, a number of delivery strategies have been developed to enable controlled spatial/temporal presentation of growth factors at the site of injury. These include, for example: lipid nanoparticle systems, ECM-inspired growth factor delivery systems, and nanofibrous structures.

6 Future Research

Various biomolecules for customization to patients are being further researched. For instance, hydrogels are being used with VEGF in fibrin gels for neural stem cell culture. In order to increase the flexibility and area that the cells are spread to, the new gels contain fibroblast growth factor-2 and bone morphogenetic protein-2 onto submicron fibrous scaffolds. Campbell et al. has showed that FGF-2 was able to persist up to 10 days and remain as active if cell culture conditions were apt [10]. Bio-printers have a goal of increased vessel formation in mice [11]. PGLA microparticles or microspheres in micrometer scale resolutions are using growth factors to regenerate inhomogeneous and complex tissues. Tarafder et al. used temporomandibular joint (TMJ) disc scaffolds to fabricate micro-precise spatiotemporal of specific growth factors. These would mimic the patients' fibrocartilage via the fabricated CTGF and TGF-beta 3 growth factors [12].

7 Key Points

1. Three-dimensional printing impact is very promising for the development of skin and wound healing.

2. The principles of three-dimensional printing have shown favorable in delivery of cells for the replication of skin anisotropy.
3. Various case studies are being performed to evaluate three-dimensional printing.

8 Conclusion

In conclusion, 3D printing has ability to enhance patient health outcomes and have a significant impact on skin reconstruction and wound healing. However, further research must be done to address limitations and to expand its use.

Quiz Questions and Answers

1. What century can three-dimensional models in dermatology be traced to?

   A. Sixteenth Century
   B. Seventeenth Century
   C. Eighteenth Century
   D. Nineteenth Century
   E. Twentieth Century

Answer: D. Nineteenth Century

2. What can three-dimensional printing improve the treatment of what in dermatology?

   A. Treatments of wounds
   B. Severe burns
   C. Dermatographia
   D. Alopecia
   E. Both A and B

Answer: E. Both A and B

3. How is skin tissue engineered?

   A. Computer-controlled cell deposition
   B. Lasers
   C. An attachment to a cell phone
   D. Skin tissue cannot be engineered
   E. None of the above

Answer: A. Computer-controlled cell deposition

References

1. Tarassoli SP, Jessop ZM, Al-Sabah A, et al. Skin tissue engineering using 3D bioprinting: an evolving research field. J Plast Reconstr Aesthet Surg. 2018;71(5):615–23.
2. Vazquez T, Forouzandeh M, Sisk M, Florez-White M, Nouri K. The modern-day moulage: incorporating three-dimensional scanning and printing to enhance dermatology education and teledermatology. J Eur Acad Dermatol Venereol. 2019;33(10):e383–4.
3. van Kogelenberg S, Yue Z, Dinoro JN, Baker CS, Wallace GG. Three-dimensional printing and cell therapy for wound repair. Adv Wound Care (New Rochelle). 2018;7(5):145–55.
4. Hrabchak C, Flynn L, Woodhouse KA. Biological skin substitutes for wound cover and closure. Expert Rev Med Devices. 2006;3(3):373–85.
5. Lee W, Debasitis JC, Lee VK, et al. Multi-layered culture of human skin fibroblasts and keratinocytes through three-dimensional freeform fabrication. Biomaterials. 2009;30(8):1587–95.
6. Bauermeister AJ, Zuriarrain A, Newman MI. Three-dimensional printing in plastic and reconstructive surgery: a systematic review. Ann Plast Surg. 2016;77(5):569–76.
7. Choi WS, Kim JH, Ahn CB, et al. Development of a multi-layer skin substitute using human hair keratinic extract-based hybrid 3D printing. Polymers (Basel). 2021;13(16).
8. Cubo N, Garcia M, Del Canizo JF, Velasco D, Jorcano JL. 3D bioprinting of functional human skin: production and in vivo analysis. Biofabrication. 2016;9(1):015006.
9. Pereira RF, Barrias CC, Granja PL, Bartolo PJ. Advanced biofabrication strategies for skin regeneration and repair. Nanomedicine (Lond). 2013;8(4):603–21.
10. Campbell PG, Miller ED, Fisher GW, Walker LM, Weiss LE. Engineered spatial patterns of FGF-2 immobilized on fibrin direct cell organization. Biomaterials. 2005;26(33):6762–70.
11. Poldervaart MT, Gremmels H, van Deventer K, et al. Prolonged presence of VEGF promotes vascularization in 3D bioprinted scaffolds with defined architecture. J Control Release. 2014;184:58–66.
12. Tarafder S, Koch A, Jun Y, Chou C, Awadallah MR, Lee CH. Micro-precise spatiotemporal delivery system embedded in 3D printing for complex tissue regeneration. Biofabrication. 2016;8(2):025003.

The Applications of Nanotechnology in Dermatology

Noreen Mohsin, Loren Elizabeth de la Caridad Hernandez, Francelia J. Eckembrecher, Daphne G. Eckembrecher, and Keyvan Nouri

Abstract Nanotechnology is a relatively new field of engineering that has led to the development of nanomedicine. Many of the benefits and risks surrounding nanotechnology concern the skin, and research over the last few decades has led to a better understanding of the potential role for nanotechnology in dermatology. As this field is rapidly evolving, practitioners must stay up to date on current research. This chapter will discuss the current uses and future direction of nanomaterials in cosmetic, diagnostic, and therapeutic dermatology.

Keywords Nanotechnology · Nanodermatology · Metal oxides · Nanocarriers · Nanoemulsion · Nanoliposomes

1 Introduction

Research on the applications of nanotechnology, the engineering of materials on the nanoscale, has been rapidly progressing over the past few decades [1]. The applications in dermatology include sunscreen, wound healing, drug-delivery, and many others. Nanoparticles are materials less than 100 nm in diameter that may have different properties than larger forms of the substance [2, 3]. These agents may be formed naturally or in the laboratory from a variety of materials, such as metals, lipids, and polymers [4]. Size, shape, or physiochemical properties can be used to classify nanoparticles, or they may be classified based on whether they are organic or inorganic [4, 5]. Inorganic nanoparticles—gold, silica, iron oxide, etc.—are being developed for intraoperative imagining of lymph nodes, tumor ablation, and many other clinical uses [5]. Organic nanoparticles—polymeric, liposomes, micelles, etc.—have

N. Mohsin (✉) · L. E. de la Caridad Hernandez · F. J. Eckembrecher · D. G. Eckembrecher · K. Nouri
Dr. Phillip Frost Department of Dermatology and Cutaneous Surgery, Miller School of Medicine, University of Miami, Miami, USA
e-mail: nmohsin@med.miami.edu

K. Nouri (ed.), *Telemedicine and Technological Advances in Dermatology*,
https://doi.org/10.1007/978-3-031-69091-4_26

a broad range of applications including drug-delivery for melanoma treatment, psoriasis treatment, and treatment of fungal and bacterial infections [5]. Nanoparticles may be used as carriers for drugs when they are formulated as nanoemulsions, nanoliposomes, quantum dots, or polymeric nanoparticle spheres [6].

2 Cosmetics

While the first nanotechnology-based cosmetic products were commercially available in 1986, the application of nanotechnology to cosmetic products is still a burgeoning area of research [7]. Due to the transparency and physical properties that prevent an increase in viscosity of the vehicle they are placed in, nanoparticles are a valuable tool in cosmetics [8]. Nanoparticles have a broad range of applications in cosmetic dermatology. Some nanomaterials have antioxidant properties, making them useful ingredients in sunscreens or skin lightening agents, and other nanomaterials have properties that make them effective in reducing wrinkles.

2.1 Sunscreen

Sunscreens contain filters that reflect or absorb ultraviolet (UV) radiation. Over a dozen types of UV filters have been approved by the U.S. Food and Drug Administration (FDA) as active ingredients of sunscreens [9]. Metal oxide nanoparticles, especially zinc oxide (ZnO) and titanium dioxide (TiO_2), are inorganic filters that offer UV protection and are the main nanoparticles in many sunscreen products [10]. Zinc oxide has been shown to protect against UV light more effectively and over a broader range of UV irradiation than titanium dioxide [11, 12]. These nanoparticles work by reflecting UV radiation and because of their size, appear translucent, which is cosmetically appealing to many patients [6].

Some groups have challenged the safety of sunscreen containing nanoparticles because of concerns of systemic absorption and potential toxicity. One study found that zinc oxide nanoparticles applied to human skin fibroblasts in cell culture resulted in cellular toxicity and another study found that zinc oxide penetrated skin [13, 14]. Many studies have shown that application of single-dose zinc oxide nanoparticles does not lead to local toxicity or skin penetration [15–18].

One group found that repeated applications of zinc oxide nanoparticles to the skin over five days did not result in stratum corneum penetration or show signs of toxicity in the epidermis [14]. In this study, zinc ions were found to penetrate the skin but were not associated with local toxicity [14]. Substantial research exists to suggest that the toxic effects of zinc oxide nanoparticles applied in vitro to skin fibroblasts do not occur when applied to intact human skin [14]. Moreover, both zinc oxide and titanium dioxide have been deemed safe and effective to use for skin protection by the FDA. Dermatologists should assure patients that using sunscreen containing zinc oxide and titanium dioxide is safe and that most research supports that the benefits of using sunscreen outweigh the potential risks.

2.2 Moisturizing Products

In recent years, pharmaceutical companies have taken an interest in using nanotechnology to create more effective moisturizing products. Rice bran oil is high in antioxidants and has been used by the cosmetic industry in sunscreen products, anti-aging products, and in treatments for skin diseases [19–21]. One study created rice brain oil nanoemulsions that showed low irritation potential in vitro and improved skin moisture in vivo [22]. Nanoemulsion is a technique that is often employed in formulating products for cosmetic dermatology because it confers increased stability and bioavailability of active ingredients [23]. This technology has the potential to be useful in treating psoriasis and atopic dermatitis, although more human studies are needed to study the efficacy of moisturizing products delivered via nanoemulsion compared to standard moisturizing products.

2.3 Skin Discoloration

Nanoparticles may be a useful addition to cosmetic products aimed at concealing uneven pigmentation in the skin, e.g. hyper- or hypo-pigmentation. Researchers have demonstrated that a spectrum of colors superior to that created by micropigments can be produced by mixing nanopigments [24]. Metal nanoparticles are especially useful in manufacturing pigments, and may be useful in reducing redness of skin [25].

2.4 Emerging Nanotechnology in Cosmetics

There are many nanoparticles that are currently being developed for cosmetic use. For example, the nanomaterial fullerene is a promising agent in cosmetic dermatology because of its antioxidant properties, which has made it a useful ingredient in sunscreens, skin lightening agents, and antiaging products [26]. These hollow spherical groupings of carbon atoms have also been shown to have benefits in treating acne vulgaris, promoting hair regrowth, and reducing wrinkles [27–32]. There are concerns, such as potential skin toxicity, that need to be further studied before this nanomaterial can be widely incorporated into cosmetic dermatology [26].

3 Diagnostic Applications of Nanoparticles

Nanoparticles have been used broadly in medicine for diagnostic purposes; for example, one group found that applying plasmonic gold nanoparticle to human nails caused a color change that allowed for detection of fungal infections [33]. Gold nanoparticles have also been engineered to assist with imaging certain cancers, including melanoma, in a non-invasive method [34]. When conjugated to melanocyte-stimulating hormone, gold nanoparticles enhanced contrast of melanoma cells in mice roughly 300% more than the control PEGylated gold nanoparticles [35].

Quantum dots, which are derived from solid semiconductor particles, may be also be useful in the detection of tumor cells because these nanoparticles are fluorescent and remain stable for long periods of time [36, 37]. They may also be used during Mohs surgery to visualize tumor tissue [36]. Although this technology is promising, these nanoparticles are derived from metals that are toxic, and more studies are needed to assess systemic absorption and risk of toxicity with these agents.

4 Therapeutic Applications of Nanoparticles

Using nanoparticles for drug delivery has many potential advantages. For example, sustained drug release, better targeting of diseased tissue, and potentially a lower risk of the drug being moved out of cells through efflux pumps due to the fact that nanoparticles are taken up by cells via endocytosis [38–40]. The vast majority of nanoparticle formulations that are FDA approved for treating cancer are liposomal systems, with the first liposomal drug, Doxil, approved in 1995 [41].

4.1 Cutaneous Neoplasm Management

Several types of nanotherapeutics have been tested in patients with metastatic melanoma [42]. In order to reduce toxicity associated with the drug formulation and non-specific distribution, nanotechnology has been applied to taxane-based drug administration [42] Nabpaclitaxel, a nanoparticle albumin-bound paclitaxel, showed promising results in a phase II clinical study [43]. In another study this drug was shown to have decreased taxane-related toxicity with increased activity against tumor cells compared to paclitaxel alone [44]. Several other phase II clinical trials have shown that albumin-stabilized paclitaxel nanoparticles improved progression-free survival compared to other chemotherapeutic agents [42, 45, 46]. However, a phase III clinical study comparing nabpaclitaxel to dacarbazine in chemotherapy-naïve patients with metastatic melanoma found no statistically significant difference in survival between the two groups [47].

Another benefit of nanotherapeutics in cancer treatment is the potential to use drugs that are unfeasible to use otherwise. For example, IL-2 is a cytokine that has been shown to have antitumor activity; however, its short half-life and severe systemic side effects limit its use [48]. One group of researchers formulated IL-2-containing nanoparticles that were conjugated to folate, and when administered to mice with melanoma grafts, this drug suppressed tumor growth and prolonged survival [48]. Similarly, siRNAs are now also being studied to treat melanoma because nanotechnology has offered a method to overcome the degradation of these agent that occurs through other methods of administration. Nanoliposomes may be used to deliver siRNAs targeting BRAF V600E and Akt3 to neoplastic cells, and one study found that this therapy inhibited growth of melanoma cells in human and mouse skin models [49].

siRNA may also be used to modify the tumor microenvironment by using a liposome-protamine-hyaluronic acid (LPH) nanoparticle-based delivery system. TGF-β has been shown to downregulate the immune system and lead to decreased efficacy of nanoparticle vaccination against melanoma [50]. In one study, mice were administered anti-TGF-β siRNA using LPH nanoparticles and then injected with a vaccine against melanoma [50]. This method decreased TGF-β levels by 50%, which increased vaccine efficacy and inhibited melanoma growth by 52% compared to the group that only received the vaccine [50].

Researchers have also discovered a way to promote the immune system to directly target melanoma cells by engineering nanoparticle vaccines created from melanoma-associated antigens [51]. Compared to the mice in the control group, vaccination of mice in the experimental groups delayed tumor growth [51]. In contrast to research on nanoparticles as carriers for chemotherapeutics, research on nanoparticle-based vaccines against cutaneous neoplasms is still in its infancy.

In addition to metastatic melanoma, nanotechnology may also be used to treat other skin cancers. One study developed fullerene nanomaterials for photodynamic treatment of squamous cell carcinomas, and reported that these nanoparticles successfully generated reactive oxygen species [52]. Another study found that using gold nanoparticles enhanced photothermal therapy used against squamous cell carcinoma in vitro and allowed for the neoplastic cells to be selectively targeted when the gold nanoparticles were conjugated to anti-epidermal growth factor receptor antibodies [53].

There are many ways in which nanoparticles can be formulated as anti-neoplastic agents. Further development of this technology to treat cutaneous neoplasms will allow for selective targeting of neoplastic cells while minimizing toxicity associated with traditional forms of these chemotherapeutics.

4.2 Wound Healing

Applying nanotechnology to wound care is promising for several reasons: (1) certain nanoparticles have been shown to have antibacterial properties, (2) nanomaterials may be incorporated into topical medications, which are ideal for wound care, (3) some nanoparticles may promote wound healing, and (4) the small size of nanoparticles increases the probability that these particles will reach their biological target at the wound site [54–56]. Nanoscaffold wound dressings mimic extracellular matrix (ECM) that has been lost during wound formation and thus promote ECM formation and fibroblast attachment, which leads to the development of healthy granulation tissue [54]. Over the past decade, development of this technology has accelerated. Silver nanoparticles are particularly of interest because they have been shown to reduce inflammation by modulating cytokines and potentially reduce scar formation [57, 58]. Additionally, silver ions have been proven to have antimicrobial characteristics [59]. One group of researchers developed a method to incorporate silver nanoparticles onto bacterial cellulose nanofibers, and this nanostructure not only demonstrated antibacterial properties, but also promoted epidermal growth and attachment without any observed cytotoxicity [60].

Nanofibers have also been developed to deliver antibiotic drugs to wound sites. For example, dual-layer nanofiber wound dressings have been shown in vitro to lead to an initial burst of antibiotic release from one layer, followed by sustained antibiotic release from the second layer [61]. Thus, nanoparticles have the potential to decrease the rates of skin infection in addition to promoting wound healing when incorporated into wound dressings. Anti-inflammatory drugs, such as indomethacin, may also be encapsulated within nanoparticles [62]. More human trials are needed to determine whether these products improve wound healing, although many animal and in vitro studies have shown that these products may lead to better outcomes for wound care than the conventional methods [54, 55].

4.3 Skin Infections

Certain nanoparticles, such as gold and silver, have been shown to have intrinsic antibacterial and antifungal properties [63, 64]. As mentioned in the section on wound healing, silver nanoparticles have been incorporated into wound dressings because of the antibacterial properties of silver ions [59]. In addition to using nanoparticles for their intrinsic antimicrobial activity, they may also be engineered to deliver antimicrobial agents.

Amphotericin B, an antifungal agent used to treat systemic fungal infections, may cause devastating toxicity that leads to discontinuation of the drug, regardless of whether the patient still has an ongoing fungal infection [65]. While a liposome based Amphotericin B formulation was created to circumvent these toxicities, there are several issues, including a high production cost and shelf-life duration, that have precluded this drug from becoming more widely used [66]. To address these issues, one group of researchers created nanoaggregates of Amphotericin B that had lower rates of systemic toxicity in mice and also demonstrated sustained release of the drug [66].

Nanotechnology has also been applied to creating more targeted antibacterial agents. Nanoencapsulation of antibiotics can be used to better target microbes while potentially avoiding antibiotic resistance mechanisms [67]. Antibiotic delivery via nanoparticles has also been shown to prolong the half-life of antibiotics and allow for sustained release of the drug [68]. One group of researchers conjugated nanoparticles loaded with vancomycin to a peptide that targeted specific tissues, including the skin, infected with *Staph aureus* [68]. The targeted nanoparticles in this study were more effective at suppressing staphylococcal infections in mice who received equivalent doses of free vancomycin or untargeted nanoparticles containing vancomycin [68]. Further development of this technology would decrease systemic toxicity by allowing for targeted drug-delivery and potentially bypass mechanisms of antibiotic resistance.

Nanovaccines are another promising area of research that may help decrease the rate of methicillin-resistant *Staph aureus* (MRSA) infections. Researchers engineered a vaccine from nanoparticles of toxins released by MRSA, and subcutaneous administration in mice was shown to be effective in reducing the number of skin lesions and bacterial count in these animals [69, 70]. This promising technology is another way that nanotechnology may help combat the rise of antibiotic resistance.

4.4 Acne Vulgaris

Delivery of topical retinoids via nanoemulsion has been studied in the treatment of acne vulgaris. As was mentioned in the section on moisturizing products, nanoemulsion allows for creation of products that have increased stability and bioavailability of active ingredients [23]. One group of researchers found that 0.1% retinol that was microencapsulated with triple nanoemulsion more effectively reduced signs of skin aging than commercially available tretinoin [71]. Another study found that the release of isotretinoin from isotretinoin-loaded nanoemulsions followed a zero-order kinetic model, which supports that this mechanism of drug-delivery allows for prolonged release of isotretinoin [72].

5 Safety Concerns

Although there is plenty of evidence that supports the potential benefits of incorporating nanotechnology into dermatology, there are still concerns regarding the side effects of nanoparticles. As discussed in the section on sunscreen, some studies have suggested that nanoparticles may be associated with toxicity from systemic absorption, while other studies found no evidence of this claim. Nanoparticles are engineered from a multitude of materials and can be manufactured by a variety of methods, and therefore broad generalizations about the safety of these materials are impractical. More studies are needed to fully understand the potential toxicity of nanomaterials.

6 Key Points

- Nanoparticles allow for creation of cosmetically appealing products due to their small size, which allows them to appear translucent and prevents them from increasing the thickness of products.
- Metal oxide nanoparticles are a major component of many sunscreen products.
- While there have been concerns regarding the safety of metal oxide nanoparticles, current research indicates that nanoparticles are safe to use and do not cause local or systemic toxicity when applied topically to intact skin.
- Delivery of products via nanoemulsion is often used in cosmetic dermatology because it confers increased stability and bioavailability of active ingredients.
- Nanotechnology may offer a non-invasive method of establishing the diagnosis of several dermatologic conditions, including melanoma.
- Nanoparticle-based drugs allow for more target delivery, which reduces systemic toxicity.
- Nanoparticles incorporated into wound dressings may be useful not only in wound healing, but also in preventing skin infections.
- Further development of nanoparticles for antimicrobial delivery may allow for more targeted drug delivery, decreased systemic toxicity, and potentially circumvent mechanisms of antibiotic resistance.

7 Conclusion

Nanoparticles have promising cosmetic, diagnostic, and therapeutic applications in the field of dermatology. The ability of nanoparticles to selectively target tissues, minimize systemic toxicity, and exhibit prolonged drug release has led to their development as antimicrobial and antineoplastic agents. Although there is abundant research that endorses nanoparticles as favorable agents, there is a scarcity of clinical trials in humans that precludes the immediate integration of nanotechnology into current therapeutic guidelines. More research is needed to further develop the applications of nanotechnology in dermatology and study the potential toxicity of these agents.

References

1. Rittner MN, Abraham T. Nanostructured materials: an overview and commercial analysis. JOM. 1998;50(1):36.
2. Roco M. Nanoparticles and nanotechnology research. J Nanopart Res. 1999;1(1):1–6.
3. DeLouise LA. Applications of nanotechnology in dermatology. J Invest Dermatol. 2012;132(3, Part 2):964–75.
4. Papakostas D, et al. Nanoparticles in dermatology. Arch Dermatol Res. 2011;303(8):533–50.
5. Anselmo AC, Mitragotri S. Nanoparticles in the clinic. Bioeng Transl Med. 2016;1(1):10–29.

6. Saraceno R, et al. Emerging applications of nanomedicine in dermatology. Skin Res Technol. 2013;19(1):e13–9.
7. Salvioni L, et al. The emerging role of nanotechnology in skincare. Adv Coll Interface Sci. 2021;293:102437.
8. Malerich SA, Krueger N, Sadick NS. Future cosmeceuticals of dermatologic importance; 2016. p. 207–12.
9. Hexsel CL, et al. Current sunscreen issues: 2007 Food and Drug Administration sunscreen labelling recommendations and combination sunscreen/insect repellent products. J Am Acad Dermatol. 2008;59(2):316–23.
10. Osmond MJ, McCall MJ. Zinc oxide nanoparticles in modern sunscreens: an analysis of potential exposure and hazard. Nanotoxicology. 2010;4(1):15–41.
11. Mitchnick MA, Fairhurst D, Pinnell SR. Microfine zinc oxide (Z-Cote) as a photostable UVA/UVB sunblock agent. J Am Acad Dermatol. 1999;40(1):85–90.
12. Pinnell SR, et al. Microfine zinc oxide is a superior sunscreen ingredient to microfine titanium dioxide. Dermatol Surg. 2000;26(4):309–14.
13. Deng Y, et al. A sunblock based on bioadhesive nanoparticles. Nat Mater. 2015;14(12):1278–85.
14. Mohammed YH, et al. Support for the safe use of zinc oxide nanoparticle sunscreens: lack of skin penetration or cellular toxicity after repeated application in volunteers. J Invest Dermatol. 2019;139(2):308–15.
15. Leite-Silva VR, et al. The effect of formulation on the penetration of coated and uncoated zinc oxide nanoparticles into the viable epidermis of human skin in vivo. Eur J Pharm Biopharm. 2013;84(2):297–308.
16. Leite-Silva VR, et al. Human skin penetration and local effects of topical nano zinc oxide after occlusion and barrier impairment. Eur J Pharm Biopharm. 2016;104:140–7.
17. Lin LL, et al. Time-correlated single photon counting for simultaneous monitoring of zinc oxide nanoparticles and NAD(P)H in intact and barrier-disrupted volunteer skin. Pharm Res. 2011;28(11):2920.
18. Leite-Silva VR, et al. Effect of flexing and massage on in vivo human skin penetration and toxicity of zinc oxide nanoparticles. Nanomedicine (Lond). 2016;11(10):1193–205.
19. Lerma-García M, et al. Composition, industrial processing and applications of rice bran γ-oryzanol. Food Chem. 2009;115(2):389–404.
20. Patel M, Naik S. Gamma-oryzanol from rice bran oil—a review. 2004.
21. Coppini D, et al. Capacitá protettiva Nei confronti delle radiazioni Solari di derivati di origine vegetable. Cosmet News. 2001;136:15–20.
22. Bernardi DS, et al. Formation and stability of oil-in-water nanoemulsions containing rice bran oil: in vitro and in vivo assessments. J Nanobiotechnol. 2011;9(1):1–9.
23. Jaiswal M, Dudhe R, Sharma PK. Nanoemulsion: an advanced mode of drug delivery system. 3 Biotech. 2015;5(2):123–7.
24. Nejad FM, Baghshahi S, Bakhtiari L. Advantages of nano pigments over micro pigments in obtaining larger spectra of colours in CMYK system. Trans Indian Ceram Soc. 2011;70(2):93–9.
25. Alfano RR, Ni X, Zevallos M. Changing skin-color perception using quantum and optical principles in cosmetic preparations. 2013, Google Patents.
26. Mousavi SZ, Nafisi S, Maibach HI. Fullerene nanoparticle in dermatological and cosmetic applications. Nanomed Nanotechnol Biol Med. 2017;13(3):1071–87.
27. Zhou Z, et al. Fullerene nanomaterials potentiate hair growth. Nanomed Nanotechnol Biol Med. 2009;5(2):202–7.
28. Inui S, et al. Inhibition of sebum production and Propionibacterium acnes lipase activity by fullerenol, a novel polyhydroxylated fullerene: potential as a therapeutic reagent for acne. J Cosmet Sci. 2012;63(4):259–65.
29. Aoshima H, et al. Antimicrobial activity of fullerenes and their hydroxylated derivatives. Biocontrol Sci. 2009;14(2):69–72.
30. Inui S, et al. Improvement of acne vulgaris by topical fullerene application: unique impact on skin care. Nanomed Nanotechnol Biol Med. 2011;7(2):238–41.

31. Kato S, et al. Defensive effects of fullerene-C60 dissolved in squalane against the 2, 4-nonadienal-induced cell injury in human skin keratinocytes HaCaT and wrinkle formation in 3D-human skin tissue model. J Biomed Nanotechnol. 2010;6(1):52–8.
32. Kato S, et al. Clinical evaluation of fullerene-C60 dissolved in squalane for anti-wrinkle cosmetics. J Nanosci Nanotechnol. 2010;10(10):6769–74.
33. Sojinrin T, et al. Plasmonic gold nanoparticles for detection of fungi and human cutaneous fungal infections. Anal Bioanal Chem. 2017;409(19):4647–58.
34. Zhu C, et al. Current progresses of functional nanomaterials for imaging diagnosis and treatment of melanoma. Curr Top Med Chem. 2019;19(27):2494–506.
35. Kim C, et al. In vivo molecular photoacoustic tomography of melanomas targeted by bioconjugated gold nanocages. ACS Nano. 2010;4(8):4559–64.
36. Boixeda P, et al. Future prospects in dermatologic applications of lasers, nanotechnology, and other new technologies. Actas Dermo-Sifiliográficas (English Edition). 2015;106(3):168–79.
37. Kim JK, Nasir A, Nelson KC. Nanotechnology and the diagnosis of cutaneous malignancies. In: Nanotechnology in dermatology. Springer; 2013. p. 127–32.
38. Shapira A, et al. Nanomedicine for targeted cancer therapy: towards the overcoming of drug resistance. Drug Resist Updates. 2011;14(3):150–63.
39. Hu C-MJ, Zhang L. Nanoparticle-based combination therapy toward overcoming drug resistance in cancer. Biochem Pharmacol. 2012;83(8):1104–11.
40. Arora HC, et al. Nanocarriers enhance doxorubicin uptake in drug-resistant ovarian cancer cells. Can Res. 2012;72(3):769–78.
41. Barenholz Y. Doxil®—the first FDA-approved nano-drug: lessons learned. J Control Release. 2012;160(2):117–34.
42. Bombelli FB, et al. The scope of nanoparticle therapies for future metastatic melanoma treatment. Lancet Oncol. 2014;15(1):e22–32.
43. Hersh EM, et al. A phase 2 clinical trial of nab-paclitaxel in previously treated and chemotherapy-naive patients with metastatic melanoma. Cancer. 2010;116(1):155–63.
44. Miele E, et al. Albumin-bound formulation of paclitaxel (Abraxane ABI-007) in the treatment of breast cancer. Int J Nanomed. 2009;4:99–105.
45. Kottschade LA, et al. A randomized phase 2 study of temozolomide and bevacizumab or nab-paclitaxel, carboplatin, and bevacizumab in patients with unresectable stage IV melanoma: a North Central Cancer Treatment Group study, N0775. Cancer. 2013;119(3):586–92.
46. Kottschade LA, et al. A phase II trial of nab-paclitaxel (ABI-007) and carboplatin in patients with unresectable stage IV melanoma: a North Central Cancer Treatment Group Study, N057E(1). Cancer. 2011;117(8):1704–10.
47. Hersh E, et al. A phase III trial of nab-paclitaxel versus dacarbazine in chemotherapy-naive patients with metastatic melanoma: a subanalysis based on BRAF status. J Clin Oncol. 2013;31(15_suppl):9030.
48. Yao H, et al. Effective melanoma immunotherapy with interleukin-2 delivered by a novel polymeric nanoparticle. Mol Cancer Ther. 2011;10(6):1082–92.
49. Tran MA, et al. Targeting V600EB-Raf and Akt3 using nanoliposomal-small interfering RNA inhibits cutaneous melanocytic lesion development. Can Res. 2008;68(18):7638–49.
50. Xu Z, et al. Nanoparticle-delivered transforming growth factor-β siRNA enhances vaccination against advanced melanoma by modifying tumor microenvironment. ACS Nano. 2014;8(4):3636–45.
51. Silva JM, et al. In vivo delivery of peptides and Toll-like receptor ligands by mannose-functionalized polymeric nanoparticles induces prophylactic and therapeutic anti-tumor immune responses in a melanoma model. J Control Release. 2015;198:91–103.
52. Serda M, et al. Developing [60] fullerene nanomaterials for better photodynamic treatment of non-melanoma skin cancers. ACS Biomater Sci Eng. 2020;6(10):5930–40.
53. El-Sayed IH, Huang X, El-Sayed MA. Selective laser photo-thermal therapy of epithelial carcinoma using anti-EGFR antibody conjugated gold nanoparticles. Cancer Lett. 2006;239(1):129–35.

54. Rajendran NK, et al. A review on nanoparticle based treatment for wound healing. J Drug Deliv Sci Technol. 2018;44:421–30.
55. Parani M, et al. Engineered nanomaterials for infection control and healing acute and chronic wounds. ACS Appl Mater Interfaces. 2016;8(16):10049–69.
56. Hamdan S, et al. Nanotechnology-driven therapeutic interventions in wound healing: potential uses and applications. ACS Cent Sci. 2017;3(3):163–75.
57. Tian J, et al. Topical delivery of silver nanoparticles promotes wound healing. ChemMedChem. 2007;2(1):129–36.
58. Kim HN, et al. Effect of orientation and density of nanotopography in dermal wound healing. Biomaterials. 2012;33(34):8782–92.
59. Lee SH, Jun B-H. Silver nanoparticles: synthesis and application for nanomedicine. Int J Mol Sci. 2019;20(4):865.
60. Wu J, et al. In situ synthesis of silver-nanoparticles/bacterial cellulose composites for slow-released antimicrobial wound dressing. Carbohyd Polym. 2014;102:762–71.
61. Zhao R, et al. Nitrofurazone-loaded electrospun PLLA/sericin-based dual-layer fiber mats for wound dressing applications. RSC Adv. 2015;5(22):16940–9.
62. Ferreira AM, et al. Bioinspired porous membranes containing polymer nanoparticles for wound healing. J Biomed Mater Res, Part A. 2014;102(12):4394–405.
63. Lohani A, et al. Nanotechnology-based cosmeceuticals. Int Scholarly Res Notices. 2014;2014.
64. Fytianos G, Rahdar A, Kyzas GZ. Nanomaterials in cosmetics: recent updates. Nanomaterials. 2020;10(5):979.
65. Laniado-Laborín R, Cabrales-Vargas MN. Amphotericin B: side effects and toxicity. Rev Iberoam Micol. 2009;26(4):223–7.
66. Zia Q, et al. Biomimetically engineered Amphotericin B nano-aggregates circumvent toxicity constraints and treat systemic fungal infection in experimental animals. Sci Rep. 2017;7(1):11873.
67. Banin E, Hughes D, Kuipers OP. Bacterial pathogens, antibiotics and antibiotic resistance. FEMS Microbiol Rev. 2017;41(3):450–2.
68. Hussain S, et al. Antibiotic-loaded nanoparticles targeted to the site of infection enhance antibacterial efficacy. Nat Biomed Eng. 2018;2(2):95–103.
69. Wei X, et al. In situ capture of bacterial toxins for antivirulence vaccination. Adv Mater (Deerfield Beach, Fla.). 2017;29(33). https://doi.org/10.1002/adma.201701644.
70. Van Giau V, An SSA, Hulme J. Recent advances in the treatment of pathogenic infections using antibiotics and nano-drug delivery vehicles. Drug Des Dev Ther. 2019;13:327–43.
71. Afornali A, et al. Triple nanoemulsion potentiates the effects of topical treatments with microencapsulated retinol and modulates biological processes related to skin aging. An Bras Dermatol. 2013;88(6):930–6.
72. Miastkowska M, et al. The kinetic study of isotretinoin release from nanoemulsion. Colloids Surf, A. 2016;510:63–8.

Stem Cell Therapy in Telemedicine and Technological Advances in Dermatology

Michael Kaiser and Evangelos V. Badiavas

Abstract The chapter will discuss the role of bone marrow and adipocyte derived stem cells in dermatology. The application of stem cells in dermatology has shown promising results in improving wound healing and reversing the cumulative damage to the skin from ultraviolet radiation. Stem cells were identified as a population of cells with progenitor capacity to become many cell types which was thought to be important in wound healing. As a better understanding of the role of stem cell therapy in cellular processes has evolved, it is apparent that a critical role stem cells play in facilitating wound healing is their ability to act in a paracrine fashion to coordinate and modulate many cutaneous signaling pathways. This shift in understanding of the way stem cells modulate the cellular microenvironment led to the recognition of Extracellular Vesicles as a vital mediator between stem cells and other cell types. EVs are recognized as the main mechanism that deliver cellular materials to target cells to coordinate wound healing following injury. In addition to recruiting and stimulating proliferation of cells, EVs play an anti-inflammatory role in dermatology which is currently being explored as an alternative method of treating conditions such as atopic dermatitis and psoriasis.

Keywords Stem cell · Exosome · Extracellular vesicle · Atopic dermatitis · Wound healing · Psoriasis

1 Introduction

Stem cells are undifferentiated precursor cells that have the capacity to generate and replace damaged or lost cells in terminal tissues. They can be obtained from harvesting embryonic structures or isolated from reservoirs such as bone marrow or adipose tissue in adults. The current body of research has focused on using stem

M. Kaiser (✉) · E. V. Badiavas
Dr. Philip Frost Department of Dermatology and Cutaneous Surgery, Miller School of Medicine, University of Miami, 1600 NW 10th Ave, Miami, FL 33136, USA
e-mail: mak320@med.miami.edu

K. Nouri (ed.), *Telemedicine and Technological Advances in Dermatology*,
https://doi.org/10.1007/978-3-031-69091-4_27

cells for wound healing therapy, chronic wounds, therapy for burn wounds, and anti-aging therapies. While stem cell therapy has yielded promising results in the field of dermatology, further understanding of the mechanism by which stem cells act therapeutically has shifted the focus to extracellular vesicles (EVs). EVs are produced by stem cells as a safer, more economical method of regulating derangements in cutaneous pathologies [1]. Extracellular vesicles are a group of endogenous structures produced by all cell types that carry signaling molecules to neighboring cells and potentiate molecular processes that serve key roles in wound healing and chronic inflammatory processes in dermatology. Understanding the role of EVs in the cellular microenvironment has shed light on a new therapeutic option for conditions such as atopic dermatitis and psoriasis as well as improving wound healing and reducing scarring.

2 Types of Stem Cells in Dermatology

2.1 *Adipocyte Derived Stem Cells (ADSC)*

Adipocyte derived stem cells (ADSC) are one of the major types of stem cells that have been examined for therapeutic application in dermatology. ADSC have gained particular interest due to the relative ease of extraction and their abundance in adipose tissue [2]. Stem cell fractions derived from adipose tissue have been termed the Stromal Vascular Fraction (SVF) and include cytokines, cellular signaling molecules such as transforming growth factor beta-1 (TGF-β1), and vascular endothelial growth factor (VEGF), both of which are thought to serve important roles in wound healing [3]. The ADSC secretome has been described and has revealed the critical role of ADSC in regulating angiogenesis and revascularization, anti-inflammatory and immunomodulatory effects, and tissue regeneration. Conditioned media collected from ADSC revealed high levels of pro-angiogenic molecules such as VEGF, granulocyte colony stimulating factor (G-CSF), and TGF-β [4]. One of the most important characteristics of ADSC is their potent immunosuppressive effect on the local cellular microenvironment. ADSC have been shown to be more potent suppressors of dendritic cells compared to Bone Marrow derived Mesenchymal Stem Cells [5]. The observed immunomodulatory effect was characterized in vitro through the reduction of dendritic cell surface markers such as CD80 and upregulation of anti-inflammatory cytokines such as Interleukin-10 (IL-10) [5, 6].

2.2 *Bone Marrow Derived Mesenchymal Stem Cells*

Bone Marrow Derived Mesenchymal Stem Cells (BM-MSC) have been characterized as excellent options for tissue repair and regeneration due to their ability to transform into a variety of cell types including bone, cartilage, tendon, and skin epithelial cells [7]. BM-MSC represent an exciting potential therapeutic option in dermatology due to their ability to engraft into injured tissue, promote angiogenesis, decrease damage from reactive oxygen species, and provide anti-inflammatory effects in the cellular microenvironment [7]. Studies have shown that BM-MSC may possess a unique ability to suppress neutrophil mediated tissue damage through the engulfment of neutrophils directly by BM-MSC and sparing excess tissue damage [8]. The ability of BM-MSC to affect angiogenesis was previously uncharacterized, however recent studies have shown that VEGF can cause BM-MSC to differentiate into endothelial cells [9]. Although the ability of BM-MSC to differentiate into a variety of different cell types was the initial therapeutic focus, there has been a shift toward understanding the modulatory and signaling roles of BM-MSCs. The main functions of secretory proteins from BM-MSC have been broadly placed into two main roles: anti-apoptosis and cellular migration [10]. Shin et al. analyzed the secretome of ADSC versus BM-MSC and found that ADSC contained more elements influencing cellular organization while BM-MSC contained more elements influencing cellular development, epithelial to mesenchymal transition, and chemotaxis [10].

3 Stem Cell Therapy in Burn Wounds

Thermal injury is a major source of morbidity and mortality in both the military and the civilian settings. Interventions that can restore perfusion, regenerate tissue, and limit scarring are areas of focus for reducing the long-term morbidity associated with burn wounds. BM-MSC therapy has been examined as a possible therapeutic option in both the acute and chronic setting for burn wounds do to their ability to positively impact tissue repair and regeneration. Mansilla et al. examined blood samples from 15 acute burn patients and 15 healthy patients and found that acute burn patients had a higher percentage of circulating MSCs which correlated directly to the size and depth of the burn injury [11]. This data combined with other studies demonstrating the downregulatory role of BM-MSC on neutrophils to minimize tissue damage suggests both an immunomodulatory role and potentially a role in tissue repair [8]. In 2005, Rasulov et al. performed one of the first studies on direct BM-MSC transplantation with skin grafting into a deep thermal wound covering 40% of a patient's face. Patient improvement was noticed in as little as three days after the first treatment, with increased vascularity of granulation tissue, decreased edema, and improved epithelialization of the treated areas [12]. Another study examined 20 patients with chronic non healing wounds were treated with a dermal collagen sponge impregnated with autologous BM-MSCs. In 18 of 20 patients (2 patients died due to unrelated issues), the wounds healed with decreased scarring and in some cases skin grafting was not required [13]. In a more recent report, Schulman et al. reported significant benefit using BM-MSCs in the treatment of deep second degree burn injuries in a dose escalation trial [14]. Among the benefits noted were rapid healing, repigmentation of burn induced leukoderma (which is often permanent), and stimulation of adnexal structure (hair) regrowth. The authors also provided data that suggest that much of these effects may have been due to delivered BM-MSC EVs.

4 Stem Cell Therapy in Photo Aging

As patients age, changes in skin are manifested as alterations in pigment, thinning and loss of elastic fibers, and wrinkling of skin all of which are not cosmetically desirable. Cumulative sun damage and genetic factors influence the way in which the skin undergoes alteration with time [15]. Structural changes that occur in the skin with age include thinning of the epidermis, flattening of the dermal–epidermal junction, alterations in collagen and elastin, and decreased subcutaneous tissue [16]. ADSCs have been a research focus for the treatment of photo aging due to the progenitor capacity and myriad of effector molecules contained within the SVF. Ultraviolet (UV) radiation is well known to cause damage to the skin, and ADSCs have been shown to combat the deleterious effects of UV radiation, prevent wrinkling, and reduce changes in pigmentation with photoaging [17]. ADSC injection has been shown to increase dermal collagen synthesis, number of fibroblasts, and dermal thickness [18]. Injection of ADSC in a murine model was found to prevent UV B induced wrinkling of exposed skin [17]. ADSCs were injected into facial skin of patients after undergoing a face lift procedure and it was found that pathologic collagen deposits were remodeled, and new collagen deposits were formed. Additionally, there was restoration of a normal elastin fiber network in the deeper dermis in treated areas [19]. This data suggests a potential reversal of solar elastosis through local injection of ADSCs. Topically applied growth factors, many of which are found in the SVF of ADSCs have been shown to reverse photo aging through increased collagen thickness and improvement of wrinkles [20]. Injection of SVF with autologous fat compared to injection of autologous ADSCs had similar results and both were found to potentiate facial rejuvenation [19, 21].

ADSCs are thought to combat photoaging through several different mechanisms. One mechanism by which ADSCs prevent photoaging is through reduction of oxidative stress and subsequent tissue damage in skin. Chronic exposure to damaging forms of UV radiation lead to DNA damage and the formation of reactive oxygen species which ultimately damage local tissues [21]. Studies have shown that ADSCs upregulate enzymes that degrade free radicals and release molecules such as IL6 that locally act as free radical scavengers [21, 22]. UV radiation and subsequent generation of reactive oxygen species has been shown to lead to decreased collagen production and elevated levels of collagen degrading enzymes (matrix metalloproteinases) which potentiate collagen degradation and epidermal thinning seen in photoaging [21, 23].

5 Extracellular Vesicles Derived from BM-MSC

While MSC based therapies offered promising results, there is considerable cost associated with growing, culturing, and transporting live cell cultures. Additionally, stem cells therapy has been associated with adverse outcomes in a murine model demonstrating possible ectopic tissue formation and pulmonary complications [24]. Initially, the therapeutic effect of stem cells was thought to be mediated through terminal differentiation of stem cells to cells of local tissues. Further investigation of MSC therapy found that less than one percent of stem cells were present in damaged tissue after one week of therapy [25–27]. Despite this seemingly low amount of stem cells present, there were positive results observed in patients treated with stem cell therapy. These findings gave rise to a theory that there was another way in which stem cell therapy potentiated tissue recovery. There is increasing data to suggest that the therapeutic effect of stem cells is through the paracrine effects of signaling molecules and immunomodulatory proteins released by stem cells.

Extracellular vesicles (EVs) are class of structures consisting of a lipid bilayer that are released from all cell types into the microenvironment. Extracellular vesicles consist mainly of exosomes and microvesicles differentiated by the size and mode of production at the cellular level. Exosomes are roughly 50–100 nm in size and are produced by cells within the endosomal system [28]. Microvesicles are greater than 100 nm in size and are produced through the outward budding of the plasma membrane [29]. While microvesicles and exosomes are produced at two distinct locations within cells, there are overlapping pathways for storage and secretion of both structures making it very difficult to molecularly distinguish these groups of secreted vesicles [30]. The uptake of EVs is often dependent on the type of cell being targeted but broadly consists of direct phagocytosis of EVs by the cell, macropinocytosis, and direct membrane fusion in a pH dependent manner [31]. EVs can also interact with cell surface receptors including major histocompatibility complexes I and II, mitogen-activated protein kinase (MAPK) activation, and potentiators of other downstream signals involved cell processes [30]. EV release is thought to be mediated by a variety of different signals including local hypoxic conditions, mechanical stimulation, changes in environmental pH, different GTPases, and Vesicle Associated membrane protein 7 (VAMP7) [32–35].

To understand the roles of EVs, McBride et al. analyzed the secretome of BM-MSC derived EVs and shed light on some of the ways in which EVs modulate wound healing and angiogenesis. Lysis of EVs followed by mass spectrometry and high-performance liquid chromatography was used to characterize the cellular cargo. Broadly the cargo of EVs could be placed into several main groups including structural elements, potentiators of cell signaling and migration, immunomodulatory agents, and finally elements that were involved in the transport of from one cell to another [36].

EVs were found to contain structural proteins such as keratin-1 and type VII collagen both of which play important roles in anchoring proteins in the basement membrane at the dermal–epidermal junction and providing structural integrity to adnexal structures within the dermis [32, 36, 37]. It has been shown that EVs can transfer collagen VII from healthy cells to cells that produce abnormal collagen VII such as in epidermolysis bullosa as well as stimulate these cells to produce normal collagen VII [38]. This study served as one of the first examples of EVs acting as transport vesicles to deliver cellular cargo to fibroblasts. This could serve as a precursor to future experiments examining using EVs purely as a delivery mechanism for cellular or pharmaceutical purposes. Using an endogenous system such as EVs as a drug delivery mechanism could be a valuable future application.

6 Extracellular Vesicles in Wound Healing

The discovery and molecular characterization of EVs has led to an increase in research into the therapeutic efficacy of EVs for cutaneous injury. While EVs can be isolated from all cell types, the main focus in this chapter will be the therapeutic role of BM-MSC derived EVs for the treatment and its potential in dermatology. Early studies into the effects of BM-MSC EVs demonstrated that EVs could potentiate crucial pathways in wound healing. Shabbir et al. found that EVs in vitro can facilitate the migration and proliferation of fibroblasts from both normal donors and in diabetic patients with chronic ulcers with fibroblasts that do not function normally [39]. Overall, studies have shown that EVs can improve the rate of wound healing and reduce scar formation [40]. There is increasing evidence that EVs potentiate their effects through modulating downstream signaling pathways such as signal transducer and activator of transcription 3 (STAT3) and extracellular signal-regulated kinase-1/2 (ERK1/2) which regulate extracellular matrix remodeling, cell proliferation, and angiogenesis [40]. It has been shown that BM- MSC derived EVs directly deliver Wnt3a, a mediator of the Wnt signaling pathway, which once delivered to fibroblasts increases fibroblast proliferation and migration [41].

BM-MSC derived EVs also play important roles in reducing inflammation and controlling neutrophil migration. EVs have been shown to decrease levels of inflammatory cytokines such tumor necrosis factor alpha (TNF-α) and IL-1β [27, 42]. Additionally many chemokines including IL-10 and hepatocyte growth factor (HGF) among others have been found within EVs suggesting an important role in immunosuppression and tissue repair and regeneration [27]. Chen et al. demonstrated that peripheral blood mononuclear cells that were cultured with EVs decreased the production of pro-inflammatory cytokines, while increasing immunosuppressive molecules such as TGF- β [42]. EVs have been shown to decrease inflammation and further tissue damage following inciting injury through preferentially increase anti-inflammatory M2 macrophages while decreasing inflammatory M1 macrophages. By upregulating STAT3 signaling, EVs potentiate M2 macrophage migration and prevent further oxidative injury from M1 macrophages [32, 43].

Another critical role of BM-MSC EVs is to promote angiogenesis and recruit cells to the site of tissue injury. A major mechanism of injury following thermal wounds is the development of a zone of stasis which is produced from coagulation and obstruction of the tissue microcirculatory system [44]. The decrease in blood flow to the damaged area leads to a delayed ischemia and further potentiates tissue damage hours to days after the initial inciting event [32]. Interventions that can restore blood flow to ischemic regions of burn wounds can prevent further injury and facilitate more rapid healing. EVs have been shown to activate VEGF receptors and stimulate angiogenesis in wounds which can lead to the restoration of blood flow and limit the progression of ischemic tissue damage [45]. EVs have been shown to promote angiogenesis in vitro through activation of the AKT/eNOS pathway facilitating the restoration of blood flow and wound closure [46]. EVs have been shown to stimulate both keratinocyte and fibroblast migration and proliferation and indirectly increase the rate of wound re-epithelialization [24, 47].

A major source of long-term morbidity in would healing is excess scarring and scar contracture that occurs over time especially in patients with second or third degree burns. EVs have been shown to reduce the formation of hypertrophic scars and limit the excess contracture that occurs with scar remodeling [48]. One of the ways in which EVs prevent excess contracture is by inhibiting the migration of myofibroblasts to the affected area [49]. BM-MSC EVs were shown to reduce levels of pro inflammatory cytokines such as TNF-α and IL6 in scar tissue and reduced collagen deposition [50].

EVs represent an acellular therapeutic option to treat acute or chronic wounds. A notable advantage to using EV based therapy over MSC based therapy is that EVs do not engraft into the wound which reduces the risk of developing long term complications such as potential secondary malignancy or graft versus host disease [24, 32]. EVs can be frozen and transported safely as their structure is relatively stable whereas live stem cell cultures are far more difficult to transport and maintain.

7 Role of Anti-inflammatory Effects of EVs in Dermatology

Given the role of EVs to modulate local cellular environments, reduce progressive and chronic inflammation, and preferentially attract populations of immune cells to an area, EVs represent a promising therapy to combat chronic inflammatory skin conditions such as atopic dermatitis (AD) and psoriasis.

Atopic Dermatitis is the most common skin disorders especially in infants affecting nearly 60% of individuals before the age of 5 [51]. The cause of AD is hypothesized to include both genetic and immune dysregulation properties. Genetically, a defect in the filaggrin protein of the epidermis impairing the epidermal barrier and leading to inflammatory reaction from cells in the dermis. This inflammatory reaction leads to pruritis which potentiates a cycle of itching and further damaging the epidermal barrier [52]. The genetic defect in AD leads to abnormal keratinocyte differentiation, decreased ceramide production, and impaired innate defense to bacteria [53]. EVs have been shown to increase ceramide levels and restore barrier function to the epidermis in patients with AD while also reducing epidermal hyperplasia and erythema [54]. AD is also associated with elevated Th2 helper T cells and increased levels of inflammatory cytokines such as TNF-α, IL4 and IL13 [55, 56]. EVs were also shown to activate genes to promote differentiation of keratinocytes and represent a potential cell free therapeutic option for patients with chronic AD [53, 54]. The potent immunosuppressive effect EVs has been examined in a murine model for AD. It was found that EVs could improve symptomatic AD through lowering levels of IgE, TNF-α, IL4, and IL23 all of which are implicated in the pathogenesis of AD [57].

Psoriasis is one of the most common chronic inflammatory skin conditions and effects nearly 4% of the population [58]. Psoriasis vulgaris, the most common form of psoriasis, is characterized as raised, scaly, red lesions which can form plaques and commonly affects the elbows, scalp, and knees [59]. Psoriasis is a derangement of keratinocyte maturation leading to abnormally rapid maturation through the epidermis. Psoriasis is mediated by potent inflammatory molecules such as TNF-α, IL-23, and IL-17 which increase immune cell infiltration and potentiate the disease process [60]. EVs from patients with psoriasis have been shown to carry inflammatory cytokines and potentiate the disease process [60]. Zhang et al. reported that in rats EVs decreased the psoriasis score in affected population by inhibiting the maturation and activation of dendritic cells and reduced levels of IL-17 and IL-23 [61]. Topically applied conditioned media from adipocyte stem cells was used to treat a patient with psoriasis of the scalp and reduced the size of the plaque and amount of scale after 2 weeks of treatment [62]. The potent anti-inflammatory properties of EVs have shown to be beneficial for chronic inflammatory conditions and could prove valuable in controlling inflammatory disease while reducing relapse rates in this population.

8 Role of Telemedicine

The increase in use of telemedicine especially within the last five years has expanded access to care and created a new opportunity for patients to receive care without incurring the lost money and time associated with traveling to appointments. These experimental treatments in dermatology using either stem cells or EVs often require meticulous follow up which can be an obstacle to patients. Routine in office treatment is a critical part of using EV therapy, and telemedicine can allow clinicians to follow patient's responses more carefully. Since a key component of treatment response in dermatology is visual, telemedicine has allowed patients to meet and converse with clinicians more often while reducing missed appointments. This more routine follow up will undoubtedly facilitate faster advancements in treatment strategies, allowing experimenters to better establish dosing regimens and dose scheduling.

9 Conclusion

Stem cell therapy represents a therapeutic modality that can improve wound healing, limit excess scarring, reverse cumulative UV damage to skin, and restore healthy collagen. While the initial therapeutic interest was rooted in the capacity of stem cells to differentiate into a variety of cell types, clinical studies suggested the paracrine signaling activity was the primary contributor to clinical improvement. Given the high cost, obstacles associated with live cell culture, and risk of long-term complications following stem cell therapy, extracellular vesicles represent a safer alternative without comprising the potential therapeutic reward.

While there is encouraging data to suggest EV therapy should have a role in dermatology, currently there are barriers to widespread use. The manufacturing process of EVs has improved but is still inefficient. Obtaining a therapeutic dose of EVs is currently laborious and time consuming. Advances in the manufacturing process will undoubtedly streamline production and once a steady supply of EVs is available opportunity of widespread application and experimentation is an exciting prospect in the future. As EV therapy becomes more mainstream it is conceivable that broader applications to other dermatologic conditions such as alopecia areata or epidermolysis bullosa become available. EVs represent an endogenous system for the packaging, transfer, and modulation of cellular pathways. Having a vehicle to deliver genetic, structural, or signaling components between cells could represent an exciting advancement in drug delivery and immunotherapy.

References

1. McBride JD, Rodriguez-Menocal L, Badiavas EV. Extracellular vesicles as biomarkers and therapeutics in dermatology: a focus on exosomes. J Invest Dermatol. 2017.
2. Bellei B, Migliano E, Picardo M. Therapeutic potential of adipose tissue-derivatives in modern dermatology. Exp Dermatol. 2022.
3. Hassan WU, Greiser U, Wang W. Role of adipose-derived stem cells in wound healing. Wound Repair Regener. 2014;22(3):313–25.
4. Rehman J, et al. Secretion of angiogenic and antiapoptotic factors by human adipose stromal cells. Circulation. 2004;109(10):1292–8.
5. Ivanova-Todorova E, et al. Adipose tissue-derived mesenchymal stem cells are more potent suppressors of dendritic cells differentiation compared to bone marrow-derived mesenchymal stem cells. Immunol Lett. 2009;126(1–2):37–42.
6. Kapur SK, Katz AJ. Review of the adipose derived stem cell secretome. Biochimie. 2013;95(12):2222–8.
7. Fu X, et al. Enhanced wound-healing quality with bone marrow mesenchymal stem cells autografting after skin injury. Wound Repair Regener. 2006;14(3):325–35.
8. Jiang D, et al. Suppression of neutrophil-mediated tissue damage—a novel skill of mesenchymal stem cells. Stem Cells. 2016;34(9):2393–406.
9. Ball SG, Shuttleworth CA, Kielty CM. Mesenchymal stem cells and neovascularization: role of platelet-derived growth factor receptors. J Cell Mol Med. 2007;11(5):1012–30.
10. Shin S, et al. Comparative proteomic analysis of the mesenchymal stem cells secretome from adipose, bone marrow, placenta and Wharton's jelly. Int J Mol Sci. 2021;22(2):845.

11. Mansilla E, et al. Bloodstream cells phenotypically identical to human mesenchymal bone marrow stem cells circulate in large amounts under the influence of acute large skin damage: new evidence for their use in regenerative medicine. In: Transplantation proceedings. Elsevier; 2006.
12. Rasulov M, et al. First experience in the use of bone marrow mesenchymal stem cells for the treatment of a patient with deep skin burns. Bull Exp Biol Med. 2005;139(1):141–4.
13. Yoshikawa T, et al. Wound therapy by marrow mesenchymal cell transplantation. Plast Reconstr Surg. 2008;121(3):860–77.
14. Schulman CI, et al. The effect of mesenchymal stem cells improves the healing of burn wounds: a phase 1 dose-escalation clinical trial. Scars Burn Heal. 2022;8:20595131211070784.
15. Bolognia JL. Aging skin. Am J Med. 1995;98(1):S99–103.
16. Fenske NA, Lober CW. Structural and functional changes of normal aging skin. J Am Acad Dermatol. 1986;15(4):571–85.
17. Kim W-S, Park B-S, Sung J-H. Protective role of adipose-derived stem cells and their soluble factors in photoaging. Arch Dermatol Res. 2009;301(5):329–36.
18. Kim JH, et al. Adipose-derived stem cells as a new therapeutic modality for ageing skin. Exp Dermatol. 2011;20(5):383–7.
19. Charles-de-Sá L, et al. Photoaged skin therapy with adipose-derived stem cells. Plast Reconstr Surg. 2020;145(6):1037e–49e.
20. Fitzpatrick RE, Rostan EF. Reversal of photodamage with topical growth factors: a pilot study. J Cosmet Laser Ther. 2003;5(1):25–34.
21. Lv J, et al. Protective roles of mesenchymal stem cells on skin photoaging: a narrative review. Tissue and Cell. 2022; 101746.
22. Rahman Z, Soory M. Antioxidant effects of glutathione and IGF in a hyperglycaemic cell culture model of fibroblasts: some actions of advanced glycaemic end products (AGE) and nicotine. Endocrine, Metabolic & Immune Disorders-Drug Targets (Formerly Current Drug Targets-Immune, Endocrine & Metabolic Disorders). 2006;6(3):279–86.
23. Sun Z, et al. Dietary Foeniculum vulgare Mill extract attenuated UVB irradiation-induced skin photoaging by activating of Nrf2 and inhibiting MAPK pathways. Phytomedicine. 2016;23(12):1273–84.
24. Bray ER, et al. Extracellular vesicles as therapeutic tools for the treatment of chronic wounds. Pharmaceutics. 2021;13(10):1543.
25. Rani S, et al. Mesenchymal stem cell-derived extracellular vesicles: toward cell-free therapeutic applications. Mol Ther. 2015;23(5):812–23.
26. Phinney DG, Pittenger MF. Concise review: MSC-derived exosomes for cell-free therapy. Stem cells. 2017;35(4):851–8.
27. Casado-Díaz A, Quesada-Gómez JM, Dorado G. Extracellular vesicles derived from mesenchymal stem cells (MSC) in regenerative medicine: applications in skin wound healing. Front Bioeng Biotechnol. 2020;8:146.
28. Chaput N, Théry C. Exosomes: immune properties and potential clinical implementations. In: Seminars in immunopathology. Springer; 2011.
29. Menck K, et al. Microvesicles in cancer: small size, large potential. Int J Mol Sci. 2020;21(15):5373.
30. Van Niel G, d'Angelo G, Raposo G. Shedding light on the cell biology of extracellular vesicles. Nat Rev Mol Cell Biol. 2018;19(4):213–28.
31. Yáñez-Mó M, et al. Biological properties of extracellular vesicles and their physiological functions. J Extracellular Vesicles. 2015;4(1):27066.
32. Kaiser M, Rodriguez-Menocal L, Badiavas EV. Role of extracellular vesicles in stem cell therapy. Curr Stem Cell Res Therapy. 2022.
33. Zhu J, et al. Myocardial reparative functions of exosomes from mesenchymal stem cells are enhanced by hypoxia treatment of the cells via transferring microRNA-210 in an nSMase2-dependent way. Artif Cells Nanomed Biotechnol. 2018;46(8):1659–70.
34. Ban J-J, et al. Low pH increases the yield of exosome isolation. Biochem Biophys Res Commun. 2015;461(1):76–9.

35. Guo S, et al. Stimulating extracellular vesicles production from engineered tissues by mechanical forces. Nano Lett. 2021;21(6):2497–504.
36. McBride JD, et al. Proteomic analysis of bone marrow-derived mesenchymal stem cell extracellular vesicles from healthy donors: implications for proliferation, angiogenesis, Wnt signaling, and the basement membrane. Stem Cell Res Ther. 2021;12(1):328.
37. Chen M, et al. Interactions of the amino-terminal noncollagenous (NC1) domain of type VII collagen with extracellular matrix components: a potential role in epidermal-dermal adherence in human skin. J Biol Chem. 1997;272(23):14516–22.
38. McBride JD, et al. Dual mechanism of type VII collagen transfer by bone marrow mesenchymal stem cell extracellular vesicles to recessive dystrophic epidermolysis bullosa fibroblasts. Biochimie. 2018;155:50–8.
39. Shabbir A, et al. Mesenchymal stem cell exosomes induce proliferation and migration of normal and chronic wound fibroblasts, and enhance angiogenesis in vitro. Stem Cells Dev. 2015;24(14):1635–47.
40. Cabral J, et al. Extracellular vesicles as modulators of wound healing. Adv Drug Deliv Rev. 2018;129:394–406.
41. McBride JD, et al. Bone marrow mesenchymal stem cell-derived CD63(+) exosomes transport Wnt3a exteriorly and enhance dermal fibroblast proliferation, migration, and angiogenesis in vitro. Stem Cells Dev. 2017;26(19):1384–98.
42. Chen W, et al. Immunomodulatory effects of mesenchymal stromal cells-derived exosome. Immunol Res. 2016;64(4):831–40.
43. Than UTT, et al. Association of extracellular membrane vesicles with cutaneous wound healing. Int J Mol Sci. 2017;18(5):956.
44. Regas FC, Ehrlich HP. Elucidating the vascular response to burns with a new rat model. J Trauma. 1992;32(5):557–63.
45. Gangadaran P, et al. Extracellular vesicles from mesenchymal stem cells activates VEGF receptors and accelerates recovery of hindlimb ischemia. J Control Release. 2017;264:112–26.
46. Yu M, et al. Exosomes derived from atorvastatin-pretreated MSC accelerate diabetic wound repair by enhancing angiogenesis via AKT/eNOS pathway. Stem Cell Res Ther. 2020;11(1):1–17.
47. Tutuianu R, et al. Human mesenchymal stromal cell-derived exosomes promote in vitro wound healing by modulating the biological properties of skin keratinocytes and fibroblasts and stimulating angiogenesis. Int J Mol Sci. 2021;22(12):6239.
48. Zhu Y-Z, et al. Extracellular vesicles derived from human adipose-derived stem cell prevent the formation of hypertrophic scar in a rabbit model. Ann Plast Surg. 2020;84(5):602.
49. Hade MD, et al. Extracellular vesicles: emerging frontiers in wound healing. Med Res Rev. 2022;42(6):2102–25.
50. Jiang L, et al. Exosomes derived from TSG-6 modified mesenchymal stromal cells attenuate scar formation during wound healing. Biochimie. 2020;177:40–9.
51. Spergel JM, Paller AS. Atopic dermatitis and the atopic march. J Allergy Clin Immunol. 2003;112(6):S118–27.
52. Berke R, Singh A, Guralnick M. Atopic dermatitis: an overview. Am Fam Physician. 2012;86(1):35–42.
53. Quiñones-Vico MI, et al. The role of exosomes derived from mesenchymal stromal cells in dermatology. Front Cell Dev Biol. 2021;9: 647012.
54. Shin K-O, et al. Exosomes from human adipose tissue-derived mesenchymal stem cells promote epidermal barrier repair by inducing de novo synthesis of ceramides in atopic dermatitis. Cells. 2020;9(3):680.
55. Kim J, Kim BE, Leung DY. Pathophysiology of atopic dermatitis: clinical implications. In: Allergy and asthma proceedings. OceanSide Publications; 2019.
56. Jacobi A, et al. Infliximab in the treatment of moderate to severe atopic dermatitis. J Am Acad Dermatol. 2005;52(3):522–6.
57. Xiong M, et al. The novel mechanisms and applications of exosomes in dermatology and cutaneous medical aesthetics. Pharmacol Res. 2021;166: 105490.

58. Griffiths CE, Barker JN. Pathogenesis and clinical features of psoriasis. The Lancet. 2007;370(9583):263–71.
59. Lowes MA, Bowcock AM, Krueger JG. Pathogenesis and therapy of psoriasis. Nature. 2007;445(7130):866–73.
60. Kim H, et al. Extracellular vesicles as potential theranostic platforms for skin diseases and aging. Pharmaceutics. 2021;13(5):760.
61. Zhang Y, et al. Exosomes derived from human umbilical cord mesenchymal stem cells alleviate psoriasis-like skin inflammation. J Interferon Cytokine Res. 2022;42(1):8–18.
62. Seetharaman R, et al. Mesenchymal stem cell conditioned media ameliorate psoriasis vulgaris: a case study. Case Rep Dermatol Med. 2019;2019.

Index

A
Access to care, 7, 9, 16, 49, 59, 84, 86, 116, 128, 153, 155, 157, 158, 162, 164, 172, 186, 187, 195, 196, 198, 220, 297, 298, 394
Aesthetic consultations, 27–30, 40
Aesthetic dermatology, 247, 329, 354, 355
Alexandrite, 34, 35, 318, 321, 322
Alopecia, 10, 12, 39, 40, 253, 255, 317, 318, 323, 324, 372
Artificial intelligence, 59, 61, 73, 74, 79, 90, 118, 179, 181, 196, 219, 220, 231, 235, 239, 248, 249, 275, 287, 288, 291, 292, 301, 306, 308
Atopic dermatitis, 20, 21, 23, 66, 244, 259, 263, 264, 291, 331, 377, 387, 388, 393

B
Barriers to care, 158, 188
Basal cell carcinoma, 9, 38, 66, 102, 104, 226, 229, 239, 254, 255, 258, 262, 281
Basal cell carcinomas, 236
Biotechnology, 329, 330, 334, 355

C
Camera, 12, 22, 28, 51–53, 62, 70, 84, 85, 87, 116, 129, 130, 173, 181, 206–210, 216, 223–225, 279
Carbon dioxide (CO_2), 36, 317–320, 322–324, 344, 354
Covid-19, 4, 6, 7, 9, 12, 17, 20, 22, 27, 49, 50, 79, 82, 84, 91, 115, 116, 121, 122, 128, 133, 137, 149, 152, 155, 156, 166, 174, 179, 180, 185, 186, 188, 199, 223, 290, 296, 303, 305, 333
Curriculum design, 119, 138, 195, 307
Cutaneous malignancy, 61, 66, 67, 69, 74

D
Data privacy and protection, 300
Dermatologic surgery, 67, 102, 105, 281
Dermatology, 3, 6–10, 15, 16, 18, 23, 27, 30, 31, 40, 41, 49, 59, 61, 63, 65, 69, 72, 74, 82, 102, 105, 106, 115, 119, 122, 127, 128, 130, 133, 137, 138, 140–142, 149, 235, 239, 259, 260, 268, 275–279, 282, 283, 291, 292, 294, 297, 308, 317, 329, 351, 367, 368, 370, 375, 381, 382, 387–389, 392, 394, 395
Dermatoscopy, 62, 64, 67, 219, 222, 223, 227
Dermo-epidermal junction, 239, 245, 255, 257
Diagnostic accuracy, 10, 21, 23, 59, 60, 62–64, 68–71, 73, 74, 103, 115, 118, 122, 140, 141, 152, 185, 187, 219, 222, 225–227, 231, 282
Digital divide, 157, 186, 188, 195, 289, 295, 307, 309
Digital health, 223, 295, 304
Digital photography, 20, 60, 62, 63, 205, 206, 208, 210–212, 215, 216
Diode, 34, 36, 37, 236, 321, 347, 354

K. Nouri (ed.), *Telemedicine and Technological Advances in Dermatology*, https://doi.org/10.1007/978-3-031-69091-4

Disparities, 23, 98, 99, 106, 122, 141, 143, 149–151, 155, 174, 175, 215, 282, 290, 296, 297, 307
Dynamic optical coherence tomography, 235

E
Electrospinning, 370
Enzymes, 330, 335–337, 340, 355, 390
Erbium
yttrium aluminum garnet (Er:YAG), 36, 317, 318, 322, 354
Ethical, legal, and social issues, 287, 289, 307, 309
Exosome, 391
Extracellular vesicle, 387, 388, 391, 392, 395

F
Flipped classroom, 137
Follow-up care, 5, 27, 30, 40, 41, 174
FST IV-VI, 153

G
Geriatric teledermatology, 186, 198
Global dermatology, 170, 174

H
Hair diseases, 49, 50, 52, 53, 133
Healthcare access, 154–157, 295
Health equity, 101
Health professions education, 164, 169
Hidradenitis suppurativa, 19, 259, 261, 264, 265, 321
High-resolution ultrasonography (HRUS), 259–268
High-resolution ultrasound, 259
Human hair keratinic extract, 370

I
Inflammatory skin conditions, 16, 18, 23, 24, 253, 259–261, 393, 394
Inflammatory skin diseases, 6, 18, 19, 235, 248
Inflammatory skin disorders, 17, 18, 259, 263–265

L
Lasers, 31–41, 106, 107, 236, 238, 242, 246, 254, 255, 317–324, 340, 344, 348, 354, 372
Line-field-confocal optical coherence tomography, 235
Live-interactive, 17, 23, 60, 62, 174, 180, 221
Live virtual visits, 186, 187

M
Machine learning, 64, 220, 221, 292, 308
Medical devices, 90, 121, 211, 212, 289, 299, 301
Medical education, 137, 208, 212, 215, 303
Melanoma, 9–11, 60, 64, 66, 68–70, 73, 118, 220, 221, 226, 229, 243, 244, 255, 257, 259, 262, 263, 276, 279–281, 376, 378, 379, 382
Metal oxides, 376, 382
Mobile, 6, 7, 17, 18, 21, 22, 30, 50, 52, 60, 62, 64, 69, 71, 74, 84, 139–141, 162, 165, 167, 168, 173, 180, 213, 219, 220, 222, 223, 226, 227, 230, 303
Mohs surgery, 59, 60, 67, 72, 103–105, 256, 378

N
Nanocarriers, 375
Nanodermatology, 375
Nanoemulsion, 376, 377, 381, 382
Nanoliposomes, 376, 379
Nanotechnology, 375–379, 381, 382
Neodymium-doped yttrium aluminum garnet (Nd:YAG), 34–38, 320–324, 354
Non invasive body contouring, 347, 350, 352
Non-invasive imaging, 235, 238, 239, 243, 253, 254, 257, 265

O
Older adults, 185–190, 192, 194–198
Optical coherence tomography, 235, 236
Optimizing care, 131

P
Papillary dermis, 245, 254–256, 322
Pathology, 80, 103, 104, 115, 116, 118–122, 142, 208, 210–212, 225,

227, 244, 275–277, 280, 282, 295, 323, 388
Patient education, 4, 9, 22, 60, 62, 80, 131, 132, 205
Photodocumentation, 206
Physical properties, 376
Pigmented lesions, 11, 35, 61, 62, 66, 69, 72, 73, 133, 140, 219, 220, 222, 228–230, 244, 309
Potassium titanyl phosphate, 34, 37, 320, 323
Psoriasis, 5, 22, 23, 66, 138, 180, 188, 225, 245, 253–256, 259, 261, 263, 264, 291, 309, 343, 346, 348, 376, 377, 387, 388, 393, 394
Pulsed dye, 318

R

Reflectance confocal microscopy, 59, 61, 72–74, 235, 238, 248, 253, 254, 257
Research, 5, 11, 72, 101, 115, 117, 119, 122, 139, 144, 150, 152, 179–183, 205, 208, 212, 215, 219, 222, 226, 227, 231, 277, 278, 282, 289, 300, 307, 309, 317, 324, 340, 341, 347, 351, 352, 367, 368, 372, 375–377, 379, 381, 382, 387, 390, 392
Ruby, 35, 36, 318, 321, 322

S

Scleroderma, 245, 265, 266
Skin cancer, 9, 10, 40, 59–61, 63–66, 68, 69, 71–74, 116, 119, 122, 140, 141, 153, 168, 186, 192, 193, 219, 226, 228–231, 235, 236, 239, 253, 254, 259, 260, 283, 291, 292, 295, 330, 337, 379
Skin neoplasms, 102, 261
Skin of color, 138, 149, 150, 181, 205, 209, 215, 216, 227, 317, 348
Skin substitute, 80, 89, 142, 369, 370
Skin tissue engineering, 367, 368
Smartphone, 4, 6, 30, 31, 51–53, 62, 64, 67, 69, 71, 90, 91, 104, 106, 118, 149, 150, 157, 162–164, 168, 169, 173, 180, 188, 206, 207, 209, 213, 214, 222, 223, 226, 230, 291, 295, 296, 299, 309
Squamous cell carcinoma, 38, 66, 226, 236, 241, 254, 255, 262, 278, 379
Stem cell, 35, 321, 330, 338–340, 344, 371, 387–391, 393–395
Store-and-forward, 3–6, 17, 23, 28, 59–62, 65, 66, 68, 70, 71, 73, 86, 91, 102, 105, 115–117, 139, 140, 162, 170, 180, 185–187, 192–196, 198, 221, 230, 290

T

Technology, 3, 4, 12, 15–18, 23, 27, 53, 59, 61–64, 66, 68, 72, 73, 79, 82, 85–87, 90, 91, 95, 97, 99, 100, 102, 104–106, 116–118, 121, 122, 127, 139, 142, 144, 156–158, 162, 165, 173–175, 179–183, 186, 188, 192, 196, 253, 277, 283, 288, 290–296, 298, 303–309, 317, 318, 324, 330, 377–381
Telecosmetics, 27–31, 40, 354
Teledermatopathology, 115–122, 163
Teledermatological surgery, 151, 153, 187, 199, 226, 230
Teledermatology, 3–8, 10–12, 17–21, 23, 30, 41, 49, 52, 56, 59–74, 82, 103, 127–134, 139, 140, 149–153, 155–158, 161, 162, 164–175, 180, 185–198, 211, 219–221, 223, 225, 226, 231, 287–292, 294, 305, 307, 309
Teledermoscopy, 62, 64, 66, 70, 72, 73, 102, 140, 144, 219–231
Tele-education, 137–144
Telehealth, 17, 21, 23, 27–30, 40, 41, 61, 64, 66, 73, 79, 80, 84–87, 89, 95, 102, 105, 128, 150–153, 174, 188, 194, 196, 211, 287–289, 304
Telemedicine, 3–12, 15–20, 22, 23, 27, 28, 30, 41, 49, 50, 52, 55, 59–62, 65, 67–69, 72–74, 79, 80, 82, 83, 86, 87, 91, 96, 99, 103–106, 116, 121, 122, 127–129, 149–152, 155–158, 161–164, 166, 169–175, 188, 189, 211, 226, 228, 287–291, 294–296, 298–300, 302–308, 394
Telepathology, 103, 104, 116–119, 121, 122, 163
Teletrichology, 10, 49, 50, 52, 53, 55, 56
Telewound, 79, 83–91
3-dimensional printing, 367, 368, 371, 372

U

Underserved, 3, 5, 12, 15, 61, 64, 86, 98, 102, 115, 119, 155–158, 162, 164,

165, 185, 198, 220, 225, 231, 288, 290, 299

W

Whole slide imaging, 116, 121, 141, 280
Wound care, 8, 9, 67, 79, 80, 82–84, 86–89, 91, 105, 187, 367, 368, 379, 380
Wound healing, 9, 34, 38, 39, 67, 68, 80, 82, 84, 85, 88, 211, 322, 335–337, 340, 345, 349, 367, 371, 372, 375, 380, 382, 387, 388, 391, 392, 395

GPSR Compliance

The European Union's (EU) General Product Safety Regulation (GPSR) is a set of rules that requires consumer products to be safe and our obligations to ensure this.

If you have any concerns about our products, you can contact us on ProductSafety@springernature.com

In case Publisher is established outside the EU, the EU authorized representative is:

Springer Nature Customer Service Center GmbH
Europaplatz 3
69115 Heidelberg, Germany

Batch number: 10756376

Printed by Printforce, the Netherlands